Dion Kagan is a writer, editor, and early career academic. He is a project officer at the Australian Research Centre for Sex, Health and Society, La Trobe University, researching stigma and disease in the Gender, Law and Drugs program. Previously, he was a lecturer in screen studies, cultural studies and gender studies at the University of Melbourne. Dion's essays and reviews have been published widely, including in *The Monthly, The Saturday Paper, The Age, The Sydney Review of Books, Meanjin* and *Kill Your Darlings*, and from 2014 to 2018 he wrote a regular longform queer column for *The Lifted Brow*. He is a former co-host of literary and culture podcast, The Rereaders.

'In this landmark study of the representation of gay men in contemporary popular culture, Dion Kagan shows how the panicked response to AIDS during the 1980s continues to haunt "post-crisis" gay life, unsettling its normalisation by resuscitating the association of homosexuality with death and disease. In a series of carefully elaborated case studies drawn from the mainstream media and informed by feminist and queer theory, Kagan traces the transformation of HIV/AIDS into a signifier of social and sexual backwardness that conflicts with the normative aspirations of neoliberal gay identities.'

Robert J. Corber, Trinity College, Connecticut, USA

'In this erudite analysis of representations of western gay life in "post-crisis" times, Dion Kagan re-activates the critical energies of early HIV cultural analysis for contemporary queer theory to ask what a "positive image" of gay life could possibly be in the current polarised environment that lurches between "progressive" attachments to clean, upstanding, respectable, sexless marrying types and the sensationalised monsters of chemsex, barebacking, HIV-positive sex and sex addiction, each of which emerge as figures of a "retrograde" sexuality we "should have grown out of by now" that effectively serve to "re-crisis" the present. Generous and expansive in its critical engagements, while sparkling throughout with astute and perceptive readings, *Positive Images* is a remarkable feat of intergenerational queer kinship that introduces an exciting new voice in sexuality scholarship.'

Kane Race, Professor in Gender and Cultural Studies, University of Sydney, Australia

'*Positive Images* should be commended for the way it astutely locates the ongoing and unresolved political consequences of the AIDS epidemic in the singularities of the moving image. Not only does Kagan give us insight into a mode of popular media production working to discipline our contact with queer histories of this crisis but he also expertly shows the particular capaciousness of using cinema as a tool for thinking through – and evidencing – such discursive regulation.'

Continuum: Journal of Media and Cultural Studies

'In *Positive Images*, Kagan undertakes a detailed study of the ways in which gay men negotiated this "post-crisis" period, that is, life after the introduction of effective antiretroviral medicines. His careful attention to cultural trends, using HIV prevention studies, queer theory, gay and lesbian studies, and television and film studies, provides a comprehensive look at how these men lived with a virus turned chronic illness, and how their lives impact gay communities today.'

Journal of Homosexuality

'*Positive Images* is original, perceptive and incisive in its critiques and is a timely analysis of contemporary representations of HIV/AIDS in popular film and media. Kagan's work is a bold propaedeutic for further inquiry into the temporality and history of AIDS and its impacts on queer and popular image-making.'

Queer Studies in Media & Popular Culture

Library of Gender and Popular Culture

From *Mad Men* to gaming culture, performance art to steampunk fashion, the presentation and representation of gender continues to saturate popular media. This series seeks to explore the intersection of gender and popular culture, engaging with a variety of texts – drawn primarily from Art, Fashion, TV, Cinema, Cultural Studies and Media Studies – as a way of considering various models for understanding the complementary relationship between 'gender identities' and 'popular culture'. By considering race, ethnicity, class, and sexual identities across a range of cultural forms, each book in the series adopts a critical stance towards issues surrounding the development of gender identities and popular and mass cultural 'products'.

For further information or enquiries, please contact the library series editors:

Claire Nally: claire.nally@northumbria.ac.uk
Angela Smith: angela.smith@sunderland.ac.uk

Advisory Board:

Dr Kate Ames, Central Queensland University, Australia

Dr Michael Higgins, University of Strathclyde, UK

Prof Åsa Kroon, Örebro University, Sweden

Dr Andrea McDonnell, Emmanuel College, USA

Dr Niall Richardson, University of Sussex, UK

Dr Jacki Willson, University of Leeds, UK

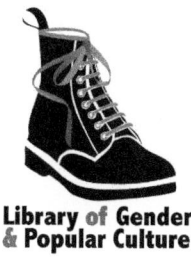

Published and forthcoming titles:

The Aesthetics of Camp: Post-Queer Gender and Popular Culture
By Anna Malinowska

Ageing Femininity on Screen: The Older Woman in Contemporary Cinema
By Niall Richardson

All-American TV Crime Drama: Feminism and Identity Politics in Law and Order: Special Victims Unit
By Sujata Moorti and Lisa Cuklanz

Bad Girls, Dirty Bodies: Sex, Performance and Safe Femininity
By Gemma Commane

Beyoncé: Celebrity Feminism in The Age of Social Media
By Kirsty Fairclough-Isaacs

Conflicting Masculinities: Men in Television Period Drama
By Katherine Byrne, Julie Anne Taddeo and James Leggott (Eds)

Fat on Film: Gender, Race and Body Size in Contemporary Hollywood Cinema
By Barbara Plotz

Fathers on Film: Paternity and Masculinity in 1990s Hollywood
By Katie Barnett

Film Bodies: Queer Feminist Encounters with Gender and Sexuality in Cinema
By Katharina Lindner

Gay Pornography: Representations of Sexuality and Masculinity
By John Mercer

Gender and Austerity in Popular Culture: Femininity, Masculinity and Recession in Film and Television
By Helen Davies and Claire O'Callaghan (Eds)

The Gendered Motorcycle: Representations in Society, Media and Popular Culture
By Esperanza Miyake

Gendering History on Screen: Women Filmmakers and Historical Films
By Julia Erhart

Girls Like This, Boys Like That: The Reproduction of Gender in Contemporary Youth Cultures
By Victoria Cann

The Gypsy Woman: Representations in Literature and Visual Culture
By Jodie Matthews

Love Wars: Television Romantic Comedy
By Mary Irwin

Masculinity in Contemporary Science Fiction Cinema: Cyborgs, Troopers and Other Men of the Future
By Marianne Kac-Vergne

Moving to the Mainstream: Women On and Off Screen in Television and Film
By Marianne Kac-Vergne and Julie Assouly (Eds)

Paradoxical Pleasures: Female Submission in Popular and Erotic Fiction
By Anna Watz

Positive Images: Gay Men and HIV/AIDS in the Culture of 'Post-Crisis'
By Dion Kagan

Queer Horror Film and Television: Sexuality and Masculinity at the Margins
By Darren Elliott-Smith

Queer Sexualities in Early Film: Cinema and Male-Male Intimacy
By Shane Brown

Steampunk: Gender and the Neo-Victorian
By Claire Nally

Television Comedy and Femininity: Queering Gender
By Rosie White

Gender and Early television: Mapping Women's Role in Emerging US and British Media, 1850–1950
By Sarah Arnold

Tweenhood: Femininity and Celebrity in Tween Popular Culture
By Melanie Kennedy

Women Who Kill: Gender and Sexuality in Film and Series of the post-Feminist Era
By David Roche and Cristelle Maury (Eds)

Wonder Woman: Feminism, Culture and the Body By Joan Ormrod

Young Women, Girls and Postfeminism in Contemporary British Film
By Sarah Hill

Bad Girls, Dirty Bodies: Sex, Performance and Safe Femininity
By Gemma Commane

Are You Not Entertained?: Mapping the Gladiator Across Visual Media
By Lindsay Steenberg

Screening Queer Memory: LGBTQ Pasts in Contemporary Film and Television
By Anamarija Horvat

"Guilty Pleasures": European Audiences and Contemporary Hollywood Romantic Comedy
By Alice Guilluy

POSITIVE IMAGES

GAY MEN & HIV/AIDS IN THE CULTURE OF 'POST-CRISIS'

DION KAGAN

BLOOMSBURY ACADEMIC
LONDON • NEW YORK • OXFORD • NEW DELHI • SYDNEY

BLOOMSBURY ACADEMIC
Bloomsbury Publishing Plc
50 Bedford Square, London, WC1B 3DP, UK
1385 Broadway, New York, NY 10018, USA
29 Earlsfort Terrace, Dublin 2, Ireland

BLOOMSBURY, BLOOMSBURY ACADEMIC and the Diana logo
are trademarks of Bloomsbury Publishing Plc

First published in Great Britain 2018 by I.B. Tauris
Paperback edition published 2022 by Bloomsbury Academic

Copyright © Dion Kagan 2018, 2022

Dion Kagan has asserted his right under the Copyright,
Designs and Patents Act, 1988, to be identified as Author of this work.

For legal purposes the Acknowledgements on pp. xv–xviii constitute an
extension of this copyright page.

Cover illustration and design: Elwyn Murray

All rights reserved. No part of this publication may be reproduced or
transmitted in any form or by any means, electronic or mechanical,
including photocopying, recording, or any information storage or retrieval
system, without prior permission in writing from the publishers.

Bloomsbury Publishing Plc does not have any control over, or responsibility for,
any third-party websites referred to or in this book. All internet addresses given
in this book were correct at the time of going to press. The author and publisher
regret any inconvenience caused if addresses have changed or sites have
ceased to exist, but can accept no responsibility for any such changes.

A catalogue record for this book is available from the British Library.

A catalog record for this book is available from the Library of Congress.

ISBN: HB: 978-1-7845-3419-6
PB: 978-1-3502-5999-7
ePDF: 978-1-8386-0899-6
eBook: 978-1-8386-0898-9

Series: Library of Gender and Popular Culture

Typeset by Newgen Knowledge Works Pvt Ltd
Printed and bound in Great Britain

To find out more about our authors and books visit
www.bloomsbury.com and sign up for our newsletters.

'The so-called phenomenon of AIDS has become very much part of the texture of the quotidian, central to our common-sense perceptions of the way the world is, and thereby to our sense of commonality... [W]e are now being urged to think of HIV seropositivity, and indeed of "AIDS itself", as a chronic condition in the order of diabetes; we are, in short, becoming persuaded that AIDS belongs to the normative rather than the extraordinary, that AIDS is chronic rather than a crisis. We have erected, perhaps in place of other erections, entire structures of intelligibility and comprehensibility on and around the pandemic, structures that themselves render AIDS normative and routine: the business of AIDS, constructed and carried on around an impossible object, has become – like genocide, nuclear terror, racism, misogyny, and heteronormativity... – business as usual'.

– William Haver, *The Body of this Death: Historicity and Sociality in the Time of AIDS* (1996).

'Depression kicked in when it occurred to me that not only was I HIV positive, but I still had to do the laundry'.

– David Caron, *The Nearness of Others: Searching for Tact and Contact in The Age of HIV* (2014).

Contents

Illustrations	xiii
Acknowledgements	xv
Series Editors' Foreword	xix
Introduction: Crisis/Post-Crisis	**1**
Belated Diagnosis	3
Crisis/Post-Crisis	7
'Post-Crisis'	14
Chapter Outline	20
Crisis Discourse	26
After Antiretrovirals	46
1 Gay Redemption: Domestication and Disavowal in The Gay 90s	**47**
'The Big A'	47
The Gay 90s Revisited	52
Abjection and AIDS	61
The Next Best Thing	63
Watering, Working and Not Wearing Much	68
Look What Happened to Me	75
Abject Lessons	83
2 Positive Men Are from Mars, Negative Men Are from Venus: Sero-melodrama in *Queer As Folk*	**89**
'Sero-melodrama'	89
How Queer is *Queer as Folk*?	93
Perfect, Except for One Thing	100
Positive Men Are from Mars, Negative Men Are from Venus	111
Melodrama, Narrative Complexity and Post-Crisis Ambivalence	122
3 Crisis Re-Runs: Barebacking, *Chemsex* and Post-Crisis Sex Panic	**125**
Chemsex	125
Déjà vu	130

xi

	What is Barebacking?	133
	The Neal Hearings	145
	'HIV Man'	147
	'Re-Crisis'	151
	Neoliberal Biopolitics and the Logic of Epidemic	157
	Ambivalent Afterlives	160
4	**AIDS Heritage in *The Line of Beauty***	164
	Queer High Pop Heritage	168
	The Heritage Debates	170
	Heritage Ga(y)ze	175
	Homeless Love	183
	Belonging	187
	Eviction	191
	AIDS Heritage and Post-Crisis	196
5	**AIDS Retrovisions: *Dallas Buyers Club* and *The Normal Heart***	201
	Turning Away	201
	Turning Back	205
	Updating Sentimental Melodrama in *Dallas Buyers Club*	209
	After the Orgy: Teleological AIDS History in *The Normal Heart*	213
	Backward/Forward	219
	Feeling Generational	222
	Notes	237
	Bibliography	267
	Film and Television References	284
	Index	287

Illustrations

1.1	Transplanted tree in *The Next Best Thing* (2000, John Schlesinger, Warner Home Video, USA)	69
1.2	Robbie (Rupert Everett) rolls out pre-grown turf in *The Next Best Thing*	69
1.3	Robbie (Rupert Everett) and Abbie (Madonna) decide to have a baby in *The Next Best Thing*	70
1.4	Safe spectacle in *The Next Best Thing*: the New Gay Man is always on the move	71
1.5	Sanitation fantasy in *The Next Best Thing*	74
1.6	Vernon (Jack Betts) in *The Next Best Thing*	76
1.7	Ashby (William Mesnik) in *The Next Best Thing*	76
1.8	The straights v the gays at Joe's funeral in *The Next Best Thing*	78
1.9	Abject dread: (from R-L) Robbie (Rupert Everett), David (Neil Patrick Harris), Abbie (Madonna) and other friends at Joe's funeral in *The Next Best Thing*	79
1.10	David (Neil Patrick Harris) struggling with his medication in *The Next Best Thing*	84
1.11	Robbie surrenders in abject defeat in *The Next Best Thing*	86
2.1	Michael (Hal Sparks) and Ben (Robert Grant) experiencing 'the now' in *Queer as Folk* (season 2, episode 7, 2000–2005, Ron Cowen and Daniel Lipman, Showtime USA)	105
2.2	'Perfect except for one thing': Ben on the dance floor in *Queer as Folk* (season 2, episode 7)	105
2.3	Ben has roid rage in *Queer as Folk* (season 3, episode 4)	113
2.4	The drama of serodiscord in *Queer as Folk* (season 3, episode 6)	115
2.5	Michael's seroconversion fantasy in *Queer as Folk* (season 3, episode 6)	117

Illustrations

3.1	'Seedy World Unravels', *Herald Sun*, 31 March 2007	148
3.2	'Dance with Death', *The Age*, 21 April 2007	155
4.1	Distortions of perspective: Nick Guest (Dan Stevens) emerges from the shadows in *The Line of Beauty*, episode 1 (2006, Saul Dibb, BBC2)	176
4.2	Toby and Nick are dwarfed by the Feddens' mansion in *The Line of Beauty* (episode 1)	176
4.3	'Is this really where you live?' Nick gawks at the house in *The Line of Beauty* (episode 1)	177
4.4	Gothic Heritage: Hawkeswood in *The Line of Beauty* (episode 1)	179
4.5	Baroque Heritage in *The Line of Beauty* (episode 1)	180
4.6	Heritage Real Estate in *The Line of Beauty* (episode 1)	180
4.7	Nick steals a glance at Toby's (Oliver Coleman) buttocks in *The Line of Beauty* (episode 1)	181
4.8	Nick watches Gerald get swamped by the media in *The Line of Beauty* (episode 3)	182
4.9	Gerald Fedden (Tim McInnerny) is enveloped by paparazzi in *The Line of Beauty* (episode 3)	182
4.10	Alone in the crowd: Nick Guest at the party at Hawkeswood in *The Line of Beauty* (episode 1)	189
4.11	The shock of class difference: Gerard greets Leo (Don Gilet) in *The Line of Beauty* (episode 1)	190
4.12	The vulnerable space of bare life in *The Line of Beauty* (episode 3)	194
4.13	Leo showering and foreshadowing in *The Line of Beauty* (episode 1)	194
5.1	Benjamin Hancock and James Welsby in the poster for *HEX* (Next Wave Festival, Melbourne: 6–11 May 2014), photo by James Brown, graphic design by Laura Summers, image courtesy of James Welsby	232
5.2	James Welsby in *HEX*, photograph by Gregory Lorenzutti, image courtesy of James Welsby	233

Acknowledgements

There are several people who were especially instrumental in the creation of this book. Brett Farmer, my first mentor and most patient advisor during this project's germinal phase. Fran Martin, omnipresent guide, a committed and practical presence from those embryonic stages and a dedicated and delicate advocate throughout. Clara Tuite, an utterly formative influence on my interests and an enduring enabler of openness and receptivity in me to transformative critical thinking. Kane Race, whose queer ideas permeated this project long before his collegial presence helped me to extend and sustain my curiosity with the territory. Jasmine McGowan, my key collaborator and foremost interlocutor on matters of queer theory, and the most unwavering of collegial intimates. Caroline Hamilton, my complete professional support network stripped of all pretences, and the most faithful friend through various office and domestic cohabitations – very affectionate thanks to you Caroline.

I'm grateful to the Gender and Popular Culture series editors, Claire Nally and Angela Smith, for their interest in and support of this project, and I could not be more grateful to Anna Coatman and Lisa Goodrum at I.B.Tauris for their commitment and patience. I will feel forever grateful to have worked with Ellena Savage, the best writer and sharpest mind I know, on edits of the final manuscript. The luminous and talented artist Elwyn Murray created an extremely handsome cover illustration and design that I love. I am thankful to all the professionals who have worked on this book including the reviewers of my proposal and draft monograph who offered excellent advice and encouragement, and to both Kane Race and Cindy Patton, whose comments on an earlier version of this project were wildly useful and emboldening.

My friends from graduate school and beyond have presented the comradeship, empathy and mischief that motivated me to persevere in the face of the relentless self-doubt and various thrashings of scholarly life. I'm

Acknowledgements

particularly grateful for the presence and good humour of workshop cronies Louise Sheedy, Romana Byrne and Alison Horbury, who have shared feedback, conference trips and high-quality late-night hilarity. For their friendship, sharpness and careful interventions on early iterations of this work I am grateful to Phillip Thiel, Emily Bitto, Caroline Hamilton and Daniel Reeders. Other friends and professional thinkers have given me support and advice that has been extremely powerful at key moments, especially Alison Huber, Max Garnery, Chris Healy, Dennis Altman, Carol D'Cruz, Alice Burgin, Kristen Tytler, Jordy Silverstein, Ryan Conrad, Crystal McKinnon, Di Sanders, Gemma Blackwood, Lucy Van, Angie Hesson, Shane Tas, Felicity Ford and Peter Van Der Merwe. I can't imagine having had the wherewithal, resources or insights to see this project through without the intellectual and professional climate afforded to me by these collaborators, mentors, employers, lovers and sympathisers.

I owe immense thanks to teaching and research academics and graduate students past and present in the School of Culture and Communication (and beyond) at the University of Melbourne. For decisive work opportunities, peership, friendship, tutelage and collaboration I am grateful to Audrey Yue, Ana Drakojlovic, Barbara Creed, Mark Pendleton, Ben Gook, Joshua Pocious, Tim Laurie, Annemarie Jagose, Wendy Haslem, Isabelle Basher, Rachael Kendrick, Stuart Richards, Sashi Nair, Katsu Suganuma, Bobby Benedicto, Aren Azuira, Lou Farris, Sara Taylor, Scott Brook, Michael Farrell, Roman Lobato, Tom Apperley, Jo Shedy, Sufern Ho, Jemma Hefter, Jessica Raschke, Peta Mayer, Jay Thompson, Michelle Smith, Romy Ash, Eddie Patterson, Lara Stevens, Robbie Fordyce, Tim Neale, Claire Henry, Amy Espeseth, Tammi Jonas, Caroline Wallace and others I have doubtlessly forgotten.

I have benefited much from the time and ideas of those who contributed insight and experience from the frontlines of HIV public health, HIV services and social sex research, particularly Colin Batrouney, Paul Kidd, Paul Byron, Henry von Doussa and Heath Paynter. Daniel Reeders has been an especially sharp and generous presence and advocate across multiple professional and knowledge fields. I am thankful to the staff and volunteers at the Victorian AIDS Council (now Thorne Harbour Health) and the Positive Living Centre in Melbourne where I worked as a volunteer for some years, and who

Acknowledgements

offered me access to their media archive. The researchers and support staff at the Australian Research Centre in Sex, Health and Society, La Trobe University – especially Gary Dowsett, Gillian Fletcher, Steven Angelides, Natalie Hendry, Andy Westle, Jeffery Grierson, Henry Von Doussa and Anthony Smith gave me valuable work and genuinely welcomed me into their supportive and inspiring research community.

I'm grateful to many artist, activist, academic and writer friends who have done work on HIV and queer life that has had a powerful influence on my thoughts and feelings. These people include Alyson Campbell, Ryan Conrad, Rohan Spong, Nic Holas, James Welsby and Benjamin Riley. There are too many important people in the Australian writing community who have worked with and befriended me during this period to list, however special mention must go to Lisa Dempster, *The Rereaders* the people of the National Young Writers' Festival and everyone at *The Lifted Brow*. Special thanks to Ellena Savage, Stephanie Van Schilt, Mel Campbell and Adam Curley.

For three and a half years this project was funded by the Australian government through an Australian **Postgraduate Award**. I have been fortunate to present portions of this research at the Cultural Studies Association of Australasia annual conferences in Sydney and Melbourne, the Australasian Society for HIV Medicine's Annual HIV/AIDS conference, the International Association for the Study of Sexuality, Culture and Society in Dublin, the Somatechnics Institute conference in Sydney, the Australasian Victorian Studies Association conference in Melbourne and to other audiences at Sydney University, the University of Melbourne and Griffith University in Brisbane. Many thanks to those that have hosted me in those institutions. And thanks to the scholarly and academic journals *Literature/Film Quarterly*, *Continuum*, *Sexualities*, *Kill Your Darlings* and *The Lifted Brow* for permission to re-publish excerpts and adapted sections from earlier versions of some of the material in this book.

I would be nowhere without the help of Judi Bernshaw, Jack Kagan and Lana Kagan, who have supported me with endless patience, sustenance, practical support and love during the slow toil through this big project. Special thanks to Julian Hobba, Laura Kelly, Michelle Dufty, Robbie McNab, Anita Fiorenza, Mitchell von Buglehall and all those

Acknowledgements

who have been charitable about making a home with me over the years. Many friends, family members and lovers have propped me up with confidence and encouragement throughout this project's lifespan. Most of them have persisted with the friendship. I am grateful to them all.

Series Editors' Foreword

AIDS entered public consciousness in the early 1980s, when it was generally misunderstood and its cause and modes of transmission remained mysterious. In 1984 medical fraternities in France and the US announced discoveries that would lead to the linking of AIDS with HIV (human immunodeficiency virus), a virus that attacks the immune system. Meanwhile, AIDS in Europe and the US was associated with homosexuals, migrants, drug users and other stigmatised communities, and widespread panic was fuelled by the popular media. The sexual dimension of this new, mysterious and frightening fatal disease stirred up a profound example of what historians of sexuality call 'sex panic'. Rock Hudson became one of the first celebrities to die from AIDS in 1985, and Freddie Mercury six years later. Media responses were scandalised, less than sympathetic and frequently conflated AIDS with the sexual practices and cultures of gay men.

But what has happened to HIV and AIDS, and to this monolithic association of the disease with homosexuality? This book is situated in the time 'after' the crisis, from the mid-1990s to the 2010s. Following the game-changing advent of lifesaving drugs known as antiretrovirals, the latter half of the 1990s were marked by a massively reduced attention to HIV/AIDS in popular media and culture. *Positive Images* addresses the representation and experience of the queer community – specifically gay men – through the popular culture of the English-speaking world during this period. It offers a corrective to this post-crisis silence, and registers the complexities of the cultural shift from the image of people dying in vast numbers, to the culture of those *living with* HIV. It also examines the increased visibility of queer life in popular culture against the fraught and unresolved legacies of the mass media panic of the AIDS crisis.

As many of the books in this series reveal, representations of gender and sexuality in film, television, digital spaces and literature can uncover

Series Editors' Foreword

how far popular culture can be a source of alternative, queer, and positive identities. Frequently, however, whilst such 'positive images' suggest increased visibility, complexity and understanding, they are also inflected with the logics of neoliberalism and homonormativity, which erodes the radical potential of sexual difference, and substitutes it with a domesticated and depoliticised gay identity.

Claire Nally and Angela Smith

Introduction

Crisis/Post-Crisis

From somewhere around the middle of the 1990s until the earlier part of the 2010s, the popular culture of the rich, English-speaking world became somewhat quiet on the subjects of HIV and AIDS. Of course, there were exceptions, and then, during the 2010s, there emerged a renewed interest in the early history of AIDS. But, generally speaking, since the introduction of antiretroviral drugs (ARVs) in 1996 – the period this book calls 'post-crisis' – things have been relatively quiet. After a very nosiy, very anxious 15 years of crisis mode responses to HIV/AIDS, Anglo-European and American popular culture went into 15 years of what Kane Race calls 'undetectable crisis'[1] – beyond the communities directly affected by it, HIV became the forgotten virus.

These years, beginning with the arrival of ARVs and concluding with the return to AIDS crisis histories in recent years, is the period that *Positive Images* takes as its principal focus. In contrast to the immense archive of literature on the media of 'The AIDS Crisis', the cultural history of HIV/AIDS in the popular culture of 'post-crisis' is a story that is yet to be comprehensively told. *Positive Images*, with its particular focus on representations of gay men and HIV/AIDS during this quieter period, starts to remedy that by asking, 'What happened to HIV/AIDS during those years?'

The relative quiet on the subject that characterised this period – the manifest absence of HIV/AIDS discussions and storytelling in the mainstream media – was by no means absolute. This is important. Were there no significant exceptions to this overall trend, like *Queer as Folk* (2000–5), *Angels in America* (2003), *The Line of Beauty* (both novel and mini-series, 2003 and 2006), various sex panics about barebacking and methamphetamine use among gay men – exceptions that all brought stories about HIV/AIDS to large audiences – this book would have scant material to consider. And yet, compared to the extraordinary scale of images and accounts of AIDS in its first 15 years, an *epidemic* (to use that now well-worn metaphor) of news reportage, film, TV, literature and photography, this second 15 was marked by absence. Now, in the fourth decade of HIV, there has been something of a popular return to HIV/AIDS as a subject of history and cultural memory. Although this return doesn't come anywhere near approximating the colossal scale of nervous, fascinated attention the disease garnered during the 1980s and early 1990s, there has been, as we shall consider in the final chapters of this book in more detail, a turn to the AIDS past: a flourishing of archival projects, visual art retrospectives, prestige period TV dramas, Oscar-winning globally popular narrative films, documentaries, remakes, remounts and cross-textual adaptations of literary and performing art works from earlier in the pandemic.

But what happened to HIV/AIDS in the intervening years? More specifically, what happened to representations of HIV/AIDS, gay men and queer life during this period? What were the legacies of the earlier moment of panicked AIDS crisis representations during these years, after the dramatic changes brought about by antiretrovirals (in the parts of the world where they became available) from around 1996 onwards? And what are the significances of these representations of 'post-crisis'? That is, how has this post-antiretrovirals period come to inform and affect the way we understand queer life and life with HIV in the present and the future? These are the main questions *Positive Images* seeks to explore.

One means to begin a consideration of these questions is by jumping straight into an example – one that is illustrative, I think, of some of this book's larger conclusions. Among the handful of popular English-speaking representations of HIV and gay men to emerge in the years after antiretrovirals was a subplot that unfolded during the fifth and sixth seasons of the

American ABC drama series *Brothers & Sisters* (2006–2011). This was a particularly quiet time for stories about HIV: after North American *Queer as Folk* finished its five-season run in 2005 there were at least five years with no HIV positive characters on American primetime television. Then, *Brothers & Sisters* introduced a new storyline in which a central character, Saul Holden (Ron Rifkin), discovers belatedly and at an advanced age that he is HIV positive and has been for a long time. As we shall see, this belatedness, the association of HIV with an older generation of gay men, and the idea of past historical incidences of naïve or dangerous sexual transmission are key dynamics in the representation of HIV and gay life in this story arc. Despite its implausibility, the HIV plot on *Brothers & Sisters* exposes assumptions around queer and AIDS history, memory, and the present and future of gay male life that starts to unravel some important themes in the logic of post-crisis representation that we will explore further in this book.

Belated Diagnosis

Brothers & Sisters was an American Sunday-night ensemble family drama that centered on the Walkers and their lives in Los Angeles and Pasadena. After remaining sexually ambiguous throughout season one and for most of season two, Saul Holden, brother of the widowed Nora Walker (Sally Field), comes out to his openly gay nephew, Kevin (Matthew Rhys). As a white man in his seventies coming out several decades after the emergence of the American gay pride movement, Saul expresses regret about the life he has spent in the closet and hopes to now live openly and honestly as a gay man. In season four, Saul is contacted by a former lover on Facebook. When he shares this with Kevin and Kevin's partner, Scotty (Luke Macfarlane), Scotty notices that the former lover's Facebook profile indicates that he is an HIV activist who has been living with HIV for many years. This information prompts Saul to admit that he's never been tested for HIV. Saul also ruefully confesses that decades earlier he'd had a series of sexual encounters without condoms because of his closettedness and because of the general ignorance about transmission and prevention in those early years of HIV/AIDS. In response to this melancholic admission of a furtive, shameful, dangerous sexual past and in spite of the fact that Saul hasn't had sex with any men since then, which has literally been decades, Kevin and Scotty encourage Saul to get tested for HIV. 'It's like spring cleaning!' Scotty says, indicating the way in which by 2010 HIV testing was well and truly a quotidian, only semi-remarkable life practice for many self- identified gay men in the places where living as an out gay man had itself become possible and even 'normal', and where regular HIV testing was widely available. Saul initially resists, quarrelling with Kevin and Scotty about this hesitancy to get tested, but eventually he relents and requests an HIV test from his doctor. In the final episode of season four, after a dramatic cliffhanger car accident that leaves Saul with a bleeding wound on his arm and another character in a coma, it is revealed that Saul is HIV positive, however medically improbable that might be after so many celibate, asymptomatic years.

There are both distinctly contemporary, 'up-to-date' and distinctly retrograde elements in this HIV plot that begin to illuminate the complex scene of post-crisis HIV representation in popular culture. Melanie Kohnen and David Oscar Harvey have noticed similar elements in the *Brothers & Sisters* plot and in the analysis that follows I have incorporated their insights.[2]

Like *Queer as Folk*, as we will see in Chapter 2, *Brothers & Sisters* calls on generational difference as a way to represent its characters' different dispositions towards gay life. Generational difference, a temporal metaphor mired in ideas about kinship, functions as a way of distinguishing Saul's from Kevin and Scotty's experiences as gay men and becomes emblematic of an imagined demarcation of past and present gay lives. More importantly, generational difference serves a broader symbolic function – one we will return to throughout this book – of understanding HIV/ AIDS through a prism of historical disparity and transformation. That a mainstream network TV drama like *Brothers & Sisters* addressed the otherwise marginal topic of HIV/ AIDS at this time may be considered progressive: it demonstrates an interest in representing marginal experience and it reiterates the important shift from earlier images of people dying from AIDS to the contemporary experience of *living* with HIV. On the other hand, *Brothers & Sisters* associates HIV with a dark and gloomy history; it cannot imagine HIV as anything but a relic from an unhappy past, and does very little to account for the experience of living with HIV today. This is illustrative of a broader trend in popular culture, as Harvey writes: 'we cannot seem to articulate or envision HIV without harkening back to its past and to previous incarnations of failing immune responses and mortality.'[3]

Saul is a member of an older generation that came of age in the heady days of the 1970s and early 1980s. This was a period of sexual liberation and lots of sex for some, but it was still very much a time of uneven social and cultural visibility, before AIDS in the 1980s and the so-called 'Gay 90s' radically augmented queer visibility, and long before the current era of queer-themed TV, equality politics and marriage reform. In contrast to Saul, Kevin and Scotty are subjects of this contemporary, post-crisis moment: open about their sexuality, settled in their partnership and expecting their own child. Their lives are oriented to the pursuit of family and the privileges of a bourgeois lifeworld. This alignment of different temporal modes – past and present, old and young, outdated and contemporary – with different life trajectories (alone vs coupled with children), different sexual modalities (promiscuous vs monogamous) and different affects (shame vs optimism; anxiety vs stability; self-hatred vs a sense of rightful entitlement) come into sharpest relief in an emotionally charged confrontation around the pressure the younger couple are putting on the older man to get tested for HIV:

SAUL: Do you have any idea what you're asking of me? Do you? This world the two of you live in, where everything is so easy and so much is possible. You have a surrogate carrying your child! You're married!
KEVIN: Technically, we're not married.
SAUL: Oh, Kevin, excuse me, I'm so sorry, you're domestic partners, whatever. When I was your age, I just hoped I wouldn't get arrested when I walked into a gay bar.

In this exchange, Saul's experience as a gay man is associated with a dark, unhappy past, while Kevin and Scotty's experience is aligned with the positive present and with a future invoked by the reference to their unborn child. Although it remains unmentioned, the event of 'The AIDS Crisis' functions as a turning point in this logic of LGBTQI+ history, a kind of historical marker dividing these two generations, albeit subtextually.

In her analysis of the show, Kohnen makes a similar observation. She argues that through this trope of generational contrast and conflict, *Brothers & Sisters* 'privileges a moralising discourse that identifies Saul's experiences as part of a shameful, oppressive past, and portrays Kevin and Scotty's life choices as exemplary, or, at the very least, as preferable and appropriate to the current historical moment.'[4] This generational tension highlights the progress *certain* gays and lesbians have made, while other queers remain associated with the oppressions of history. As we will see throughout *Positive Images*, popular memories of AIDS are frequently recruited to this teleology of progress from the shameful closeted past to the proud, visible LGBTQI+ present. What this teleology tends to overlook is that increased visibility and other forms of 'progress' have developed alongside a narrow 'normalising' of queer life – a shift registered in popular culture by the increased presence of white, upwardly mobile, cis gay monogamous couples like Kevin and Scotty on our screens, an image that has become the iconic representation of a new way of being gay, a privatised, life-styled, domestically-oriented 'new homonormativity'.[5]

A 'behind the scenes' discussion of this story arc featuring writer-director David Marshall Grant and actor Ron Rifkin reiterates the generational and temporal logic informing this HIV plot development. Grant says that:

> what we were so invested [in was] this notion of *the generational divide* in terms of the experience of being gay. And, to have grown up gay when you are seventy now, is a very different experience to being gay now [sic]… So, for Ron's character to come out was a huge thing for him. And then we wanted to take it *to its next conclusion* – well, not conclusion, the next possible story – which is, what if, after all these years, he had never been tested, and found out that he was HIV positive.[6]

Beyond Grant's emphasis on a 'generational divide', there is an awkward temporal shift from describing Saul who is 'seventy now' to 'being gay now' that privileges a certain form of gayness – the one embodied by Kevin and Scotty – as the form more comfortably aligned with the present. The implication is that the older character, Saul, is not actually 'being gay now'. Grant's suggestion, then qualified, that HIV would be the 'logical conclusion' for a gay man of Ron's vintage, reveals an alignment of HIV with the past.

Introduction

The storyline of Kevin and Scotty as parents is also, as Kohnen points out, 'another example of how reproductive futurism shapes current modes of queer visibility.'[7] We'll return to queer futurism and its relationship with HIV/AIDS later in this chapter and in the next. For now, it is enough to point out that through the character of Saul, HIV/AIDS takes on a temporal dimension that is *negatively valued*. Via Saul, HIV falls outside of the norms of contemporary gay life and becomes a 'reprehensible reminder of a past that gays and lesbians should leave behind.'[8] Saul's tension with his nephew is organised around a logic of historical difference in which HIV/AIDS and the queer past are pitted against the present and against the norms of '"positive images" of HIV negative men.'[9] Queer identifications and practices that fall outside of the Kevin and Scotty paradigm don't fit with the current model of how to be gay; HIV positive gay men are throwbacks to the past.

There are by now a very large number of critiques of the 'homonormalisation' of queer life and representation in contemporary culture, particularly in the privileged Global North. These critiques have developed for at least the last fifteen years and we will consider some of them in more detail shortly. If we include the history of HIV and AIDS representation alongside these critiques, it becomes clear that after antiretrovirals, HIV/AIDS has increasingly become a signifier of *backwardness* in popular culture. This logic is evident in *Brothers & Sisters* and, in some or other fashion it haunts all of the examples of post-crisis cultural production considered in this book. 'Haunting' is a useful metaphor because it evokes a troubling, unresolved presence, something from the past that both persists in and disturbs the present – a 'ghost' that rattles and clashes with the priorities of that present and that many would prefer to ignore, forget or exorcise. Before we consider these hauntings as they manifest in artifacts of post-crisis culture, we must first return to both the history of HIV/AIDS and the transformations that have taken place since the advent of ARVs in 1996.

Crisis/Post-Crisis

The extraordinary scale of the public sex panic around the AIDS crisis of the 1980s and early 1990s was unprecedented. Like all chronicled chapters in the history of epidemic disease – plague, typhoid, cholera, syphilis – the representation of AIDS drew on a large, pre-existing archive of frightening images. But, unlike previous epidemics, HIV/AIDS became visible in images and language at a historical moment when communication technologies could produce, reproduce and distribute those messages more vividly and more extensively than ever before. Reflecting on this time, David Caron writes that 'the metaphorical power of all infectious diseases, especially if they are new, mysterious, and lethal, found itself multiplied in the case of AIDS.'[10] This was an epidemic of the media age. In 1987 Paula Treichler pithily dubbed this explosion of AIDS images and storytelling an 'epidemic of signification.'[11] Some years later, Lee Edelman called it 'The Plague of Discourse.'[12] Now able to be mediated through an unprecedented number of new broadcasting avenues and consumed at myriad sites of reception, the alarm bells set off by a sexual epidemic were amplified loudly.

Western gay men living in urban gay epicentres were the first groups publicly associated with AIDS and thus, from the beginning, the story of AIDS was tied to old and new stories about homosexual men and homosexual sex. When HIV/AIDS first entered the official medical and scientific record in 1981, it was labelled 'Gay Related Immune Deficiency' (GRID). So, although there is nothing inherently meaningful about a virus,[13] particular conditions of history and ecology meant that the meanings that emerged around HIV/AIDS hitched their wagon to pre-existing ideas about modern identarian homosexuality.

This irresistible, reasonable-seeming association between an already perceived-to-be pathological sexuality and a mysterious and almost certainly fatal sexuality transmitted disease became very difficult to prise apart. A decade after the first reports of 'GRID', feminist philosopher Judith Butler wrote that 'throughout the media's hysterical and homophobic response to the illness there is a tactical construction of a continuity between the polluted states of the homosexual by virtue of the boundary-trespass that *is* homosexuality and the disease as a specific modality of homosexual pollution.'[14] Gay activist and historian Jeffrey Weeks was able to look back at the first decade of HIV and similarly declare that AIDS and male homosexuality had become 'intertwined in a difficult and complicated history.'[15] One might even suggest that male homosexuality had almost become unthinkable by that time without the presence and meanings associated with AIDS. 'Anyone writing on homosexuality, especially male homosexuality', Weeks wrote, 'does so under the shadow of HIV infection and AIDS… [for] it is surely undeniable that a major part of the symbolic power of "AIDS" stems from its association with a still stigmatised sexuality and an unpopular sexual minority in the industrialised countries of the "advanced" west.'[16] To generalise what by then had become a central observation in the emerging scholarly and activist field of AIDS cultural criticism: during the first decade of the AIDS crisis (and in many instances beyond), public discourses from scientific research journals to tabloid reports to blockbuster Hollywood movies represented AIDS as 'the disease of gayness itself'.[17] Many years on, we continue to live with the complex and stigmatising legacies of this conflation.

Now, more than three and a half decades into the global pandemic, the conditions surrounding HIV/AIDS are almost unrecognisably transformed. For People Living with HIV (PLWHIV)[18], the meaning and experience of HIV changed radically around 1996, the year that saw the advent of Highly Active Antiretroviral Therapies (HAART). A life-prolonging medical treatment, HAART was announced at the 1996 International AIDS conference in Vancouver, provoking discussions of 'the end of AIDS' and heralding the so-called 'post-AIDS' era.[19] Where a positive diagnosis had previously promised almost certain and sometimes precipitate death, now, where access to HIV testing, ARVs and other optimal health and welfare conditions became available, PLWHIV could anticipate living healthy, 'normal' lives. Though it would be wrong to assume that this is the case for all people affected by the disease worldwide, now, in many places, treatment discourses encourage us to think in terms of 'HIV' instead of 'AIDS.' Rather than a spectacularly terrifying death sentence, HIV is understood as a chronic but manageable illness.

The shifts brought about by these life-saving medical interventions completely altered the epidemiological, political and cultural scripting of HIV/AIDS and its temporalities.[20] In the rich, industrialised countries of the Global North, the apocalyptic rhetoric that once characterised AIDS discussions appears to be all but gone. HIV is more quietly interweaved into the fabric of social and cultural life, and much of the time it remains concealed from broader public view – an 'undetectable' crisis. In Australia, for example, long-time AIDS activist and academic Denis Altman wrote in *The Monthly* in 2007 that HIV/AIDS was at 'the margins of our attention'.[21] Five years later the same magazine reiterated this theme of cultural invisibility in an article titled 'A Quiet Anniversary: AIDS 30 Years on'.[22]

In such parts of the privileged Global North like Australia where drugs have been longer available and better distributed, there has been something of a 'normalisation' of HIV, a diminution of its once terrifying status and a kind of incorporation of it into institutional, social norms. David Herkt describes this fittingly when he writes that, after 1996 'HIV/AIDS gradually became a setting, not an emphasis. It retreated into the omnipresent background static of an acceptable medical circumstance.'[23] Though this isn't necessarily a unique historical trajectory for epidemic diseases, in the case of HIV it did happen considerably quickly – the relatively recent epidemiological conditions of 'crisis' becoming a fast-receding historical past, whereas HIV in the present becomes quotidian, even banal in some quarters. From the extraordinary, spectacular position it once held in public discussions, HIV/ AIDS has faded, superseded by the urgency of newer viral threats like Ebola, Zika and of course now Covid-19. In this sense, we have learned to live with HIV.

And yet this isn't the full story. The shift in perceptions as we have moved from 'AIDS crisis' to 'post-crisis' and the effect this shift has had on representations of HIV and AIDS and male homosexuality is not a simple story of a fatal disease becoming a manageable one and thus becoming 'normal.' These transformations are a complicated, non-linear tale. HIV has been domesticated, but in complex, ambivalent and paradoxical ways, with implications for how *all* sexualities are understood and experienced. My aim in *Positive Images* is to unearth and think through some of these implications.

Like HIV, male homosexuality is something our culture has also seemingly become more accustomed to living with, again in fraught and uneven ways. From the 'Gay 90s' onwards, images of benign and easily digestible types of gay men proliferated across pop cultural forms. While during the AIDS crisis male homosexuality was widely characterised in the media as polluting, promiscuous and disease-spreading, the 'positive images' of the last 20 to 30 years have become far more likely to portray gay men as squeaky clean, asexual or monogamous, life- and love-affirming.

Introduction

Positive Images examines this transformed, post-crisis media landscape in parts of the Global North and in artifacts of global Anglophone popular culture. What kind of transformed images has this new cultural landscape generated, and what are the implications of these images for our understandings of (homo)sexuality and epidemic disease? What has changed in the shift away from AIDS-as-crisis to the calmer, more mundane landscape of post-crisis? And what are the legacies of the panicked, rhetorically inflated discourses of the crisis years? If AIDS and gayness were once tangled in an inextricable metaphorical embrace, how do we understand the relationship between HIV and male homosexuality now? *Positive Images* responds to these questions through a close analysis of popular English-speaking media texts that represent gay men and HIV/AIDS in or from within this transformed cultural moment. It offers the first dedicated cultural history of the years since 1996, albeit with a necessarily specific focus on key moments, key texts and particular debates. Taking my cue from an earlier archive of (predominantly North American) critical responses to AIDS representation, I look mostly to 'the popular' and 'the mainstream' as a lens through which to consider the cultural politics of this period. Of course, there are other methods to answer such questions. However, my examination of American, British and Australian texts from across a range of widely-consumed media forms, including narrative cinema, documentary, popular fiction, cable TV, news coverage and pornography, highlights the continued – albeit transformed – presence of 'crisis' in the new landscape of 'post-crisis', the uneasy relationship between these two historical moments, and some of the main ways this relationship is grappled with in popular culture.

In this context, then, 'positive images' has at least two meanings. For this book's specific focus of study it refers to representations of gay men who are HIV positive or whose lives are touched in significant ways by their living in the era of HIV. At the same time, 'positive images' is a nod to the idea of prideful, progressive representations of queer people that emerged from the 'politics of representation' debates in gay and lesbian studies and activist circles during the late 1970s and 1980s, and crossed over into mainstream media production and reception in the 1990s. Drawing inspiration from feminist criticism, early waves of gay and lesbian media scholarship identified the stereotypes on display in popular culture, charging the culture industries with a history of queer exclusion and calling for greater visibility and 'accuracy' in the representation of queer sexualities. Pioneering works like Richard Dyer's *Gays and Film* (1977) and Vitto Russo's *The Celluloid Closet* (1981) identified (and tended to denounce) representations that reinforced homophobia. These critiques were largely aligned with the aims of anti-homophobic movements including organisations like the still-active US Gay and Lesbian Alliance Against Defamation (GLAAD), formed in New York in 1985 to protest against defamatory and sensationalised coverage of AIDS in the *New York Post*. Drawing on the energies and sentiments of 1970s gay pride and affirmation politics, this strand of activist, scholarly and cultural work yearned to replace 'negative images' with 'positive' ones. The history of this impulse is tied in interesting ways to the history of AIDS representation.

Dyer, who has remained a key figure in debates about queer representation, has explained that the 'positive images' ideal has tended to imply three attributes of representation: 'thereness', 'goodness' and 'realness':

> Thereness insist[s] on the fact of our existence; goodness, assert[s] our worth and that of our life-styles; and realness, show[s] what we were in fact like.[24]

However, as Dyer contends, thereness and goodness can sometimes be at odds with realness. Though a campaign for prideful representation is understandable given the dominance of homophobia in western media culture throughout modernity, the conventions that have become the mainstay of the positive images agenda – smiling faces, happy endings and stories of success – don't always reflect the material realities of queer lives.[25] Positive images have tended to disavow a consciousness of the negative states and feelings that have constituted queer life, both historically and now. They may also set up a further set of unrealistic norms that are irrelevant or unreachable for most queer people. Nonetheless, to a large extent the positive images rationale has fixed the standards of judgement for the representations of queer sexualities and genders in popular culture. It has become a key criterion informing the entire enterprise of producing and consuming images of queer people: Are they positive or negative images? Are they accurate representations or stereotypes?

The conventions of positive images have also become implicated in and emblematic of the now widespread politics of queer liberalism and the rights-based political agendas of mainstream LGBTQI+ organisations. Ellis Hanson alluded to this when he somewhat acerbically described 'positive images' as

> representations of sexual minorities as normal, happy, intelligent, kind, sexually well-adjusted, professionally adept, politically correct ladies and gentlemen who have no doubt earned all those elusive civil rights for which we have all been clamouring.[26]

In other words, positive images represent both impossible ideals and restrictive norms. As we shall see, the move toward the neoliberal normative has become a core thematic trajectory in post-crisis image culture's migration from the traumatic geography of AIDS crisis to the new landscapes of the post – as it has in mainstream contemporary gay and lesbian politics and cultural production more generally. 'Positive images', then, in both of the senses of the term as I have explained it here, frequently denotes a gay and/or an HIV 'positive' agenda for representation dominated by homonormative images of gay and lesbian life in neoliberal times, at the expense of other, queerer and more marginal identities and lives.

So, although this book is part of the tradition of critical examinations of the politics of representation, it is probably clear by now that *Positive Images* is more consciously aligned with the political, theoretical and cultural interventions of queer theory and queer politics. 'Queer' has tended to be more suspicious of the desire for and implications of normativity that has become implicit to and complicit with positive images. The politics of queer critique sit somewhat uneasily with the positive images agenda. And yet, both traditions are motivated by the ongoing conviction that, as Dyer famously put it, 'representation matters'.[27] Representation, especially popular representation, provides us with the stories, symbols and myths through which we are able to understand and participate in a common culture, including what it means and how it feels to inhabit a sexed, gendered and erotically coded body. Representation – literature, film, TV, digital media, *all media* – are a symbolic and imaginative reservoir out of which we fashion our sense of identity, community and relationality. And representation has material effects: 'how we are seen', Dyer explains, 'determines in part how we are treated; how we treat others is based on how we see them [and] such seeing comes from representation.'[28] I remain convinced that closely considering representations and people's uses of and responses to them can reveal important things about the way we live, particularly the way we comprehend and experience sexuality. Therefore I draw on the methods of close textual analysis, informed by feminist, queer, poststructuralist and post-Foucauldian theories of language, meaning and ideology. Some people criticise this approach because of a supposed 'gulf between cultural or textual analysis, on the one hand, and social or political effect, on the other.'[29] However, I have ongoing faith in the capacity for ideologically attuned textual analysis to highlight the broader cultural and social contexts from which those texts emerge, and in which they themselves constitute cultural events with a range of effects. As Robert Stam explains, culture is 'spread out over a broad discursive continuum' within which 'texts are embedded in a social matrix and where they have consequences in the world.'[30]

This is as much the case for disease as it is for sexuality. The conviction that representation matters has been central to humanities and social sciences interventions into HIV/AIDS and remains of utmost important to the lived experience, understanding and management of HIV. 'AIDS' and 'HIV' cannot be understood separately from the ways in which they are represented. This has been a pivotal axiom for AIDS cultural criticism since the early 1980s and cultural work on HIV remains of ongoing importance. Beyond its interest to readers curious about sexuality and gender in popular media then, this book's cultural history of positive images since the transformative medical interventions of 1996 may, I hope, be relevant to readers in other professional contexts like public health, activism, medical and scientific research, stigma reduction, disease prevention and the myriad other community and professional practices concerned with HIV.

'Post-Crisis'

The term 'post-crisis' originates from the field of AIDS social research where it was first used to describe the transformed conditions surrounding the epidemic among gay men in the developed world. In Australia, the term evolved out of Gary Dowsett's formulation of 'post-AIDS', introduced at a health promotion conference in Sydney in 1995. Dowsett intended 'post-AIDS' to describe a cluster of changes including the advent of ARVs and the perception that HIV was no longer a crisis, which he observed was the dominant feeling among many American and Australian gay men at that time.[31] Debate about the usefulness of 'post-AIDS' and its potentially misleading implication that HIV/AIDS was over gave rise to 'post-crisis' as an alternative term.[32] For many social researchers, peer educators, health promoters, policymakers and others across the HIV/ AIDS sector, the notion of post-crisis came to operate as a kind of umbrella description of the evolving conditions of the epidemic among gay men and men who have sex with men (MSM) in the post-ARVs universe (regardless of whether this term was explicitly used or not).

Appropriating this concept from these contexts, I suggest we put 'post-crisis' to use as a category of culture and representation. As a periodising framework, 'post-crisis' describes the cultural re-scripting of HIV/AIDS from a state of crisis to one of chronicity that has acted as a backdrop to new representations of HIV and AIDS and male homosexuality. I have pinpointed the advent of ARVs (*c* .1996) as a turning point to help identify distinctions between 'crisis' and 'post-crisis' as historical and cultural moments with different representational schema – although we shouldn't over-determine the impact of medical technologies as a single culture-altering factor or as a precise historical point around which large scale epidemiological, somatechnical changes and shifts in meaning and representation have occurred.[33] Certainly, the centrality of drugs, other technologies of disease prevention and the medicalisation of HIV management in the scene of post-crisis cannot be understated. Indeed, the frequent *lack* of images of pharmaceutical drugs and explorations of treatment issues related to living with HIV in popular culture has been one of this culture's most striking absences. However, placing too much emphasis on the advent of ARVs may risk overlooking other important factors: it risks reinforcing a 'technological determinism' that ignores the complicated pre-existing assemblages into which new health technologies arrive. Culture and science are not discrete or opposing domains. On this matter I agree with Kane Race who wonders if 'the desire to keep things completely separate doesn't reproduce the notion of the social and the biomedical as independent and discrete spheres – as though the social were not affected by the products of capitalised medicine and as though these products were not the outcome of specific social practices and frames of reference.' I share Race's conviction that, when it comes to HIV, 'we need an account of this moment that situates it in terms of a broader politics of knowledge and consumption – a politics that cuts across commercial and socio-sexual domains.'[34]

Alongside the dramatic changes wrought by the advent of ARVs there have been other major technological, social and epidemiological transformations. These include: the rapid and widespread incorporation of safer sex practices between 1984 and 1994 that led to a steep decline in HIV in gay male populations;[35] emotional and political burnout among first-wave AIDS activists; various makeovers in the roles and anatomy of AIDS Service Organisations (ASOs);[36] the ascendance of neoliberal strategies of HIV management including the regulation of HIV positive health through the lens of the viral load test;[37] new debates about new technologies of HIV prevention including rapid testing, treatment as prevention (TasP), which includes the deployment of undetectable HIV viral load as a preventative measure against onward transmissions and the use of pre-exposure prophylaxis (PrEP, commonly known in some places by its commercial drug name, 'Truvada') among at-risk populations, one of the most controversial of these developments. These are all complex phenomena and contexts that warrant dedicated discussions of their own. *Positive Images* takes popular cultural as its focus. The critical examination of biomedical and other scientific literature on HIV has been an extremely productive tradition in AIDS cultural criticism. As I shall discuss shortly in more detail, the contention that scientific and medical knowledge and practices are construed in accordance with pre-existing or emergent metaphoric and linguistic – and hence ideological – structures has been a central preoccupation in this field. Virology, immunology and epidemiology are no less metaphor-free than other scientific languages. Scientific knowledge is never neutral or pure, which makes critical analyses of medical practice, scientific idioms and the reception of new technologies crucial.

For example, Race has written of the way in which medical discourses around 'patient compliance' with ARVs, viral load testing and other technologies of HIV management work to operationalise 'a new field of normativity around health and consumption, in which the moral worth of subjects is *exemplified* in relation to a generalised sense of medical prescription.'[38] In other words, HIV positive people may be deemed good citizens if they comply with the prevailing instructions of medical and scientific authorities. HIV is a life field in which the dynamic flows of technology and behaviour are constantly shifting; debate and critical analysis of these flows is key to understanding and intervening in the ever-evolving landscapes of the pandemic. However, I leave the critique of HIV biomedicine, treatment technology and other scientific, juridical and regulatory responses to HIV in the capable hands of other researchers.[39] The sphere of 'culture' is by no means separate from these domains, and yet looking too far beyond the texts and contexts of fictional and documentary media has been beyond the scope of this project.

The most recent UNAIDS global and regional statistics on AIDS and HIV reported good and bad news. At the time of writing, the number of new HIV notifications per year has decreased in most parts of the world, including western and Central Africa, Eastern and Southern Africa, Asia and the Pacific. However, in parts of North Africa and the Middle East they have increased. The global uptake of antiretroviral therapies continues to increase globally, in the millions, and AIDS-related deaths continue to decrease in almost all parts of the world, with the exception of parts of Eastern Europe and Central Asia.[40] The character of HIV/AIDS epidemics are so varied internationally as to make global generalisations almost impossible. And yet, the news from most places is good enough to have supported a new language of ambition and optimism ('ending HIV'; 'getting to zero'; 'AIDS free generation') among recent global UNAIDS initiatives. It is also still fair to say that, although things are much better in many places, the rich world is faring better and has been for much longer. 'Post-crisis' certainly began as, and in many ways remains, a phenomenon of the privileged Global North.

There has also been and remains a tendency in these richer parts of the world to imagine that 'AIDS' is something happening elsewhere. From the perspective of many westerners, the epicentres of 'AIDS crisis' moved sometime around the turn of the millennium from the proximate, visible urban gay enclaves of San Francisco, New York, Paris, London and Sydney ('back') to the remote continents of Africa and South Asia. Along the lines of poverty and privilege upon which the global pandemic plays out, HIV/AIDS went from being a 'gay disease' to a 'problem in the global south' – two notions that are both fantasies of quarantine. This 'thirdworldisation'[41] of

HIV and AIDS has been largely synchronous with a withdrawal of media interest in HIV/AIDS in the Global North, and the atmosphere of silence that this disinterest has shaped.

It is important to also emphasise that the privileged conditions of Anglo-American and European post-crisis mean different things in different parts of these worlds. The different histories of different responses to HIV/AIDS in the US, Canada, Europe, the UK and Australia make it impossible to reduce 'English speaking' representations of post-crisis to one monolithic category. For example, in Australia, official public health responses to HIV/AIDS in partnership with affected communities happened more quickly than in America and the UK.[42] Post-crisis signifies differently in these different places precisely because of their different histories and I have tried to remain attentive to the local contexts of the various texts under consideration, placing them within their specific geopolitical and historical contexts of production and reception, as well as within the larger, global flows of representation in which they circulate.

As all of these texts will also illustrate, 'crisis/post-crisis' is not a neat, well-behaved temporal schema. In post-crisis culture there are frequent re-eruptions of the modes and moods of 'AIDS-as-crisis'. Like 'postmodernity', 'postfeminism' and other 'post' formulations that identify and characterise cultural change over time, post-crisis indicates both a continuation from and a break with the past. Indeed, this temporal mobility is a key feature of post-crisis culture – it frequently manifests a puzzling vacillation between the historical and discursive atmospheres of crisis and (the as-yet-unfinished) post. So, while I suggest that this temporal logic (crisis/post-crisis) may be a useful framework to start unpacking contemporary images of gay men and/with HIV/AIDS, I stress from the outset that the periods it delineates is not a neat distinction nor a reified historical fact.

If the logic of crisis/post-crisis plays out in this way – as an ongoing temporal dialectic, a movement backwards and forwards and backwards again – one of its effects is that later, post-crisis treatments of HIV/AIDS remain haunted by the legacies of the anxious, phobic early responses to HIV/AIDS. Inter Intergenerational tension and trauma, 'ghost stories', hauntings,[43] 'traumatic unremembering'[44] and 'temporal hiccups'[45] are all metaphors that have been used to think about the contours, effects and affects of these legacies, and the way in which the past continues to inflect and interrupt the present. In many of these metaphors, the past presents itself as a challenge or a negative feeling, but this, also, is not always the case. *Positive Images* raises the provocation of how a traumatic past may be mobilised and managed in contemporary culture in *both* enabling and disruptive ways – how it is unremembered in steadfast gestures of progress and privilege, or revisited and honoured as a reminder of identity and of survival in the present as well as in the past; how crisis memory is used in particular to bolster the dominant narratives of gay life under neoliberalism, and how it may also radically undermine them. As we saw earlier, in the example of *Brothers & Sisters*, popular culture after antiretrovirals frequently struggles to contain the modes of gay life with which HIV/AIDS has become associated by rendering them as antiquated or anachronistic. This desire to render HIV a figure of the past in turn helps to shape the terms of contemporary representations of gay life and its normative aspirations.

In other words, how we are oriented to the queer past and the dispositions we are encouraged to assume in relation to the gay experience of AIDS are key to understanding gay life in the present. If we are living post-crisis, where we are less anxious about AIDS and are encouraged to think in terms of 'management', 'treatment', 'chronicity' and 'living with HIV', we nonetheless remain haunted by the afterlives of AIDS-as-crisis. *Positive Images* is particularly interested in the ways in which what Roger Hallas calls the 'toxic ideology of dominant AIDS representation'[46] continues to infect representation in the era of ARVs in identifiable but sometimes unpredictable ways: in modes of amnesia and disavowal; in new but uncannily familiar spectacles of diseased sexual outlaws drawn in opposition to normative, healthy personhood in neoliberal society; in nostalgic or reparative and highly affective modes. The afterlives of the AIDS crisis suggest that it remains important to revisit and re-appraise what I call 'crisis discourse' – the rhetorically inflated, spectacular images of gay men as diseased others – which I will describe in more detail in the second half of this chapter.

Reflecting this temporal logic of crisis/post-crisis, representations of gay men and with HIV in the cultural landscape of post-crisis tend to vacillate between the extraordinary and the mundane. This is one my central arguments: that within a landscape that incorporates

HIV into the fabric of the quotidian (albeit ambivalently) there emerge awkward eruptions of the phobic legacies of AIDS crisis, or 'crisis discourse'. This tension, or dialectic, has emerged from the patterns of recent history. As we shall see in many of this book's case studies, male homosexuality and HIV/AIDS can signify as spectacular – unintelligible, radically other, a site of anxiety and disgust, a site of fascination or edgy titillation, something in need of containment and management – *and* as perfectly normal – mundane, easy to assimilate, part of the rhythms of the everyday. Healthy/pathological, deviant/normal, extraordinary/mundane, crisis/post-crisis: these *dialectics of post-crisis* manifest in a range of ways, and have a range of ramifications for queer masculinities, gay male sexual practices and HIV management. A central unresolvable paradox – the extraordinary/mundane – is at the heart of how we imagine gay men and HIV in contemporary popular culture.

The dialectic of the extraordinary/mundane may also be applied, and is in some ways the effect of, an ongoing anxiety underwriting the production and reception of (homo)sexual difference in popular culture. Ron Becker has called this 'heterosexual panic'.[47] A recalibrated version of Eve Sedgwick's 'homosexual panic',[48] Becker's formulation helps to explain the discomfort informing the production and reception of queer images in a culture 'not only uncertain about the ontology of sexual identity but also uncertain about heterosexuality's moral authority'.[49] Heterosexual or 'straight panic' he explains, 'describes what happens when heterosexual men and women, still insecure about the boundary between gay and straight, confront an increasingly accepted homosexuality.'[50] In this somewhat progressive, somewhat reactionary climate, images of homosexuality may be either sexual spectacles or mundane artifacts of commodity culture, or both. When HIV/AIDS enters the purview of queer images, as we shall see, it can redouble this ambivalence, creating particular challenges for gay male representability.

Chapter Outline

Each chapter of this book examines the tensions of post-crisis representation as they inhere in representative case studies. These are organised roughly chronologically as a means of historicising a trajectory 'out of' the spectacular moment of crisis toward a quotidian, normative post. This historical approach requires that we begin in the second half of this introductory chapter with a return to the 'origins' moment of this cultural history – the AIDS crisis – in order to identify and re-appraise its core narratives and rhetorics. 'Nothing has made gay men more visible than AIDS', Leo Bersani wrote in 1995; 'if we are looked at more than we have ever been looked at before – for the most part proudly by ourselves, sympathetically or malevolently by straight America – it is because AIDS has made us fascinating.'[51] AIDS panic thrust male homosexuality into the spotlight of mass culture more so than ever before, offering lurid images and outlandish stories to produce a particularly monstrous fantasy of homosexuality. Underwriting this epidemic of signification was a particular ideological narrative about the recklessness, culpability and sexual otherness of gay men. Simon Watney famously called this 'the spectacle of AIDS.'[52] It was a powerful and pervasive public campaign of sexual scapegoating that emerged partly in response to the terrifying meaninglessness of HIV.[53] In *Positive Images*, I often refer to this historically particular (but temporally mobile) spectacle via the shorthand 'crisis discourse.' A rich account of crisis discourse already exists in the archive of AIDS cultural criticism; for readers who are new to this field, the overview of crisis discourse that follows these chapter outlines should offer an acquaintance not only with the key features of this discourse, but with key works in that field.

The politics of representation debates described above began to really flourish during 'the Gay 90s.' These responded to the increase in images of queers in American and other English-speaking popular cultures – images that were significantly contoured by the AIDS crisis. Chapter 1 argues that a new queer stereotype, 'the New Gay Man',[54] emerged as a significant figure of popular culture at this time – a white, bourgeois, domesticated image of gayness that was a sympathetic and frequently comedic appendage to the plots and settings of American cinema and TV sitcoms. I argue that the New Gay Man came to exist through what I suggest was a ritual *disavowal* of AIDS crisis signification across popular culture. He was a figure that directly reacted to and substituted for the polluting, promiscuous hedonist 'faggot' so widely advertised in AIDS crisis discourse. As an 'illustrative example, I consider the Hollywood gay man/ straight woman 'buddy comedy', *The Next Best Thing* (2000). This critically loathed and largely forgotten film has received virtually no scholarly attention. However, as Chapter 1 attempts to show, the visual and narrative conventions that this film uses to frame the figure of the New Gay Man are instructive: they typify the disavowals at work in the immediate popular response to the scene of post-crisis, a symptom of that culture's traumatised response to the previous decade's crisis. *The Next Best Thing* redeems male homosexuality for popular consumption through the reproduction of an anachronistic AIDS other, a repository of difference against which to plot out space for the emergence of a new normal.

Chapter 2 examines the gay male body positive and the issues faced by serodiscordant couples as they were dramatised in the globally popular TV series, *Queer as Folk* (Showtime, 2000–5). In this case study the dualistic tension between 'AIDS' and normativity exist together *within* the body of the PLWHIV, rather than as polar forces in the diegesis. 'Serodiscordant' refers to a relationship in which one partner is HIV positive and the other is HIV negative. *Queer as Folk* offered a long-term narrative concerning the overcoming of serodiscord as a melodramatic obstacle in the relationship of two central characters, Michael and Ben. I argue that the discourse of 'HIV polarity'[55] that is exploited as a source of drama in *Queer as Folk*'s melodrama of serodifference is one that relies on the binary metaphor of gendered heteropolarity as a means to articulate the 'problem' of serodiscord. I also argue that the treatment of HIV in the series reflects neoliberal shifts in the reception of the pandemic from a public crisis inspiring collective action and communities of care to one of a discreet, largely invisible, individualised health management exercise.[56] The trajectory of Michael and Ben's relationship towards committed domesticity and their participation in the political battle for the package of rights associated with same-sex marriage reflects and reinforces this broader cultural shift in both the official culture of the epidemic and in the mainstream of LGBTQI+ politics. In *Queer as Folk*, the drama of living with HIV, or what I have dubbed 'sero-melodrama', reflects these larger trends. All of the above make *Queer as Folk* an emblematic post-crisis text.

Chapter 3 moves from the American and global context of fictionalised depictions of post-crisis gay life to the nailbiting anxiety aroused in discussions of the controversial practice of anal sex without condoms, or 'barebacking'. The recurrent sex panics around barebacking and other 'epidemics' of adventurous sex and drug use among gay men have become something of a paradigmatic site for illustrating the tension in post-crisis representation between the extraordinary and the mundane. On the one hand, barebacking entered the culture as a spectacular, outré sexual practice: enigmatic, irrational, a source of anxiety and a behaviour calling for regulatory intervention – almost the literal opposite of the carefully cultivated 1990s 'positive image.' Early discussions of barebacking and 'the barebacker' recalled and recalibrated the images and affects of crisis discourse. That is, they updated the idioms of the AIDS crisis to accommodate a set of new circumstances and practices. Chapter 3 examines the sex panics surrounding the VICE media documentary *Chemsex*, and in the media coverage of a high-profile legal case of the reckless infection of persons with HIV, part of an alleged 'epidemic' of barebacking and bug chasing. In these sex panics, barebacking became a site of the recrudescence of the logics of crisis discourse, and the re-emergence of one of its key figures, the 'AIDS Monster'. Resembling other panics about gay male sex and drug practices across the globe, the Australian case shows how the resurrection of crisis discourses may function to discipline gay men as individualised managers of HIV risk in the transformed contexts of the pandemic.

Sex panic is only one of the numerous modes through which the representation of barebacking has played out. As new practices and technologies of HIV prevention have entered the scene, and, as the market for porn depictions of 'raw sex' has developed exponentially, 'bareback' has become something of a mundane signifier. Competing representations of barebacking expose further layers of paradox in post-crisis culture and these paradoxes help to explain why the practice of sex without condoms remains an ongoing source of prurient fascination, erotic investment and anxiety. Moving to one side of the popular mainstream, but hopefully in order to shed more light on it, Chapter 3 also considers the literature of 'barebacking sexology', a large archive of research across social, scientific and humanities disciplines that sought to investigate the various practices associated with condomless sex. Barebacking sexology exhibits an ongoing obsession with charting and taxonomising gay male sexual practices. Alongside the vernaculars of porn and pop culture, I suggest that barebacking sexology itself became a discursive site of authoritative knowledge production or 'sex talk' like those identified by Foucault in *The History of Sexuality* (1976).[57] These authoritative sciences of sexuality have implications for how we understand and practise homosexuality and HIV in the post-crisis era.

Recent years have witnessed AIDS crisis memorialising in books, memoirs, exhibitions, archival and historical projects. Significant public AIDS histories have emerged in documentary, narrative and digital/archival forms, with American-centric and gay male-centric stories heavily dominating the global narrative of AIDS history. Culturally, the disease that once signified urgency and 'nowness' has shifted, in the Global North at least, to being associated with the past. The last two chapters of *Positive Images* turn more explicitly to AIDS memory and this increased interest in the history of AIDS. Two early small-screen examples of this trend were HBO's *Angels in America* (2003) and the BBC's *The Line of Beauty* (2006), both adapted from multi-award-winning literary and theatrical sources, and both set in the earlier moment of the AIDS Crisis. In Chapter 4 I look at BBC2's *The Line of Beauty*, a three-part adaptation of Alan Hollinghurst's Booker award–winning novel of the same name (2004) and an early example of such AIDS memorialising. *The Line of Beauty* is produced in the generic style of Anglophilic heritage cinema, a genre that has often been accused of colluding with reactionary, nostalgic, nationalist conservative agendas. Drawing on more recent, revisionist critical understandings of both heritage and nostalgia, I argue that BBC2's adaptation uses heritage style to present a critical history of the socially conservative elite of Thatcher's Britain, offering a revisionist queer British national history of AIDS that confronts the lethal ideology of crisis discourse and its implicatedness in the birth of neoliberal economic and social life. As an early entry in a burgeoning archive of popular AIDS histories, *The Line of Beauty* demonstrates post-crisis culture's complicated relationship with the AIDS past. As we shall see, it offers a range of 'backwards feelings'[58] that have become characteristic of post-crisis culture's unresolved relationship with the AIDS past.

In 2011, the HIV/AIDS epidemic turned thirty. Coinciding with this anniversary there emerged a pronounced retrospective trend in documentary filmmaking starting with the appearance of several AIDS crisis documentaries in 2011 and 2012, including *We Were Here* (2011), *Vito* (2011), *How to Survive a Plague* (2012) and *United in Anger* (2012). This trend extended to globally distributed Hollywood films in *Dallas Buyers Club* (2013), to prestige American cable TV in HBO's *The Normal Heart* (2014), and to national Anglophone cinemas in Australia, Canada and the UK. These popular AIDS histories raise questions about representation, custodianship, domination and silencing in popular histories. They have raised questions about the relationship between looking backward and the current circumstances of sexuality and HIV, how these histories are re-signified and 'used' in the present-day contexts of LGBTQI+ politics and culture.

Positive Images concludes by reflecting on this backwards turn in AIDS cultural production. The boom in AIDS memory practices requires another book-length consideration, but here I offer some preliminary reflections on how recent turns to AIDS history both sustain and break with the representational trends of post-crisis culture identified earlier in the book. These cultural memories of the gay experience of AIDS are a complex 'archive of feelings', to borrow Ann Cvetkovich's description of trauma and lesbian public cultures[59]– they offer amnesiac, nostalgic and reparative tendencies that effect both our present-day capacity to grasp the phenomenon of HIV/AIDS, and shape the contours of contemporary queer movements and their futures by narrativising their pasts.

Before we turn to this past, a brief note about the objects of scrutiny in this book. *Positive Images* is largely limited to works that are popular, mainstream and western. By 'western', I mean culture rather than geography; that is, cultural production that originated in the wealthy, developed, English-speaking countries of the Northern Hemisphere and/or Australia and New Zealand, although it may circulate globally. 'Mainstream' is a contested term. I use it here to denote a focus on media artifacts that are widely and popularly consumed rather than produced by and for a minority queer market. Such a designation does not exclude texts that are gay-authored, like Alan Hollinghurst's novel, *The Line of Beauty*, for example. Nor does it exclude media like *Queer as Folk*, consumed by large queer as well as non-queer audiences. However, with some minor exceptions, it *does* exclude fringe and subcultural works, and works made for and consumed by a predominantly queer audience – say, for example, in queer film festivals, activist spaces or artistic communities. In many instances these other texts offer richer and more varied narratives about queer life and HIV, however these have remained beyond the scope of this book. In *Positive Images* I have tried to examine some of the few popular HIV/AIDS texts from the years since 1996 in a bid to illustrate larger patterns in post-crisis culture. But before we move on to these, we must first return to the 1980s.

Crisis Discourse

The Greek origins of the word 'epidemic' – *epidêmos* – signifies the arrival of a foreigner.[60] This neatly encapsulates the 'otherness' around which the genres of early AIDS representation were organised. Whether soliciting horror, fascination, pathos or a combination thereof, the spectacular idiom of AIDS crisis discourse was oriented toward allaying (and exploiting) fears of the sexual, racial, national, class, ethnic and other differences of the groups first associated with the disease: gay men, people who inject drugs and their sexual partners, African, Asian and Haitian migrants, African-Americans and sex workers. Personifying AIDS – that is, connecting it to *types* of people – was a means of symbolically and psychically cordoning it off from the white, middle-class, suburban, sexually decorous heterosexual 'general population.' Though disease rarely respects those fantasies of difference, this well-worn strategy of imaginatively 'quarantining' it among people already classed as 'others' has a long genealogy in the history of sexually transmitted and epidemic disease.

The first reports of a cluster of Pneumocystis pneumonia (PCP, a form of pneumonia that can lead to lung infections in people with weak immune systems) in five gay men in Los Angeles in 1981 led to the labels 'Gay-Related Immune Deficiency' (GRID), 'Gay Compromise Syndrome', 'Gay Cancer' and 'Community-Acquired Immune Dysfunction'.[61] 'GRID' became 'Acquired Immune Deficiency Syndrome' or 'AIDS' in 1982 after clusters of Kaposi's sarcoma (KS, a cancer that causes usually purple lesions to grow in the skin) and PCP were also reported among other groups including Haitians, haemophiliacs, blood transfusion recipients and children born to possibly infected mothers. Nonetheless, the symbolic nexus between AIDS and male homosexuality intensified not only in the hysteria of the ensuing decade but also in the supposedly rational spaces of medicine and epidemiology.

This nexus also became the heart of what I call 'crisis discourse.' By 'crisis discourse', I mean narratives and metaphors across official, documentary and fictional genres that contributed to the general construction of AIDS as a gay disease. Less than a decade after homosexuality had been removed from the pathology category in American psychiatric literature, AIDS 're-medicalised' homosexuality.[62] The ideas that helped form initial understandings of the human immunodeficiency virus were thus shaped by phobic attitudes toward same-sex desire, anal eroticism and the supposedly amoral, promiscuous sexual culture of gay liberation. At the heart of these rhetorical constructions was the organising cultural fantasy of the homosexual as progenitor, conveyor and embodiment of disease. This was not necessarily a new idea. The cultural construction of 'gay AIDS' was based on a 'characterological' model of disease that itself drew on an eclectic history of pre-existing traditions, including the image-rich archive of earlier epidemics, the degenerate figures of the *fin-de-siècle* Decadent novel and concepts from the archive of late nineteenth and early twentieth-century sexology. These historical figures of disease, monstrosity and sexual pathology were repackaged in contemporary media forms, especially science fiction, horror and melodrama – key genres for imagining frightening forms of otherness.

Crisis discourses' lurid fixation with male homosexuality is perhaps most comprehensively explored in Simon Watney's seminal work of AIDS cultural criticism, *Policing Desire* (1987). *Policing Desire* explains the ways that the representation of gay men and 'AIDS victims' as monstrous others was part of a larger and longer history of safeguarding The Family and The Home and their attendant institutions of marriage, parenthood and property.[63] Drawing on Foucault's formulations on bourgeois governmentality, Watney suggested that the spectacular castigation of homosexual men in AIDS crisis media was grounded in the ideo-logic of modern familialism. In Foucault's influential theory, the modern family is the 'privileged instrument for the government of the population.'[64] The 'spectacle of AIDS', Watney argued, was part of this mode of modern governance. The image of the corrupt/ing homosexual body could be mobilised as a means of domestic surveillance and identity regulation: 'Homosexuality has lately come to occupy a most peculiar and centrally privileged position in the government of the home – homosexuality ideologically constructed as a regulative admonitory sign… the axiomatic identification of AIDS as a sign and symptom of homosexual behaviour reconfirms the passionately held view of "the family" as a uniquely vulnerable institution.'[65] As the title of Watney's book, *Policing Desire*, implies, the spectacle of AIDS helped to regulate and reinforce the institutions of family life and the heteronormative sexual and gender identities these institutions depend on.

Policing Desire not only addressed the iconography of AIDS representation but the technologies of vision within which it was framed and the psychoanalytic models of identification that attend these structures of looking. In psychic terms, the two modes through which the processes of identification operate are the 'substantive mode', where one recognises themselves in relationship of resemblance to the other, and the 'transitive mode', where identification operates as a recognition of the self as different. The body of the homosexual 'AIDS victim' could only ever enter public visibility in the mode of the latter, 'upon the strictly enforced condition that any possibility of identification with it is scrupulously refused.' This configuration of the gaze structures the way in which audiences were encouraged to see and respond to images of PWA.[66] In the spectacle of AIDS, the homosexual body was subjected to 'extremes of casual cruel violent indifference, like the bodies of aliens, sliced open to the frightened yet fascinated gaze of uncomprehending social pathologists…. "disposed of", like so much rubbish, like the trash it was in life.'[67] The sexual other becomes hyper-visible, hyper-surveilled and utterly dehumanised in order that it may demarcate the viewing Self from the Not-Self.

Revisiting Watney's argument with the benefit of hindsight, there is a way in which the ideological spectacle of AIDS crisis discourse *already* inhabits the dialectic of the extraordinary/mundane that characterises postcrisis culture. If, as Watney argues, crisis discourse becomes a technology for the disciplining of the modern white bourgeois subject, then it is already a mundane discourse. Although on the one hand the excess and amplified emotion of the spectacle of AIDS seems extraordinary, in as far as it resembles the spectacles of sexual otherness that have helped reinforce sexual norms throughout modernity it is ideological business-as-usual, a conventional modern strategy of governing populations, part of what Foucault and others since have called 'biopolitics.' The spectacle of AIDS was largely consumed in the home, in the space of the domestic and the everyday, the chief distribution sites of modern social and sexual norms. So, AIDS panic, like other contemporary sex panics, is as *quotidian* as the regime of modern familialism is quotidian. And yet, it was also a moment of heightened, excessive discourse and imagery – an affectively explosive, ferocious instance of the public policing of private lives, which circulated an unprecedented number of images of gay male bodies, gay life and gay death. In this sense, crisis discourse was already both mundane and spectacular.

AIDS and Metaphor

For readers interested in the body of intellectual work responding to popular representations of the AIDS crisis, a frequent starting point is American intellectual Susan Sontag's groundbreaking book, *AIDS and its Metaphors* (1989). For Sontag as for many others, the early association of AIDS with already-stigmatised minorities like queers, migrants and drug users became central to its treatment in public discussions. In particular, the perceived 'culpability' of these groups was linked to the resurrection of the long-dormant biblical metaphor of 'plague', the 'highest standard of collective calamity, evil, scourge.'[68] Baptist pastor and televangelist Jerry Falwell, for example, described AIDS as 'God's judgment on a society that does not live by His rules.'[69] Outspoken moralists like Senator Jesse Helms and Pat Buchanan, Senior Advisor to President Ronald Reagan, infamously used the concept of plague to account for AIDS. With its logic of (sexual) guilt and blame, the plague metaphor re-circulated the idea of disease as a form of divine punishment.[70]

AIDS and its Metaphors was a rejoinder to Sontag's earlier 1978 work, *Illness as Metaphor*, in which she examined the metaphors that describe cancer and tuberculosis. If cancer had been the central object of disease metaphorisation throughout the twentieth century, AIDS 'banalised cancer':[71] AIDS, Sontag wrote, 'is a disease whose charge of stigmatisation, whose capacity to create spoiled identities, is far greater.'[72] Sontag's core argument that the representation of disease is riddled with metaphor became a foundational concept in AIDS cultural criticism and remains influencial today. However a problem among Sontag's critics was her idealisation of science and the medicine. Both AIDS activists and scholars have been suspicious of the truth claim of science, which they have argued, are themselves dependent on metaphors.[73] As Paula Treicheler had already argued by the time *AIDS and its Metaphors* was published, scientific constructions of HIV and AIDS are based 'not upon objective, scientifically determined "really" but upon what we are told about this reality: that is, upon *prior* social constructions routinely produced within the discourses of biomedical science.'[74] Medicine and science are always in some way political. Sontag's bid to 'abstain from' and 'retire' metaphors from discussions of disease[75] was a second problem for AIDS cultural critics. And yet, 'one would be hard-pressed' as David Caron writes, 'to find a single discourse, whether popular or scientific, literary or technical, oppressive or resistant, that has been able to engage HIV and AIDS without the use of metaphors.'[76]

In this sense, AIDS cultural criticism is strongly influenced by poststructuralist theories about the omnipresence of metaphoric thinking. Whereas the classic, Aristotelian model of metaphorisation understands it as a process of substitution (giving the thing a name that belongs to something else), poststructuralism came to understand metaphor as a part of the logic of language itself. In his pioneering study of metaphor, Hawkes argued that 'all languages contain deeply embedded metaphorical structures which covertly influence overt meaning.'[77] Later, Lakoff and Johnson argued that language systems are both saturated and defined by tropic (that is, metaphoric) thinking: 'most of our ordinary conceptual system is metaphorical in nature'; 'metaphor is not just a matter of language… of mere words… on the contrary, human *thought processes* are largely metaphorical.'[78] Because of the pervasiveness of metaphoric thinking *within* the structures of language and thought, metaphors 'make us' rather than the other way around. The social and semantic processes by which disease acquires meanings are therefore unavoidable: 'no matter how much we may desire to resist treating illness as metaphor,' Treichler writes, 'illness *is* metaphor.'[79] For most AIDS cultural critics there is no 'HIV' or 'AIDS' outside of metaphor.

That we can only comprehend HIV and AIDS through their figuration in language and images remains a central axiom for AIDS cultural criticism and for this book. As Douglas Crimp, in the much-quoted introduction to a special edition of the journal *October* titled 'AIDS: Cultural Analysis, Cultural Activism', writes:

> AIDS does not exist apart from the practices that conceptualise it, represent it, and respond to it. We know AIDS only in and through these practices. This assertion does not contest the existence of viruses, antibodies, infections, or transmission routes. Least of all does it contest the reality of illness, suffering and death. What is *does* contest is the notion that there is an underlying reality of AIDS, upon which are constructed the representations, or the culture, or the politics of AIDS.[80]

Notice that Crimp is careful not to imply that disease is *only* metaphor – disease is an inescapably material phenomenon, hurting and frequently killing the bodies that suffer it. And yet this doesn't alter the need to identify and intervene in the metaphors used to describe disease, for disease is *both* a material and a linguistic reality. This urgent need to address representations of AIDS became a rallying call for both critics in the humanities and activists. If we can identify toxic metaphors and their locatedness in structures of power we may be ourselves empowered to critique and reformulate them – so goes the logic of these interventions. The *October* special issue was a formative, agenda-setting publication for cultural studies of HIV/AIDS. Republished as a book, it included essays by Crimp, Watney, Bersani, Treichler and Gregg Bordowitz, among others, who became key figures in this field. It assembled theories from psychoanalysis, Marxist and post-Marxist thought, Structuralist semiotics and Foucauldian genealogical analysis. However interdisciplinary in methods and multi-(con)textual in their sites of analysis (the biomedical, the epidemiological, news media, HIV prevention campaigns, photographs of PWA), all of the *October* essays are unified on one front: they regard disease discourse *not* as a separate or second-order reality but, rather, as a site of struggle; representations of AIDS mediate – they affect and are affected by – our experience and understanding of reality.

Queer

If poststructuralist theories of metaphoric thinking were influential for early AIDS cultural criticism, so too were poststructuralist thought and AIDS cultural criticism influential to the queer theory that emerged in the 1990s and beyond. Although it is not frequently acknowledged now, early ideas in queer theory were significantly informed by the activist and academic response to HIV/AIDS. Queer thought has, in turn, been central to cultural studies of AIDS. In her field-defining 1996 primer, *Queer Theory*, Annemarie Jagose explains how the exigencies and materialities of AIDS came to influence developments in queer theory. Queer's emphasis on the deconstruction of identity, its critique of an essentialising, ethnic model of gay and lesbian identity and its interest in emphasising sexual practices over sexual identities are all theoretical tendencies with antecedents in community responses to AIDS, coalitional AIDS activism and safer sex discourse. AIDS cultural criticism saw itself as inseparable from these 'in yer face' activist projects and from the 'urgent need to resist dominant constructions of HIV/AIDS'.[81]

For example, the demographic map of HIV transmissions functioned as something of an incitement to the types of anti-normative and identity denaturalising approaches pursued by queer theorists because it plainly demonstrates that people's actual sexual desires and practices very often disrespect the social boundaries of marriage, monogamy, the family, the supposed coherence of sexual identity categories like 'heterosexual' and 'homosexual' and the hierarchical classifications of gender, race and nation that attempt to regulate and segregate the private spheres of sexuality.[82] As Shoumatoff writes, HIV/AIDS has the potential to make all 'private indiscretions' public; it is 'like a swallow dye pill illuminating all the *liaisons dangereuses*, the thousands upon thousands of marital, premarital, extramarital, interracial, and homosexual encounters that must have taken place for it to spread as far as it has.'[83] Cindy Patton calls this 'the queer paradigm.' Regardless of exposure routes, she argues, the AIDS 'mark of perversion' transforms all of the infected into '"queers".'[84]

Since the beginning of the twenty-first century, work in queer studies has turned increasingly to the ascendance of neoliberalism – what Lisa Duggan describes as 'the brand name for the form of procorporate, "free market," anti-"big government" rhetoric shaping US policy and dominating international financial institutions since the early 1980s.'[85] This is important to mention here for two reasons: first, neoliberalism in its various formations is a prevailing political economy, inseparable from culture in the mostly western nations where HIV post-crisis can be said to manifest; and, therefore, to a large extent, neoliberalism *is* the culture of post-crisis. For example, the biopolitical scene of HIV, particularly among gay men and MSM, reflects neoliberalism's prioritisation of particular forms of sociality and personhood: individualism, entrepreneurship and the rational, responsible subject. Race has written of the way in which medical discourses around 'patient compliance' with ARVs, viral load testing and other technologies of HIV management have operationalised 'a new field of normativity around health and consumption, in which the moral worth of subjects is *exemplified* in relation to a generalised sense of medical prescription.'[86] Second, the politics of neoliberalism are intimately connected to queer liberalisms or what is more commonly called 'homonormativity.' Duggan famously described 'the new homonormativity' as 'the sexual politics of neoliberalism.' Homonormativity describes the most visible and dominant form of contemporary LGBTQI+ politics in the Global North, a politics that, in Duggan's much quoted words, 'does not contest dominant heteronormative assumptions and institutions but upholds and sustains them while promising the possibility of a demobilised gay constituency and a privatised, depoliticised gay culture anchored in domesticity and consumption.'[87] As we shall see in Chapter 2's discussion of HIV positivity and serodiscord in *Queer as Folk*, the personal and relational dramas of living with HIV have been privatised and depoliticised under the conditions of neoliberalism. In Chapter 3's examination of bareback panic, the folk devils of post-crisis AIDS spectacle are part of the disciplinary apparatus of individualised, neoliberal epidemic management. In Chapter 4, we return to the moment of British AIDS crisis and the birthplace of Thatcherite neoliberalism in *The Line of Beauty*, wherein all forms of personhood and intimacy, including romance and kinship, are subsumed to the logic of the neoliberal marketplace. In many ways the entire history of AIDS is coterminous with the history of neoliberalism. As we shall see throughout *Positive Images*, post-crisis representations are significantly shaped by and interpreted through the ideological, economic and affective–interrelational logics of neoliberal culture.

Characterology and the Legible Body

Because those first affected by HIV/AIDS were seen to be representatives of already despised or feared, marginalised social groups, HIV infection was perceived to be the manifestation of an innate predisposition to illness, a 'symbolic extension of some imagined inner essence of being, manifesting itself as disease.'[88] Sontag called this the 'characterological predisposition to illness'.[89] Jackie Stacey calls it 'textual body discourse'. Its spurious logic is that individuals have brought about their own suffering due to pre-existing imbalances in character. Cancer, for example, is attributed to 'psychological defeat', 'internalised rage' and 'emotional defeat'. In this understanding, disease is 'simply the language of the psyche writ large on the body'.[90]

An exemplary case of characterological thinking in the context of AIDS is the work of popular American healer and 'New Thought' writer Louise Hay. For Hay, the physical symptoms of illness – anything from colds to cancer – are outward signs of an inner problem, the body 'speaking' its sublimated grievances in destructive ways: 'I believe we create every so called "illness" in our body.' Hay began a support group for six HIV positive men in 1985 that became a national phenomenon following appearances on *The Oprah Winfrey Show* and *Donahue* in 1988 and, subsequently, almost a thousand positive men became involved in Hay's group. In her book, *You Can Heal Your Life*, published in 1984, which has since sold more than 35 million copies in 30 languages and was adapted into a film, Hay wrote that the 'probable cause' of AIDS is 'feeling defenceless and hopeless. Nobody cares. A strong belief in not being good enough. Denial of the self. Sexual guilt.'[91] Dangerously, Hay's diagnosis re-orients what in fact may have been (and may remain) the likely *effects* of an HIV diagnosis – feelings of sexual guilt, loneliness – as its causes.[92]

Characterological logic can also be extrapolated from the individual to the (risk) group. Hay, again, demonstrates this when she writes that gay men

> have created a culture that places tremendous emphasis on youth and beauty.... [T]he feelings inside have been totally disregarded… only the body counts… Because of the way gay people often treat other gays… the experience of getting old is something to dread. It is almost better to die than to get old. And AIDS is a disease that often kills.[93]

Drawing on the homophobic idea that gay men can't help being 'lethal narcissists',[94] Hay all but states that gay culture itself causes AIDS. According to Sontag, the characterological model has been central to modern attributions of illness,[95] although in the case of HIV, the metaphors we use to describe and understand immunity and the immune system seem to have strengthened its explanatory power.[96]

Characterological thinking about disease also echoes nineteenth and early twentieth-century medico-sexological models of homosexual inversion, where sexuality is understood as the innate property of bodies. It is now virtually axiomatic among historians of sexuality to argue that the nineteenth century gave birth to the modern idea of 'sexuality' itself, and that the way we tend to understand sexuality today – as a core, organic property of the body – developed at this time. This way of thinking was particularly evident in the model of homosexual 'inversion' – the idea that the homosexual was an 'invert' whose sexual nature was the result of a mysterious inversion of their inner 'nature' relative to the outward expression of gender. Karl Ulrichs, for example, argued that same-sex desiring people had the soul of the other sex's body trapped within them. In the literature of nineteenth century sexology, sexuality developed as an essential, morphological function of the body – something innate that not only determines a person's sexual desires but their social disposition, moral character and life trajectory.

The 'innate qualities' attributed to homosexual bodies by classic sexologists like Richard von Kraft-Ebbing and Havelock Ellis included a number of characteristics that we may still recognise in certain representations today – things like a sexually masochistic drive, the idea of homosexual desires as something contagious, an imagined constitutional weakness of the homosexual body, and the legibility of sexual perversity on the body's surface. This last quality – that sexual difference/ deviance was somehow perceptible from observing the body – was a defining idea of nineteenth century sexology. Edelman calls this 'homographesis' – the 'disciplinary and projective fantasy that homosexuality is visibly, morphologically, or semiotically, written on the flesh.'[97] This idea that (homo)sexuality can be detected on the body's surface (in the way a man looks, the way a woman talks, and so on), enables those looking to imagine they can detect the presence of a sexual deviant and therefore police the boundaries between heterosexual and homosexual bodies.[98]

The logic of homographesis was echoed powerfully in AIDS crisis discourses. AIDS representations were similarly fascinated with the revelatory stories that could be told by the body. They partake in this same cultural imperative to understand deviant bodies as 'inherently textual', as 'bodies that might well bear a hallmark that could, and must, be read.'[99] This imperative to read sexual difference and sexual guilt in the stories told by the body couldn't have been more shockingly illustrated by the media's obsession with the clinical indications of 'full blown AIDS'. Despite the fact that, as Patton sensibly pointed out, HIV itself 'cannot reasonably be rendered as a surface phenomenon,'[100] KS and wasting, the iconic 'signs' of HIV, were obsessed over in the visual imagery of crisis discourse.[101] 'We want a stigma of AIDS', Patton argued, and 'since HIV cannot be visualised as "on the body", it is represented... in the figure of the forlorn, wasted person with AIDS'.[102] The broad range of clinical manifestations of HIV/AIDS seemed to bolster this sexological, characterological way of thinking. As Roberta McGrath describes, HIV infection at this time was understood to:

> create a body which turns upon itself, killing not through a single disease, but through an accumulation of our most feared diseases.... These diseases not only mark the body on the outside, but dissolve it from within. This is total war waged on the body... [A]lthough various modes of transmission are recognised, HIV has been represented as fundamentally sexually transmitted. Thus HIV is the link between sex and death.[103]

In the spectacle of the AIDS-ravaged body, 'homographic' or 'characterological' logic reads visible symptoms as signs of an 'interior essence'. The media's fascination with the emaciated, KS-lesioned body during the 80s and 90s is powerful evidence of our culture's anxious yearning to read both sexual deviance and disease on the body.

Epidemic Histories and Literary Genealogies

For historians of infectious and sexually transmitted diseases, it was 'almost impossible to watch the AIDS epidemic without experiencing a sense of déjà vu'.[104] While Sontag pointed to the metaphorical revival of bubonic plague metaphors, others have noted the ways in which crisis discourse drew also from the cultural archives of cholera, syphilis and leprosy.

HIV is not 'contagious' – it is potentially transmissible through very specific, intimate forms of contact with bodily fluids including blood and semen. In spite of this, an exposure/contamination/corruption theory of AIDS became part of its early mythology. This recalls the history of leprosy, which, like AIDS, was initially feared to be highly infectious, possibly due to the quick and devastating physical deterioration it can cause.[105] Actually, both diseases are far less easily transmissible than originally supposed. It's hardly incidental that same-sex desire has long been imagined in terms of 'contagion' – that is, as something one can 'catch' through contact with someone who is lesbian or gay. This is another mainstay of modern homophobic constructions of homosexuality that crosses over with the historical archive of disease representations: the concept that queer/diseased spaces are places where one is at high risk of being seduced and/or infected. This idea relies again on the metaphor of contagion but also the spatial metaphor of the 'cesspool' – an image that featured prolifically in the culture surrounding outbreaks of cholera in the nineteenth and twentieth centuries. Cholera was thought to emerge from 'infected' atmospheres – poor living conditions and unwholesome environments, miasma, effusions emerging from something unclean. Choleric bacteria can thrive in pools of still water and hence the 'disease-carrying atmosphere came to be identified with urban rather than rural squalor, and with garbage, rot [and] the proximity of cemeteries.'[106] In the early days of HIV/AIDS and well beyond, urban gay enclaves and places where gay men met for sex like beats and bathhouses became fertile territory for choleric cesspool metaphors – they are spaces imaged as capable of nurturing both perverse sexualities and transmissible disease.

Perhaps more so than cholera or the plague, the iconography of syphilis offered the most thorough precedent for AIDS representations. In western literature and culture the syphilitic has appeared as a figure of sexual excess, frequently associated with adultery, promiscuity and prostitution. The homosexual PWA recalled the syphilitic because of their associations with decadence, sexual recklessness, effeminacy and disease as the imagined punishment for such wantonness. Sander Gilman pointed out that the iconography of syphilis was pervasive in American news media images of PWA: these depicted the 'AIDS victim' as alone, isolated, melancholic and tarred with the stigmata of bodily sores.[107]

Leo Bersani identified further important connections between syphilis in the late nineteenth century and AIDS in the twentieth. In his controversial and extremely influential 1988 essay, 'Is the Rectum a Grave?', Bersani argued that the notorious hyper-promiscuity of gay men recalled the nineteenth century portrayal of Victorian prostitutes as the 'contaminated vessels' of syphilitic contagion. Common to the depiction of both figures is the image of sexual passivity and the trope of insatiable female sexuality as itself intrinsically contaminated. That is, both gay men and the historical figure of the prostitute were imagined as capable of having sex with an endless number of partners and to therefore enact a potentially endless number of disease transmissions. 'Promiscuity in this fantasy', Bersani writes, is central: 'far from merely increasing the risk of infection, [promiscuity] is the sign of infection. Women and gay men spread their legs with an unquenchable appetite for destruction.'[108]

More pointedly, Bersani also argues that the conflation of homosexuality and AIDS had more to do with 'the kinds of sex involved' than homosexuality per se. Anal sex, he argued, was the central and most important source of anxiety and unease in AIDS crisis discourses: the '"black hole" in the mythology of "AIDS".'[109] 'Is the Rectum a Grave?' drew attention to a central image lodged in the unconscious of crisis discourses: the 'seductive and intolerable image of a grown man, legs high in the air, unable to refuse the suicidal ecstasy of being a woman.'[110] Like the syphilitic prostitute, the gay man appeared to welcome passivity and penetration, to desire getting fucked. Passivity, the 'fantasy of female sexuality as intrinsically diseased'[111] and the imagined fatality of (receptive) anal sex all come together in this image. The potential of HIV to *appear to* literalise the connection between passive penetration and biological death, Bersani argued, 'reinforced the heterosexual association of anal sex with a self-annihilation originally and primarily identified with the fantasmatic mystery of an insatiable, unstoppable female sexuality.'[112]

Getting fucked threatens a further, symbolic death – the death of phallic masculinity. Identifying as a male in our culture requires the prioritisation of the penis as the central, legitimate organ of male eroticism. The anus, on the other hand, is associated with feminine passivity, and, as even the most amateur Freudian will tell you, feminine passivity is the antithesis of phallic masculinity. According to the binary logic of heterosexual difference, in which masculinity and femininity are bound to a socially prescribed active/passive opposition (men do; women are done to), to be fucked is to be placed in the position of the feminine and hence to lose one's claim to authentic (that is, phallic) masculinity. This is the received cultural wisdom at the heart of anal anxiety. As Brett Farmer explains, 'the act of anal intercourse… avows a structure of passivity that is antithetical to patriarchal fantasies of male phallic dominance and authority.'[113] Therefore, the anal zone features strongly in the cultural imagination as a symbol of sexual docility, of penetrability.

HIV/AIDS may have exacerbated taboos surrounding anal sex, but, on the other hand, it also provided the context for a more complex valuation and politicisation of anality. In a more enabling, radical move, Bersani also pointed out that part of the unconscious pleasure of getting fucked was in fact to do with *taking pleasure in* the symbolic execution of phallic masculinity. As Brian Pronger puts it, 'Getting fucked is the deepest violation of masculinity in our culture. Enjoying being fucked is the acceptance of that violation, it is the ecstatic sexual experience in which the violation of masculinity becomes incarnate.'[114] This radical flipside to the cultural conflation of anal penetration and death became one of the most discussed propositions in Bersani's provocative essay: the pleasure taken in anality, he argued, is a form of *jouissance*, a rapturous, orgasmic kind of pleasure linked to a psychic division and splitting of the self, a self-shattering, and a shattering of the masculine subject. Like the Victorian prostitute from the archive of syphilis, the promiscuous gay man was presented as a penetrated, passive figure, bringing about the symbolic death of masculinity and also, in the age of HIV, wilfully exposing himself to literal death. But, paradoxically, because it enacts a potent threat to phallic masculinity, anality becomes a means through which gay men may contest masculinity norms – and crisis discourses, as Bersani pointed out, brought this contestation into sharp relief.

As we shall see, the post-crisis context has given rise to further developments in and recalibrations of the nexus between queer masculinities, anal sex and epidemic disease – in ways that, again, are both enabling and reactionary, extraordinary and mundane. In Chapter 3 these complex, paradoxical resonances make a historical reappearance in the heightened discussions of barebacking in the 2000s. One example: in certain barebacking practices and representations, including some varieties of bareback porn, a new brand of gay male bottomhood, the 'power bottom', performs a masculinity powerful enough to endure endless arse-poundings and buckets of cum. Rather than the wilful embrace of feminisation, the power bottom is enthusiastically re-masculinised by his ability to 'take it like a man'.[115]

The deaths of high profile gay male celebrity-artists like Freddie Mercury, Liberace and Rudolf Nureyev, among an almost endless and devastating catalogue of other less famous gay artists, were further 'evidence' associating homosexuality and the disease known as 'AIDS'. Likewise, AIDS brought about some notorious unclosetings, invoking a thematics of secrets, scandal, the closet, celebrity, entertainment and art in popular cultural storytelling.

Rock Hudson was the first and undoubtedly the most spectacular of these unclosetings. The outing of Rock as both a homosexual and as the 'face of AIDS' is frequently regarded as a turning point in public discussions of HIV/AIDS. It was the moment when Americans 'took notice of AIDS' because it signified widely as a moment of 'viral leakage', violating the fantasy of a quarantined homosexual 'risk group' separate from the 'broader' (i.e. heterosexual) population.[116] Tabloid images of the Hollywood icon of wholesome beefcake masculinity juxtaposed with later images of Hudson wearing the stigmata of KS and wasting – the legible 'signs' of AIDS – did much to suture the narrative of homosexuality's uncloseting with the visual symptomatology and iconography of AIDS. 'Closeted through all these years of his celebrity,' explains Richard Meyer, 'Rock Hudson's secret finally registers, Dorian Gray-like, on the surface of his body.' If AIDS was able to make a previously and shamefully secret homosexuality visible and 'verifiable' at the level of the body, so the logic goes, 'homosexuality supplants HIV as the origin and aetiology of Rock Husdon's illness.'[117] The Rock scandal is a good illustration of Sontag's characterological thinking and of the sexological model of disease/sexuality that Edelman calls 'homographesis': a diseased/homosexual essence emerges from within the person, materialising like stigmata on the surface of their flesh. Rock's unclosetting illustrated the media's obsession with the storytelling capacities of the body of the homosexual PWA; and the iconographies associated with the actor both before and after he became the face of AIDS have had legacies in the visual culture of post-crisis, as we'll see in the next chapter.

Introduction

Meyer's reference to the literary figure of Dorian Gray here in the case of Rock Hudson is also worthy of some further attention because of its prevalence in crisis discourse. Dorian Gray crops up in AIDS crisis culture, and across AIDS cultural criticism a striking number of times. The recurring story structure linking homosexuality and AIDS through a narrative of crime and punishment is a structure that recalls Oscar Wilde's iconic novelisation of veiled homosexuality, *The Picture of Dorian Gray* (1895), in seemingly uncanny ways. Of course, there are other novelistic genealogies for the representation of AIDS, Particularly in the nineteenth- and twentieth-century literatures of syphilis, which associated the disease with gifted, emotional or spiritual individuals and heightened, feverish states of creativity. However, Wilde's neo-gothic novelisation of the fall and punishment of a beautiful, narcissistic young man provided a handy narrative structure for imagining AIDS allegorically – as a punishment or a moral lesson. Dorian Gray made a famously Faustian bargain to preserve his youth and physical beauty. Safe from the ravages of corporeality and mentored by literary history's most charismatic queer tutor, Lord Henry Wotton, Dorian pursued a career of sensory experience, pleasure, and 'meaningless' artifice that corrupted him morally and spiritually. Wilde's novel provides all the elements of what would come to constitute a sort of neo-gothic mythology of AIDS crisis discourses: a vain and egotistical (queer) anti-hero whose lethal narcissism leads him to self-destruction, unspeakable secrets, decadence, drug and sex addiction, the visual inscription of sin/disease at the level of the body, and a fatal(istic) conclusion foreshadowed from the outset.

The Picture of Dorian Gray is probably the most influential late nineteenth-century work to forge and popularise the stereotypical link between art, decadence and homosexuality. The novel became a cultural touchstone for burgeoning definitions of 'the homosexual' that grew up around the figure of Wilde and the Wilde trials in the 1890s and is frequently read as a coded representation of homosexuality, particularly via the figures of the aesthete and the dandy, whose style and self-production had become central to burgeoning *fin de sciecle* taxonomies of homosexuality.[118]

Beyond its famous association of creativity and homosexuality, *Dorian Gray* offers a 'novelistic logic' in which death becomes the 'truth' or 'essence' of gay subjecthood.[119] Dorian's trajectory towards self-destruction, foreshadowed in the novel's first scene, distils fatality as the quintessence of the homosexual subject, offering a powerful narrative form for the 'deep cultural idea about the lethal character of male homosexuality.'[120] AIDS representations reiterate this narrative. If 'AIDS has helped to concretise a mythical link between gay sex and death',[121] and if 'AIDS has served either to confirm the truth of gay identity as death or death wish',[122] this is because these tropes have been central to cultural fantasies of same-sex desire throughout modernity. Linking narcissism and fear of ageing with sexual perversity, Dorian's wish that the painting grow old in his stead is a sort of death wish: the secrets of perverse desire, disease and inner depravity would inevitably reveal themselves on his body, just as they did in the case of Rock Hudson, who, like Dorian Gray, ends his story, as Wilde puts it, 'withered, wrinkled, and loathsome of visage'.[123] Because of its simple allegorical structure, its long association with 'the love that dare not speak its name', and its teleological linkage of male homosexuality and fatality, Wilde's fable of Dorian Gray became a sort of mythic ur-narrative of crisis discourse.

For example, the resonances of the Dorian myth are evident in another spectacular and widely circulated story of gay sexual licence, moral abandon and death: the notorious 'Patient Zero' story. A kind of HIV/AIDS 'typhoid Mary', Patient Zero entered public folklore as 'The Man who bought AIDS to North America'.[124] This idea originated in *And the Band Played On*, the 1988 docudrama by gay journalist Randy Shilts that became the most popular work of AIDS journalism, selling over 700,000 copies.[125] In that book, Shilts identified a French-Canadian airline steward, Gaëtan Dugas, as one of the first men in North America to develop AIDS. Shilts' account was based on Auerbach and Darrow's 'cluster myth' (1984),[126] in which forty men identified as among the first few hundred diagnosed with AIDS in the US were linked to each other by sexual contact tracing. Dugas was supposedly at the center of the cluster and therefore implicated in (and blamed for) the infection of gay men in New York, Los Angeles, and San Francisco before an infectious disease specialist from the public health department tracked him down. Shilts' book portrayed Dugas as a charming, handsome sexual athlete who averaged hundreds of sex partners a year: a reckless, deliberate infector who refused to stop having unprotected sex despite being warned to do so by a doctor. *And the Band Played On* drew Dugas as a kind of Narcissus who could cast a fatal spell over his lovers, a Dorian Gray figure whose erotic/aesthetic appeal masked an insatiable, bloodthirsty sociopathology. Later researchers discredited the cluster hypothesis,[127] however, 'Patient Zero' had already became a mythic figure of AIDS mythology, a 'superspreader.' James Miller described Shilts' Patient Zero as 'a nightmarish personification of motiveless malignity' and 'a Bad Fairy out of Walt Disney, the sort of *National Enquirer* alien that inquiring minds don't want to know'; he is what HIV would look like 'if HIV had a human face, a pretty face'.[128] In some ways, Patient Zero also seemed to personify an apparent link between the sexual licence of 70s gay liberation and AIDS in the 80s. As we'll see in Chapters 3 and 4, the Dorian Myth has had explicit and oblique afterlives in the universe of post-crisis representation.

Meaninglessness

'Nothing could be more meaningless than a virus', Judith Williamson wrote; '[i]t has no point, no purpose, no plan; it is part of no scheme, carries no inherent significance.'[129] Nevertheless, HIV was quickly enveloped in a superabundance of stories that endowed it with meaning, giving it narrative structure and shape, infusing and encircling it with an excess of signification. Stories – with their beginnings, middles and ends, their morals and meanings – have the unique capacity to work against meaningless. The threat of abject meaninglessness, however, remains. 'Even as AIDS is invested with meanings through these structures', Williamson explains, 'that meaninglessness which is thereby negated lurks ominously at the edges of perception, at once a threat, and a constant spur, to the formation of explanatory fictions.'[130]

Queers and queerness may also have a privileged relationship with meaninglessness. As Edelman argues in his polemic work, *No Future: Queer Theory and the Death Drive* (2005), queerness – symbolically, psychically, and sometimes politically – signifies the very undoing of that which society deems most meaningful: reproduction and The Child. *No Future* infamously argues that to become socially meaningful one must lodge an intention to participate in 'reproductive futurity', the structure that fixes intelligibility to the teleological reproduction of kinship structures via The Child. If 'the biological fact of heterosexual procreation bestows the imprimatur of meaning-production on heterogenital relations,' Edelman writes,[131] then queerness is a force opposed: queerness *undoes* meaning and is therefore meaning-less. Reproductive futurity, Edelman argues, is the 'underlying structure of the political', but also of the psychic/Symbolic. It is governed by the 'fantasy of achieving Symbolic closure through the marriage of identity to futurity in order to realise the social subject,'[132] the possibility of the future embodied in the promise offered by The Child. Queerness, on the other hand, exists in the space of the negative, the meaningless, the refusal of this social order. Queerness is opposition to reproductive heterosexuality; it embodies the 'death drive, intransigent *jouissance*… sexuality's implication in the senseless pulsations of that drive.' Queerness, Edelman writes, is constituted through 'its insistence on repetition, its stubborn denial of teleology, its resistance to determinations of meaning… and, above all, its rejection of spiritualisation through marriage to reproductive futurism.'[133]

Much of the same could be said about a virus, particularly a fatal one. The terrifying meaningless of both queerness and of a sexually transmitted disease seem to line up quite neatly because both reject the 'metaphysics of meaning on which heteroreproduction takes its stand.'[134] Crisis discourse's proliferation of storytelling (of which the homosexual stories about AIDS are but one chapter) can be understood as a defensive psychic response to these universe-threatening forms of meaninglessness. As we'll see in Chapter 1, post-crisis culture has continued to invent ways to escape this spectre of meaningless.

Melodrama

By the mid-1990s, an alternative set of images of HIV/AIDS had emerged: Benetton ads depicted sympathetic PLWHA, celebrities wore red ribbons to the Oscars and HIV-positive characters appeared on prime-time American soap operas. In 1993 there was *Philadelphia*, the AIDS melodrama par excellence, which re-wrought the public story of gay men and AIDS as a heroic battle against prejudice and a lesson in tolerance and liberal pluralism. For many, these more 'positive images' signalled a progressive consciousness and tolerance-raising shift, community-authored and activist-driven images of people *living* with HIV/AIDS that redressed some of the violence of earlier AIDS discourses and did much to reduce HIV stigma. Others, such as Daniel Harris, viewed these positive images as a 'kitschification' of the pandemic, a co-optation of it by the market in patronising, reductive and sentimental images. These genres of sentimentality transformed PLWHA into heroes and martyrs – 'living Hallmark sympathy card[s]' – through morally simplistic narratives, infantilisation and the erasure of unpalatable sexual practices.[135]

In the 'coming-home-to-die' genre,[136] for example – films like *An Early Frost* (1985), *Our Sons* (1991), *A Place for Annie* (1994), *It's My Party* (1996), and *One Night Stand* (1997) – the generally gay male PLWHA became a 'sacrificial other', an object of pity who dies or represses elements of himself in order to make living (and mourning) easier for those around them. According to Hart, the sacrificial PWA is an heir to the legacy of the female other of 1950s and 60s melodrama, the classic example of which is Stella Dallas from Douglas Sirk's eponymous 1937 film. An object of pity, antipathy and counter-identification, Stella Dallas is tragically eviscerated from the narrative in order that it may conclude.[137] Though gentler than the monstrous otherness produced in horror and science fiction AIDS films, these images still ensured the viewer would not identify with the victim of AIDS: 'the contamination of sickness and death could remain visibly contained in the vessel of the emaciated, dying body of a person with AIDS.'[138] Aspects of this sentimental approach continue twenty years on, as we'll see in Chapter 5's discussion of *Dallas Buyers Club*: the PLWHA as a heroic figure and a spokesperson for tolerance and awareness, but still isolated, marked visibly by KS and wasting, and thus a human object lesson in pity for the viewer.

Philadelphia exemplifies the compromises entailed by the sentimental gaze of AIDS social realism. On the one hand, the Academy Award–winning film dramatised the stigma concentrated around the gay male PLWHA to a huge American and global audience, and most accounts of the film are liberal celebrations claiming that it increased HIV/AIDS awareness. On the other hand, critics have also described the film as a case study in 'sentimental nationalism', 'de-homosexualising' strategies, and the erasure, privatisation and theatricalisation of the political rage and organised public response to official government negligence.[139] The sanitising of AIDS in the film was achieved in part by the casting of a white homosexual hero played by American icon of boy-next-door wholesomeness, Tom Hanks. His character, Andy Beckett, was made sympathetic through a number of means, including his sexual guilt, his giving up of an active sex life after his diagnosis, his battle against unsympathetic institutions, and his alliance with the initially homophobic African-American lawyer, Joe Miller (Denzel Washington), who learns tolerance through liberal sympathy. A scene of Andy kissing his long-term partner, Miguel (Antonio Banderas), was infamously left on the cutting room floor.[140] This desexualising, as we'll see in the next chapter, is a key strategy of redeeming gayness for popular audiences. As Robert Corber argues, *Philadelphia* constructs gay men as objects of the 'sentimental gaze', a liberal alternative to the forms of nationalism that violently exclude racial and sexual minorities. Sentimentality operates as a form of mass-mediated pedagogy and a technology of citizenship that mediates gender, race, sexual and class conflict; images of minority suffering and death promote understanding and pity as a means of incorporation into the nation, but this incorporation is largely symbolic, and its dependence on pity reduces freedom to the absence of suffering.[141]

After Antiretrovirals

Since the advent of ARVs in 1996, much has changed. As we shall see in the chapters that follow, the transformed contexts of post-crisis give rise to new modes of representation, and, as I will argue, a dialectic of the spectacular/ mundane that is the effect of the historical encounter between the crisis vision of AIDS as a gay disease and the ambivalent 'normalisation' of HIV in the current culture.

If the dominant image in crisis discourse was of the contagious homosexual, the ideological enemy of the family, or an object of pity and mourning for it, in the 'Gay 90s' a domesticated gay man appears and takes his place. Chapter 1 examines this figure, the 'New Gay Man', who adopts a more palatable role as best friend to heterosexual women and willing aid to the narrative priorities of reproductive futures. This post-crisis archetype becomes a key figure in the development of neoliberal and neoconservative homosexualities. As we shall see, the New Gay Man must make sacrifices and renunciations, including the repudiation of sex and a disavowal of the psychic and symbolic spectre of queer meaninglessness in order to be allowed back into the family house.

1

Gay Redemption

Domestication and Disavowal in The Gay 90s

'The Big A'

VICKIE: You don't even know, I'm sitting here... maybe... probably dying of AIDS. And I'm totally alone. [*pauses*]. You don't understand, every day, all day, it's all that I think about, OK? Every time I sneeze, it's like I'm four sneezes away from the hospice. And it's like it's not even happening to me, it's like I'm watching it on some crappy show like *Melrose Place* or some shit, right? And I'm the new character, I'm the H-I-V/AIDS character, and I live in the building and I teach everybody that 'It's OK to be near me, it's OK to talk to me!' And then I die... And there's everybody at my funeral wearing halter-tops or chokers or some shit like that.

LELAINA: [*Laughing anxiously*] Vickie, stop, OK? Just stop. You're freaking out. And you know what? You're gonna have to deal with the results. Whatever they are, we're gonna have to deal with them... just like we've dealt with everything else.

VICKIE: This isn't like everything else.

LELAINA: I know that, all right? But it's gonna be OK, you know? I know it's gonna be OK. [*Pauses*]. *Melrose Place* is a really good show.

Reality Bites, Dir. Ben Stiller, 1994

Reality Bites is an American romantic comedy-drama tracing the post-college fortunes of four twenty-somethings in Houston, Texas in the early 1990s. It revolves around an aspiring videographer, Lelaina Pierce (Winona Ryder), who documents her friend's disenchanted 'slacker' lives. After a series of quirky episodes developing the familiar predicaments of so-called Gen X-ers, the film establishes a more conventional love triangle in which Lelaina's affections are divided between slick TV executive Michael (Ben Stiller) and disaffected grunge rock artist Troy (Ethan Hawke), two men whose differences come to emblematise her own (and Gen X's) internal conflicts between pragmatism and idealism, conventional life choices and high-minded, artistic ones.

Perhaps due to the film's generous lashings of television trivia and its close association with the Generation X moment in global Anglo-American popular culture, *Reality Bites* became somewhat iconic. This is a little ironic given the film itself repeatedly ironises its own patchwork of pop-cultural references. In any case, my interest here is not in whether this cultural touchstone accurately captured the moods and lifestyles of Generation X, but in the way it depicted HIV/AIDS and gay male life, two themes that are marginal to the central heterosexual romance narrative but whose treatment provides an instructive glimpse at a broader set of trends in mainstream American film and television of the 1990s that I wish to re-examine in this chapter.

Reality Bites has two supporting characters, Vickie and Sammie. Vickie (Janeane Garofalo) is Lelaina's sassy, quick-witted housemate and best friend, and the reluctant assistant manager of clothing store The Gap. She has a series of dry one-liners and one-night stands before confronting her fears of HIV/AIDS and of being alone, twin phobias that are conflated under the sign of promiscuity. Early on we see Vickie adding to a long list of names of the men she has slept with in a notebook by her bed. Later we see her through the lens of Lelaina's documentary camera, announcing her arrival at a medical centre: 'The free clinic AIDS test!' she announces with faux excitement, 'The rite of passage for our generation. We're so lucky!' Shortly after, in the tragi-comic confession quoted above, Vickie admits that she is terrified she could be HIV positive. *Reality Bites* doesn't indicate whether or not Vickie has been practising safer sex, but this is somewhat immaterial. Given the pervasive images of PWAs[1] in 1980s and early 1990s mass culture as figures of merciless isolation,[2] and the highly publicised conflation of HIV/AIDS with promiscuity, we can recognise, if not perhaps share, Vickie's fears. In light of these associations, it's no surprise that Vickie's fear of AIDS is associated with her fear of being alone.

These fears are presented as universal, for Gen X at least: as Vickie says, the test is 'a rite of passage for our generation'. In the universe of *Reality Bites*, HIV is a fact of life, a 'biting reality', and Vickie's confession expresses its place in the emotional landscape of her world. Tellingly, she frames her confession through the ironic citation of popular TV soap opera, *Melrose Place* (1992–99), the 1990s standard-bearer for titillating sex drama and over-the-top plot twists. The TV reference bespeaks a knowing awareness of the way in which popular screen images of AIDS and HIV/AIDS awareness-raising discourses were, by this time, dominated by the generic conventions of melodrama[3] and 'kitsch sentiment', as Daniel Harris's provocative essay, 'The Kitschification of AIDS' later catalogued.[4] Vickie's AIDS speech gestures – however faintly – to Harris's critique of the liberal, sentimental gaze of mainstream US culture that offers tokenistic and morally simplistic, 'politically correct' minority representations, wrapped up in commercial agendas and resulting in portraits of romanticised pity and martyrdom. The *Melrose Place* reference also reflects the way in which, more broadly, the conventions of popular media culture (re)frame the fears and fantasies of everyday life.

But for all this self-awareness, *Reality Bites* itself, as we shall see, goes on to rehearse similarly reductive conventions. Lelaina's other friend Sammy (Steve Zahn) is a character whose main attribute is that he is gay. Unlike the rest of the cast, Sammy has neither romantic interest nor sexual encounters. He functions mostly as comic relief and he has scarcely a sub-plot to call his own apart from a brief sequence in which he comes out of the closet. Before this there is a comedic 'rehearsal' scene in which Sammy and Vickie read from dummy scripts, emphasising the 'scriptedness' of the coming out scene. The film then cuts to a dejected Sammy sitting outside his mother's house where the 'real' emotional fallout is documented by Lelaina's camera. Sammy says

> Well, I came out to her and… she's still a little bit upset. But you know [*pauses*]. You know, I think the real reason… I've been

celibate for so long isn't really because I'm that terrified of The Big A... but because I can't really start my life... without being honest about who I am [cut].

Given Sammy is gay and given the fears expressed by Vickie we might assume that 'The Big A' is a reference to AIDS. But it may also refer to anal sex given that Sammy says he has been celibate. Either way, in this brief sexual confession, *something* is unmentionable. Moreover, in spite of the self-aware parody in the coming out rehearsal scene, this is, ironically, the only character development – the only scene – that Sammy gets: Lelaina cuts her documentary right at the point where Sammy seems about to open up and tell his story.

I open this discussion of HIV/AIDS and 'The Gay 90s' with this example because it very clearly iterates a broader trend in popular culture from the time. In *Reality Bites* the presence of a gay male character is not a big deal, yet he doesn't get a plot of his own besides the dramatic disclosure of his sexuality. Sammy's predicament exemplifies a broader tendency in the emerging positive images of the 1990s, which is to portray homosexuality almost exclusively in what Dennis Allen calls 'narratives of disclosure.' Narratives of disclosure, Allen explains, are 'continually substituted for any possible narrative, romantic or otherwise, predicated on such a sexuality'; beyond the revelation of homosexuality, there is no actual gay drama.[5] Funnily enough, Allen identifies the example of Matt Fielding (Doug Savant), the resident gay character on *Melrose Place*, the very show that Vickie references in *Reality Bites*. For Allen, homosexuality in *Melrose Place* is an 'endlessly repeated story',[6] and Matt is constantly relegated to the role of 'accomplice to the machinations of other characters.'[7] The coming out vignette serves as an epistemological support to the imperatives of the enveloping heterosexually-oriented narrative; it creates a space for the participation of a queer character but prevents them from rupturing either the development or the closure of the over-arching heterosexual plot. As Scott Paulin writes, this 'practice of denotation, linked as it is to a discourse of "coming out", implies a greater willingness to acknowledge that gay men and lesbians exist, [however] it does not necessarily imply a greater commitment to challenging the ideology that privileges heterosexuality in the first place.'[8] Sammy's narrative inconsequence is neatly conveyed by

Gay Redemption

Lelaina's exasperated question to him later in the film: 'Sammy, what are you even doing here? You don't even live here!' Plotless and sexless (and apparently homeless), Sammy exemplifies a broader 1990s trend of recruiting queer characters to secondary and supporting roles in hetero-oriented narratives, and, importantly, the quarantining of them from other queer people and from acting on their sexual desires.

The phenomenon of a desexualised gay character who is restricted to a narrative of disclosure was particularly ubiquitous in the 1990s and there is a substantial archive of criticism, both popular and scholarly, on these avowedly 'positive images'. But what if we were to return to this moment in modern gay representation and ask afresh about the role of AIDS in these images? How is this figure of gay male celibacy informed by the lurid AIDS crisis discourses discussed in the previous chapter? What happens if we attempt to bring the unspeakable 'Big A' from the margins of narrative consciousness to the centre of the analysis?

As will become clear in this chapter, Sammy's euphemistic reference is a useful clue to a broader cultural project of *AIDS disavowal*. The displacement of the drama of AIDS from Sammy to Vickie in *Reality Bites* – from celibate gay man to sexually active straight woman – is part of the mechanisms of a historically particular cultural trend that I call 'Gay Redemption.' The conventions of Gay Redemption permit gay male characters to enter mass culture on the proviso that they remain sexually inactive. These strategies became widespread in the 1990s[9] and remain prevalent in contemporary entertainment culture. Looking back, it seems increasingly clear that the specific forms of narrative containment that surrounded this sexually unthreatening queer figure operated to disavow the particular sexual anxieties aroused by HIV/AIDS. This 'New Gay Man', as Shugart calls him,[10] emerges with particular visual, narrative, performance and casting conventions developed specifically to accommodate these disavowals.

In the remainder of this chapter we will make several returns. First, we'll return to the Gay 90s, to the birthplace of the New Gay Man and his original contexts of production and reception. Here, as we shall see, certain modes of characterisation, embodiment and narrative role (or lack thereof) operated as a reversal or a denial of the meanings (and meaninglessness) surrounding 'AIDS' that emerged in the previous decade. Second, we'll return briefly to the literature of (also predominantly 1990s) post-feminism and its examination of the psychic mechanisms of disavowal and abjection. In the tradition of Robin Wood's use of Freud's 'Return of the Repressed' formulation as a model for thinking psychically and politically about the meanings of the monster in 1970s horror movies, I use post-feminist ideas about abjection and disavowal to analyse the symbolic meanings of the domesticated gay man of 1990s romantic comedy and family melodrama.[11] Finally, we'll return to unearth an almost entirely un-investigated example of this archetype in the cinematic flop, *The Next Best Thing* (2000), a monstrous genre hybrid buried in critical loathing and box office un-success, but a thoroughly instructive example of Hollywood Gay Redemption conventions nonetheless. This film's New Gay Man – played by patron saint of Gay Redemption, Rupert Everett – both breaks with and reaffirms the generic regulations imposed on this archetype, bringing its mechanisms and their attendant contradictions into relief. With HIV/AIDS lurking at the margins of the film's narrative, *The Next Best Thing* neatly demonstrates the processes through which the New Gay Man is constructed via rituals of symbolic purification, including domestic labour, the obsessive eradication of dirt, the symbolic burial of the AIDS body and the renunciation of the PLWHIV.[12] These processes of disavowal become key imperatives in an aspirational narrative labouring toward normative life, what Edelman calls 'reproductive futurity' – the 'mandate by which our political institutions compel the collective reproduction of the Child'[13] and through which politics remain beholden to heteronormative visions of the future, achievable only via an endless struggle against the meaninglessness associated with the 'queer'.

The Gay 90s Revisited

> I want to be let back in the house.
> Sammy, *Reality Bites*

During the 1990s the archive of openly queer characters grew exponentially in Hollywood and other national cinemas. Sympathetic gay male characters like Sammy appeared in box office hits like *Philadelphia* (1993), *The Birdcage* (1996) and *In and Out* (1997). Later in the decade, the gay man/straight woman 'buddy' formula emerged as a popular sub-genre of romantic comedy with films including *My Best Friend's Wedding* (1997), *The Object of My Affection* (1998) and *The Next Best Thing* (2000).

TV was even more prolific than Hollywood in its manufacturing of sexually unthreatening gay male characters. The secondary-but-permanent gay character became a staple of 1990s dramas and situation comedies, including *NYPD Blue*, *Chicago Hope*, *ER*, *Mad About You* and *Roseanne*. Eventually queer protagonists became central characters in, for example, *Ellen* (1994–1998) and *Dawson's Creek* (1998–2003). The decade was dubbed 'the Gay 90s' by Jess Cagle in *Entertainment Weekly* in 1994.[14]

Across American entertainment culture, queerness became chic – albeit a very celibate kind of chic. Virtually without exception, the queer characters populating the Hollywood landscape were either chastely single or in committed, monogamous but sexually non-demonstrative relationships. In 1998, a critic in *The Advocate* wrote that 'nobody can get laid':

> Homosexuals are allowed to exist as long as they never have (homo)sex… Rupert Everett in *My Best Friend's Wedding* and Greg Kinnear in *As Good as It Gets* had a very dry white season… *The Object of My Affection* creates a universe in which the casual acceptance of gays in a straight world is unquestioned, and that's certainly refreshing. But you are asked to believe that an attractive man like Paul Rudd could come out of a four-year relationship with another man, move in with a strange woman, and never have so much as a phone call from any gay person he's ever met. Not to mention sex.[15]

The absence of sex was so consistent and conspicuous that, as Paulin suggests, the celibate male homosexual 'may well be the dominant cultural representation of the gay man in the mid-90s'.[16]

On TV, too, the ever-multiplying queer characters rarely entered intimate relationships. If they were coupled, they tended to appear for a single episode or narrative arc, disappearing before the quandary of how to avoid depicting sex was posed.[17] Later in the decade, romantic relationships began to appear more frequently, though these tended to nestle queer couplehood in the reassuring contexts of bourgeois good taste, cultural and financial capital and the sexual dignity earned through proximity to monogamy, family and material privilege. They were also overwhelmingly white, as Ron Becker's study of American TV's archive of queer characters reports: in the 1990s, more than 50 per cent of America's TV queers were white, with very few Latino, African American or Asian American queers.[18]

The most enduring case in point was Will (Eric McCormack) of NBC's enormously popular *Will and Grace* (1998–2006) who was in a dynamic buddy coupling with TV's first out 'fag hag', Grace (Debra Messing). In fact, NBC capitalised on *Will and Grace*'s sexlessness, advertising the relationship as 'a kind of friendship that's possible between a man and a woman when sex doesn't get in the way.'[19] The earlier icon of gay celibacy was of course *Melrose Place*'s Matt, whose chastity was especially conspicuous in the shamelessly horny soap known for its endless assignations and philandering. Matt became the subject of an *Advocate* cover feature in December 1994 which posed the question: 'Why can't this man get laid?' In response, *Melrose Place* creator and producer, Darren Star, acknowledged that 'the nature of television and advertising is such that we cannot permit Matt to have real physical relationships onscreen like the other characters.'[20]

The commercial rationale Star cites was certainly a major factor contributing to this proscription of gay sex onscreen. Becker explains primetime's easily assimilable gays through an account of TV audience demographics. The types of queers on TV, he argues, tended to reflect the 'quality demographic' they were being pitched at: '[i]nstead of images of nelly queens or motorcycle dykes, we are presented with images of white, affluent, trend-setting, Perrier-drinking, frequent-flier using, PhD.-holding consumer citizens with far more income to spend than they know what to do with.'[21] Becker calls the psycho-graphic market to which queer TV content was being pitched 'slumpies' ('socially minded, urban-minded professionals'), a '"hip", "sophisticated", urban-minded, white, college-educated' audience with 'liberal attitudes, disposable income, and a distinctly edgy and ironic sensibility.'[22] For this prized demographic, the inclusion of 'a gay neighbour, a lesbian sister, or some queer plot twist' was a signifier of quality or risqué television, making gay-themed content a 'shrewd business decision.'[23] This business of targeting slumpies and a smaller but no less prized, upscale queer viewership was happening alongside the development of narrowcasting in the media industries, the mainstreaming of the gay rights movement, multiculturalism and the increasing currency of political correctness.[24]

Because the mainstream appearance of out homosexual characters was at this time still novel, these characters were scrutinised by scholars, critics and audiences. In some camps the very presence of 'positive images' were celebrated for augmenting the project of queer visibility in its own right, echoing the activist mantras of GLAAD and other organisations, and the 'representation matters' principle of gay and lesbian identity politics. Others were more ambivalent.

For example, Aronson and Kimmel saw the celibate gay man of 1990s Hollywood cinema as a figure who had to renounce his sexuality as a curative response to a 'crisis of heterosexuality' in the social landscape of post-feminism.[25] American romance narrative, they argue, had long depended on the idea of the transformative power of women's love and its ability to lure the errant man back to the conjugal realm. After second wave feminism, however, this convention stopped working because contemporary women were no longer considered pure or virtuous enough to transform the wayward male.[26] It was thus, they argued, that a different 'Angel of the House' was required – either a child or a gay man. The celibate gay thus became a spokesperson for the future of the family: an instructor, chaperone, aid or restorative agent to hetero-disequilibria, teaching straight women how to maintain their relationships, their families, and to 'reset their priorities so that domestic bliss takes priority over career hustles.'[27] These gay role models often materialised in anticipation of a wedding, playing a rejuvenating role in the tired marriage plot. For example, *Four Weddings and a Funeral* (1993) offered a devoted same-sex relationship that heterosexuals could only envy. The characters Gareth (Simon Callow) and Matthew (John Hannah) modelled commitment and functionality as a foil for the doddering incompetency of heterosexual characters Charles (Hugh Grant) and Carrie (Andy McDowell). As another romantically muddled character declares: 'if we can't be like Gareth and Matthew then we might as well give up.'

Shugart offers an emphatic feminist critique of these figures, whom she views as ultimately more oppressive of women than they are of gay men. Considering the straight woman–gay man buddy comedies, she proposes that if we view these friendships as a kind of romantic pairing then they actually show how gay men come to enjoy the privileges of the patriarchal dividend,[28] shoring up heterosexual male privilege, while their female friends are without 'truly reciprocal privileges'.[29] The New Gay Man – a term that Shugart coins – re-inhabits a hierarchical gendered power relation by voicing a rational, paternal, instructive discourse; 'their control over these women ultimately… manifests in their control over female sexuality'.[30] In particular, she argues, the unprecedented and unlimited 'sexual access' they have to their female friends is 'tantamount to a degree of sexual entitlement that is, notably, no longer readily available to heterosexual men'.[31] Though Shugart leaves little room to consider relationships between gay men and straight women as fertile sites for imagining spaces outside of patriarchy – stripping the feminist and queer viewing pleasures of these films – her attention to the heterosexualising of these gay male figures is valuable. If the safe eroticism of the buddy coupling is a response to a perceived crisis in the status of heterosexuality, as Aaronson and Kimmel also propose, and a potential means of repairing that heterosexuality (and hence shoring up male privilege), then its stripping away of queer sexual desires surely involves some degree of effeminophobia, if not misogyny. In theories of masculinity, effeminophobia is a key part of the reproduction of hegemonic masculinities;[32] and, as we saw in the previous chapter, passivity was a particularly anxious component of the image of the gay male PWA in crisis discourse. As we shall see in more detail shortly, a particularly AIDS-inflected strain of effeminophobia haunted positive images of gay men in the 1990s.

The now-familiar trope of the celibate gay male friend as an aid to heterosexual romance reached its most glaring apotheosis in the mid-noughties lifestyle makeover show, *Queer Eye for the Straight Guy* (2003–7). In *Queer Eye* the gay male 'Fab Five', a team of neoliberal lifestyle experts, are put to work as micro-managerial advisors on the intimate, personal and presentational practices of an ideal contemporary straight male lifestyle, and, ultimately, the 'perfection of heterosexual romance'.[33] *Queer Eye* was a very blunt example of the gay man's renunciation of desire. At the close of each episode, the Fab Five sit in a studio watching their straight-male makeover subject seducing his female paramour – literally becoming spectators of the heterosexual romance that they themselves helped to bring about. Here, as Bateman writes, 'Queer men are positioned comfortably outside the spectacle; they are onlookers, accomplices, facilitators, but alas, not participants'.[34] Gay desire is sublimated into cultural and aesthetic expertise aimed at supporting the project of heterosexuality, redeeming the straight man from errant lifestyling.

Bateman makes a key connection between the domestication strategies of *Queer Eye* and the spectacle of AIDS in previous decades. The neutering of queer desire in this show is noteworthy, he writes,

> when we take into account our culture's recent antipathy towards and terror of the gay body expressed through countless moral panics over AIDS… [A]fter years of stigmatising and quarantining the gay body, straight culture has finally found an aspect of homosexuality to which it wants to be exposed. The gay man can now be absolutely infectious, absolutely contagious, so long as we are speaking of his fashion sense and not his pathological desire.[35]

As the Introduction outlined, the widely circulated spectacle of AIDS involved images of male homosexualities so corrupted by hedonism, promiscuity and a charactorological predisposition to illness, that they came to stand in for the then-fatal sexually transmitted disease itself. Other contemporary representations, like the homosexual serial killer film *Cruising* (1980), had presented gay men as insatiable, risk-addled urban sexual adventurers, alongside the queer self-authored literature and political rhetoric of gay liberation from the 1970s onwards that celebrated promiscuity as an affirmative political act. But, by the 1990s, the dominant image of male homosexuality was one of innocence, celibacy and domesticity. If gay male bodies were sites that triggered anxiety, then the asexual, domesticated gay male archetype that emerged in 1990s representations was the solution. If the 'spectacle of AIDS' had publicised the homosexual as the ideological enemy of the family – against which the bourgeois Self identifies – then the redemptive capacities of the New Gay Man could, alternatively, be embraced as the solution to the family's problems.

I don't claim to be the first to forge this connection between AIDS crisis imagery and the New Gay Man. For example, in his 1996 analysis of the erotic thriller *Single White Female* (1992), Paulin suggested that desexualising could be a strategy designed, consciously or otherwise, to divert cultural anxieties about AIDS.[36] 'Fear of disease', he hypothesised, has 'dictated the permissible parameters within which gays may be represented.'[37] He pointed to the way this particular film worked overtime to disavow an active gay male sexuality through 'subtle and unspoken absences, presented as if natural and unremarkable'. 'It seems inevitable', he wrote, 'that this progression toward colonising and sanitising the homosexual, and in particular the body of the gay male, is linked to cultural anxieties about AIDS'. Noting the increase in queer characters in popular culture, Paulin posited that 'in order to be sympathetic, a gay male character must reassure an AIDS-phobic audience that he is not contaminated and will not be an agent of infection.'[38] A decade later, Becker suggests that the caginess of advertisers around queer TV content in the 1990s was linked to AIDS discourses and anti-gay rhetoric from the 1980s: 'Advertisers and network executives had good reason to consider it a highly divisive issue – something to be carefully avoided in an era still dominated by broadcasting principles.'[39] More than another decade later still, this connection between AIDS and the emergence of a desexualised, domesticated gay archetype demands further reflection. Through what visual conventions are 'positive images' purified of AIDS signification? What narrative limitations are imposed by this ritual disavowal of sexual signifiers? And what are its ideological implications? How has this popular image come to inform gay representation and gay politics in the post-antiretrovirals – that is, the 'post-crisis' – landscape?

The New Gay Man both replaces and renounces the construction of homosexuality in crisis discourse as monolithically, narcissistically sexual, as the ideological enemy of the family, and as a source of contagion and death. Quite the contrary, Gay Redemption narratives champion the adult prioritisation of relationships, superseding vanity, ambition and sexual gratification. As a by-product of this, the New Gay Man also tends to react against many of the perceived negative social effects of feminism, gay liberation, radical queer politics and AIDS activisms. Like the neo femme fatales of 1980s and 1990s feminist backlash films, the New Gay Man is a figure of reactionary sexual politics.[40] As we'll see in the forthcoming case study, he is compelled to distance himself from queerness and become a footman in service to the narrative priorities of reproductive futurity.

Before we move on, two brief but important points. Firstly, the domesticated, celibate homosexual figure was not entirely or only an invention of the 1990s. In addition to cinematic precursors, like the homosexual best friend in *Darling* (1965), the archetype has an older genealogy in English literary culture. For example, the 'odd' bachelors in the Victorian-era works of William Thackeray, Henry James and Daphne Du Maurier that Eve Sedgwick described as 'distinctly circumscribed', 'often marginalised', and, crucially, 'housebroken by the severing of ... [their] connection with a discourse of genital sexuality'.[41] These figures, Sedgwick notes, are often associated with the maintenance of the domestic sphere.

Secondly, it should be acknowledged that queer cultural histories have a tendency to themselves overdetermine readings of celibacy as sexual repression. This colludes, as Benjamin Kahan argues, with a logic in which representations of queers 'not engaging in sex is capitulating to homophobic forces'.[42] Riffing on Foucault's famous 1976 critique of 'the repressive hypothesis', Kahan calls this 'the expressive hypothesis': a dichotomy inherited from the 1980s 'sex wars' between anti-pornography and pro-sex feminists and the cultural battlegrounds fought around AIDS between the poles of 'censorship and conservative politics, on the one hand, and expression and oppositional liberal politics, on the other'.[43] Labouring under this dichotomy, Kahan observes that in queer studies we tend to write celibacy 'under the sign of censorship... as an alibi or "beard" for the "obscenity" of homosexuality'.[44] The 'crusade against censorship [among sex positive feminist and queer activists, for example] left no room for sexuality without a normative aspiration to sexual acts.' Consequently, queer readings habitually identify celibacies as 'repressed', 'latent', 'closeted' or 'reluctant' homosexualities;[45] 'sex and sexuality are conflated, as there is no sexual expression without sex.' Kahan suggests instead that celibacy may be reconceived *as sexuality* rather than as absence, as powerfully anachronistic and indeterminate through its failure to align with 'modern frameworks of determined and determinate sexuality'.[46] I'm very sympathetic to this reading of celibacy as 'an organisation of pleasure' and I don't wish to reproduce another queer cultural history that is, by-default, a history of sexual failure. Nonetheless, I'm reluctant to give too much hermeneutic leverage to a recuperative reading of celibacy in the case of the New Gay Man, because, as the case study to come will hopefully illustrate, this would obscure the very *sexually-loaded* mechanisms of disavowal (of pleasure, of AIDS and AIDS signification) that he instantiates. The New Gay Man operates as a figure or sexual redemption precisely through his prophylactic distance from active intimacy and pleasure, and the queer cultures surrounding it.

If this was an anxious after-effect of the exponential visibility of diseased homosexualities in AIDS discourse, then it speaks directly to the psychic process of disavowal and abjection. Drawing on the psychoanalytically-informed ideas of post-feminist scholars including Mary Douglas,[47] Julia Kristeva,[48] Elizabeth Grosz[49] and Judith Butler,[50] I suggest that we may think about the New Gay Man as an archetype produced through the work of a cultural disavowal that aims to erase the spectre of AIDS and its attendant connotations: promiscuity, hedonism, feminisation, isolation, narcissism, contagion and death. The efforts required to regulate these absences produces a new subject of contemporary gay masculinity, sporting an image that is desexualised, domesticated, often masculinised and generally endowed with the hallmarks of bourgeois, white (hetero-) normative personhood. As Butler argues, repudiation is actually one of the constitutive processes of identity construction:[51] 'certain exclusions and foreclosures institute the subject and persist as the permanent or constitutive spectre of its own destabilisation.'[52] A discursive prohibition – in this case the rendering unspeakable of AIDS – becomes the constitutive precondition of a new sexual persona. The denial of one thing (AIDS) produces another (the New Gay Man).

And yet, as Kristeva's theory of abjection reminds us, spectres can never be buried entirely. Indeed, the significance of these spectres is reaffirmed through the efforts required to purge them. Jackie Stacey describes this process very eloquently when she writes that:

> A layering of cultural disavowals erases the categories in question but simultaneously confirms their significance…. While the force of people's fear may require that these categories be euphemised, displaced or substituted, the necessity of such strategies leads directly back to the prohibitive imperatives of that fear.[53]

The absence/presence of AIDS produces a new unspeakable and the New Gay Man becomes a figure of high anxiety. Shortly, we will move on to a detailed analysis of *The Next Best Thing*, which illustrates precisely how these processes operate at the level of cinematic language. However, first, a brief elaboration of these psychic and social processes of disavowal – and how they may be deployed as cultural reading practices – is required.

Abjection and AIDS

'Abjection' is a term famously developed by Julia Kristeva in *Powers of Horror* (1982) to describe the border between order and (pre-symbolic) disorder. The abject describes those things that threaten psychic and social boundaries, disturbing stability or identity, and – crucially – disturbing meaning. Kristeva's theory of abjection proposes that the attainment of 'proper' subjectivity and sociality requires the expulsion of the improper, the unclean and the disorderly. For the individual, abjection describes a pre-linguistic moment at which we separate from, or recognise a boundary between, our own and our mother's body. Culturally, it refers to the process of creating a demarcation between what is considered human and what is considered animal, between culture and that which precedes it. In psycho-analytic literature, this principle of expulsion goes back to *Totem and Taboo* (1913) in which Freud argued that civilisation is founded on the exclusion of 'impure' attachments, particularly incest.[54] For Kristeva, abjection is the primal effort to separate ourselves from the animal: 'by way of abjection, primitive societies have marked out a precise area of their culture in order to remove it from the threatening world of animals or animalism, which were imagined as representatives of sex and murder.'[55]

The abject thus has to do with all that is repudiated: 'what disturbs identity, system, order. What does not respect borders, positions, rules';[56] that which may break down meaning because it draws attention to an indistinction between subject and object, or between self and other. This is why bodily fluids – blood, faeces, sweat and mucus – are frequently described as abject. They remind us of the body's permeability and can elicit a visceral horror or disgust response. According to Kristeva, this response is pre-linguistic and is associated with the routine disavowal of material reminders of death. If we react with disgust to excretion or menstruation, for example, it is because they confront us with the materiality of (our own) death. Kristeva writes:

> A wound with blood and pus, or the sickly, acrid smell of sweat, of decay, does not *signify* death. In the presence of signified death – a flat encephalograph, for instance – I would understand, react, or accept. No, [...] refuse and corpses *show me* what I permanently thrust aside in order to live. These body

> fluids, this defilement, this shit are what life withstands, hardly and with difficulty, on the part of death. There, I am at the border of my condition as a living being.[57]

The sick or dying body demands an acknowledgment of mortality that threatens to collapse the boundaries between life and death, sickness and health. In the context of HIV/AIDS, an entire inventory of abject bodily detritus comes to the fore: blood, semen and saliva as potential fluids of transmission; sweat, lesions, mucus, shit and tears as potential by-products of infection.

Being recognised as a meaningful, intelligible subject is at issue here: the delimitation of a 'clean' and 'proper' body is a condition of the subject's constitution as a speaking subject.[58] As we saw in the previous chapter, HIV/AIDS and queerness threatens the subject with an abject loss of meaning.[59] The abject must thus be repudiated in order that one remains an intelligible subject.

Part of what has made Kristeva's work on abjection so capacious is that she doesn't distinguish between the social and the psychic. Abjection has therefore, been used as a framework to describe processes of social exclusion and discrimination, and has been especially useful in feminist and queer theory, and in theories of social stigma.[60] Both Iris Marion Young[61] and Judith Butler have drawn on Kristeva to show how 'the repudiation of bodies for their sex, sexuality and/or color is an "expulsion" followed by a "repulsion" that founds and consolidates culturally hegemonic identities.'[62] The ascription of the abject to the bodies of social others is a process of social and sexual regulation and exclusion. The 'dreaded identification'[63] with the abject is especially salient in the case of HIV/AIDS where the combination of (homo)sexual or racial difference and death (especially prior to the advent of ARVs) signifies a double form of abjection: 'the corpse threatens the ego from *outside*, sexual difference challenges the ego from *within*.'[64]

Julia Epstein has explored how metaphors of immunity in discussions of AIDS may produce both 'border anxiety'[65] and a category crisis.[66] The immune system is the metaphorical locus of bodily health and also of autonomy, she writes, an imagined 'walled apparatus of differentiation between the immune and the compromised.'[67] Epstein argues that the terror of collapsing boundaries between the normal and abnormal are enhanced in the case of AIDS because HIV attacks the immune system, allowing infections to encroach on corporeal sovereignty.[68]

As we shall see next, the New Gay Man is a function of the process of the abjection of HIV and AIDS metaphors, a subject constituted through their disavowal. And yet, as Kristeva tells us, the abject does not let go. What is excluded always 'hovers at the borders of our existence, threatening the apparently settled unity of the subject with disruption and possible dissolution.'[69] As Stacey puts it, the abject 'haunts the subject with stories from the border of the self, both guaranteeing its existence and yet affirming its end'.[70]

So, if the disavowal of spectres never ensures their obliteration entirely then we must work continuously at this displacement. As Butler explains, 'the production, exclusion and repudiation of abjected spectres' is actually central to the work of cohering identity; it is, in fact, 'the repeated repudiation by which the subject installs its boundary and constructs the claim to its "integrity"'.[71] For Butler, the figure of abjection 'is not a buried identification that is left behind in a forgotten past, but an identification that must be leveled and buried again and again, the compulsive repudiation by which the subject incessantly sustains his/her boundary.'[72] Action and repetition are fundamental to this process: the subject must work, continuously and indefinitely, at the project of disavowal despite the impossibility of ever excluding those psychically reviled elements with any finality.

In the next section of this chapter I show how cinematic strategies in *The Next Best Thing*, including characterisation, narrative, *mise en scène*, intertextuality and the cinematic gaze work together at this project of redemption through renunciation. If the subject needs to work constantly and anxiously to maintain 'a certain level of mastery over the abject', to 'keep it in check and at a distance in order to define itself as a subject,'[73] then the New Gay Man is a case in point: to be redeemed of the stigma of HIV/AIDS and become both visible and intelligible as a subject, the New Gay Man must work.

The Next Best Thing

> It was a sickly script about a nasty humourless woman and her flubby gay best friend.... Funny, supportive, great dress sense, everything a man was not.... He gave up the awkward subject of sex years ago when all his friends died.... These two highly

> revolting people decided by page twenty-three to go ahead and have a baby.
>
> Rupert Everett[74]

The Next Best Thing (2000) was a second-rate attempt to extend and cash in on the success of the gay man–straight woman buddy genre. While *Will and Grace* continued to enthrall viewers and collect Emmy awards well into 2006, *The Next Best Thing* was loathed by critics and was a complete box office write-off. Its progenitor, *My Best Friend's Wedding* (1997), however, had been extremely successful, grossing US$286.9 million.[75] It too co-starred Everett as George, a dashing, witty, gay male best friend and sidekick to the central female character, Jules (Julia Roberts). Her editor and confidant, George was so 'sleek, stylish, and radiant with charisma' (the character's own words) that he made the New Gay Man type iconic. Everett became one of the first openly gay Hollywood celebrities and an international sex symbol.

What made *My Best Friend's Wedding*'s George so appealing? Susan Bordo (2000) suggests it was his difference from heterosexual men. As the film's 'moral centre' and the 'best-adjusted, happiest person in it,'[76] George was a 'stolen delight for straight women', speaking 'directly' and 'powerfully' to them.[77] A Cary Grant–like figure, he poses very little sexual threat, to women and to straight men, and recalls a lost gentlemanliness from the era of Classical Hollywood cinema.

My Best Friend's Wedding ends with Roberts on the phone to Everett being counselled for the loss of her love object. *The Next Best Thing* opens with Madonna's character, Abbie, doing the same. Cowering behind a pot plant, Abbie calls Robert for emergency guidance as she watches her now ex-boyfriend Kevin (Michael Vartan) packing his belongings. He's leaving her, but not because Abbie is anything less than perfect. Indeed, Abbie is *too* perfect. Her character is introduced via Kevin's break-up speech:

> It's not you it's me. I mean you're great! You're smart, you're beautiful, you're a good cook, and you're a great lay. I'm just not ready, alright. I'm not there yet…you're *way* too much for me right now. I wanna date less complicated women.

Abbie's perfection recalls Aronson and Kimmel's examination of the problems faced by the post-feminist heroine of contemporary Hollywood romance and capitalises on Madonna's superdiva star persona. Indeed, both Abbie and Robbie are apparently flawless; but despite perfect bodies and glamorous, successful LA lifestyles, neither have been lucky in love.

And Abbie's biological clock is ticking. She's upset about the missed opportunity to create a family ('I feel like Kevin was my last chance for a *normal* life' / 'I'd like to have a family at some point... before it's too late'). Robbert and Abbie then attend the funeral of a friend who has died from HIV/AIDS, an instructive scene that I will discuss in more detail shortly. Afterwards, they console themselves with an indulgent Independence Day spent by a pool that belongs to Robert's rich queer clients, Vernon and Ashby. After one too many poolside martinis, the raucous celebration turns raunchy, bringing about *The Next Best Thing*'s 'wacky' premise: a drunken sexual encounter turns Robbie and Abbie into prospective parents and they decide to go ahead and forge a family together.

The film skips forward through six years of child-rearing and domestic co-habitation to their son Sam's (Malcolm Stumpf) birthday party. It also shifts here from camp buddy comedy to family melodrama, attempting to dramatise the tensions that emerge in this new configuration of American family. The romance of platonic co-habitation is now interrupted by some predictable problems: Robert is dating a strapping cardiologist (Mark Valley), Abbie is jealous and quietly aching for her own lover ('Dear God, please hook me up!'), and their son Sam begins to wonder why his parents don't share a bedroom. Torn by the allegedly incompatible demands of parenting and a burgeoning gay relationship, Robert soon dumps his boyfriend in order to prioritise fatherhood. Abbie then begins dating a fetching investment banker, Ben (Benjamin Bratt), and, in an ironic reversal, Robert becomes increasingly jealous and possessive. Domestic disorder ensues. Abbie and Ben decamp with Sam, and the fluffy romantic comedy turned tart family melodrama turns again – this time into a *Kramer Vs Kramer*–style courtroom drama. Desperate to grasp custody of Sam, Robert attempts to manipulate legal process and in the midst of this it is revealed that he is not actually Sam's biological father – in fact it was Kevin – which severs Robert of any custody entitlement. Abbie's lawyer exploits a series of 'pervert tropes' to characterise Robert as a licentious, promiscuous, drug-taking faggot. Abbie gets full custody of Sam. *The Next*

Best Thing ends with a broken Robert reunited with his lost son thanks to Abbie's compassion and the promise of a potential rapprochement between the now estranged friends.

'Congratulations, not only is *The Next Best Thing* The Worst This Year, it also hits high on The Worst of All Time' punned one critic.[78] Another summarised the prevailing critical consensus when he wrote that:

> the newly pop-culture-friendly gay man/straight woman paradigm – rendered invariably as a wellspring of waggish repartee and mutual you-go-girl empathy – reaches a hall-of-mirrors dead end with real-life tag team Rupert Everett and Madonna… [B]oth are shrill, maudlin, narcissistic creatures who speak in wilted epigrams. Whether in screwball-gaysploitation or issue-of-the-week mode, the movie… favours crude dramatic devices over even the most basic character psychology.[79]

Other critics described it as 'disingenuous [and] emotionally deficient,'[80] 'a garage sale of gay issues, harnessed to a plot as exhausted as a junkman's horse,'[81] and 'so weirdly acted, shot, edited, directed, written and scored you can't believe it's happening – though, on a gut level, it is enjoyable in the way that certain forms of masochism are enjoyable.'[82]

Queer critics found the film disappointing, unfunny and expressed frustration with its promise of an unconventional family narrative on the one hand, and its re-hashing of the most threadbare gay stereotypes on the other. *The Next Best Thing* is 'an unsubtle cinematic plea for the viability of the alternative family,'[83] wrote Kendrick. Foreshadowing Becker's critique of the positive images of the 1990s, he hypothesised that 'Hollywood seems incapable of imagining an alternative family outside of a straight white woman and a gay white man… "alternative" is becoming just as stubbornly unflinching in its construction as "traditional." Critics reiterated the complaint about the sexlessness of mainstream images of gay men, even though Robert does have a relationship, including a brief, frigid scene that acts as evidence of a sex life. The *San Francisco Chronicle* wondered: 'If Abbie gets her squeeze, why not Robert? The movie brushes off the question when Robert tells a hunky cardiologist that he's too involved in fathering to be somebody's partner.' Indeed, why should there be such an intractable conflict between these aspects of his life? The critic blamed studio economics: 'If Everett were to kiss a man, as Madonna does, *The Next Best Thing* would be rated R instead of PG-13, and Paramount's profit margin would start disappearing'. The most central convention of the post-crisis Gay Redemption narrative remains: to present Robert as a sympathetic protagonist he must renounce queer desire.

In the cultural and industrial climate in which the film came to exist, the struggle to invent a generic template that accommodates an extended role for the New Gay Man, whilst maintaining the visual and narrative containment that his presence demanded, seems to have miserably failed. The film's unsuccessful meshing of genres (lurching from camp buddy comedy to family melodrama to court room drama) and the affective incoherence this generates may ultimately have been what made *The Next Best Thing* such an abject artifact of popular culture.

With the exception of Shugart's feminist critique of the buddy films, there is no sustained criticism of *The Next Best Thing*. This is no great surprise. However, I suggest that the failed attempt to extend the narrative of the sexless gay male archetype of the 1990s in this film makes *The Next Best Thing* worthy of further attention. Indeed, a close examination will, I argue, indicate that the film is an exemplary study in the narrative containment of the New Gay Man that brings his relationship with – and the disavowal of – AIDS signification into sharp relief. Robert/Everett not only renounces sex, but a range of narrative, visual and performance strategies (that may not at first glance seem to be doing the work of disavowal) function here to domesticate the gay man while abjecting 'the queer'. These strategies are:

(1) a hyper-visualisation of the desirable but sexually unthreatening male body;
(2) a ritual cleansing of the gay body through scenes of work, sanitation and wholesome activity;
(3) a severance of the gay character from queer friends, lovers and community; and, most saliently,
(4) the contrasting of the New Gay Man with other queer characters who are selfish narcissists, Production Code–era stereotypes, HIV positive or dead.

These strategies reveal much about the way the representation of gay men in the popular culture of the 1990s was underwritten by a logic of AIDS disavowal. Everett's New Gay Man is aggressively delineated from the gay male PLHIV and all he represents, and this is central to the film's attempt to produce him as sympathetic, safe and a viable candidate for a narrative straining toward reproductive futurity. Robert may not be the *best* candidate (i.e. a straight man) but he can be the *next best* given his renunciation of and safe distance from queer culture and its clutch of polluting qualities: childishness, vanity, self-absorption, self-pity, bitchiness, sex, drugs and abject meaninglessness – all qualities that, as we shall see, the film brings together under the sign of 'HIV'.

Watering, Working and Not Wearing Much

When we're introduced to him in the film's opening sequence, Robert is overseeing the re-landscaping of a large Hollywood yard. In this scene of sweaty labour, Robert, a landscape designer, is energetic, robust, commanding and competent. As the opening credits roll, he is pictured from above, monitoring the transplantation of a well-established palm tree into a hole in the earth (see Figure 1.1). He looks rugged, his muscular arms exposed, his body athletic; the camera admires Everett's tall, burly physique, establishing a safe erotic gaze that will continue throughout the film.

However, the transplantation of an already-grown tree symbolically undermines the classic 'fertile male' metaphor, introducing the idea of imitation or importation. This idea is boosted in the next shot, which shows Robert on his hands and knees pressing pre-grown, rollout turf into the ground (see Figure 1.2), the crawl position also conjuring the bottom position in male-male sex. So, although at the outset the New Gay Man appears to possess what are considered traditionally manly qualities, the 'naturalness' of his masculinity is subtly undermined. A gardener who oversees the placement of plants grown elsewhere is reduced to a secondary role. This foreshadows the film's nasty biological twist: though Robert proves to be a capable and loving father, the 'seed' was planted by a straight man (Kevin).

This trope of artificiality is picked up again when Abbie expresses her desire to have children. 'This is the twenty-first century', Robert says, 'just go out and buy yourself some nice frozen ivy-league sperm, swish it around in a test tube and [gulps] bottoms up!' When Abbie replies that she doesn't want to have a baby 'that way', he replies, 'well then, go to China

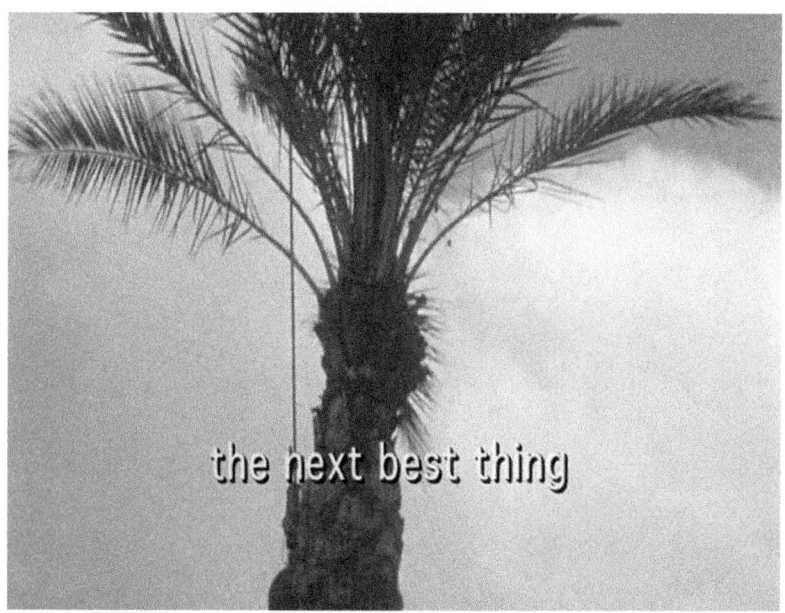

Figure 1.1 Transplanted tree in *The Next Best Thing* (2000)

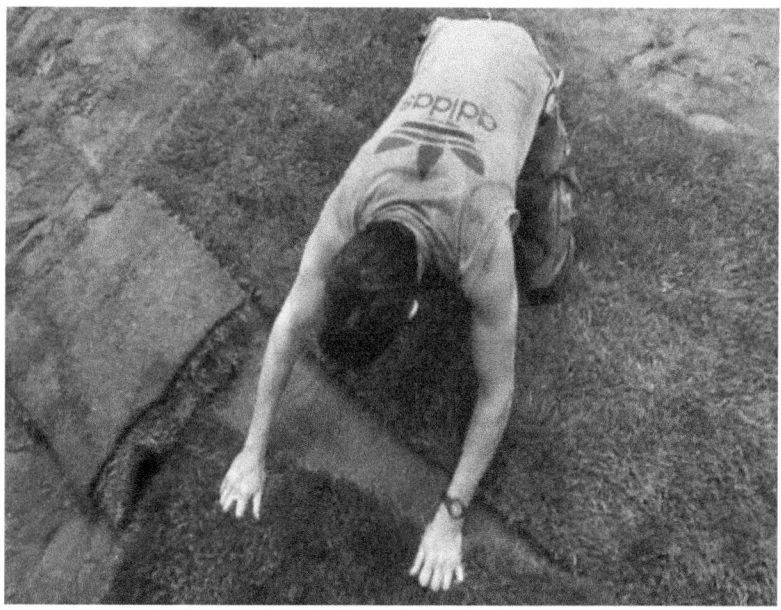

Figure 1.2 Robbie (Rupert Everett) rolls out pre-grown turf in *The Next Best Thing*

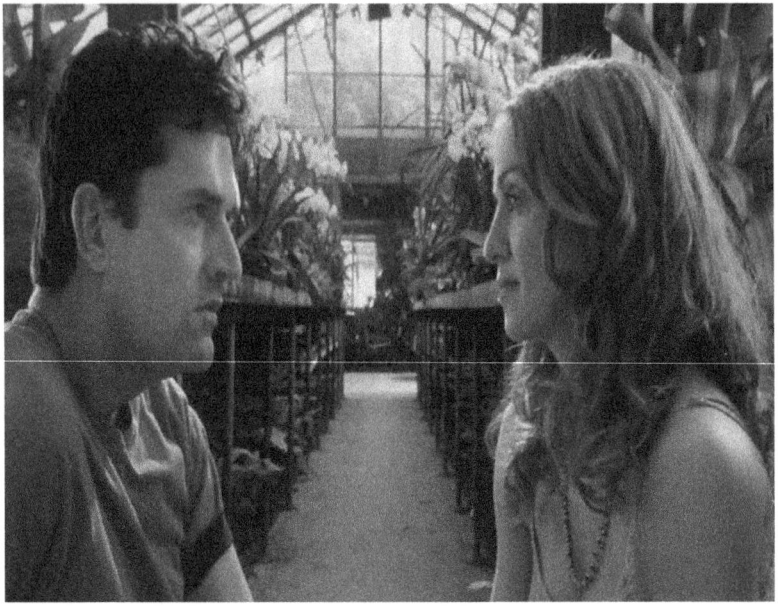

Figure 1.3 Robbie (Rupert Everett) and Abbie (Madonna) decide to have a baby in *The Next Best Thing*

and *buy* one.' These references – transplantation, IVF, trans-national adoption – further distance Robert from reproduction configured as natural. When Abbie reveals her pregnancy she finds Robert in a greenhouse (see Figure 1.3), another metaphor for fabricated growing conditions. The New Gay Man's 'naturalness,' a quality linked ideologically to normative, heterosexual, cis-male fatherhood via conventionally recognised biological reproduction, is undermined. These severings of the queer character from biological reproduction is one of the film's most anxious acts, cordoning off homosexuality from an infecting relationship to straight reproductivity. Given we ultimately discover Robert did not father Sam biologically, did the best friends even have sex to begin with? These subtle underminings increasingly distance Robert from 'authentic' father-hood, positioning him as a degraded or second-order father and man.

Somewhat paradoxically then, the cultural project of Gay Redemption in *The Next Best Thing* operates precisely via the characterisation of Robert

Gay Redemption

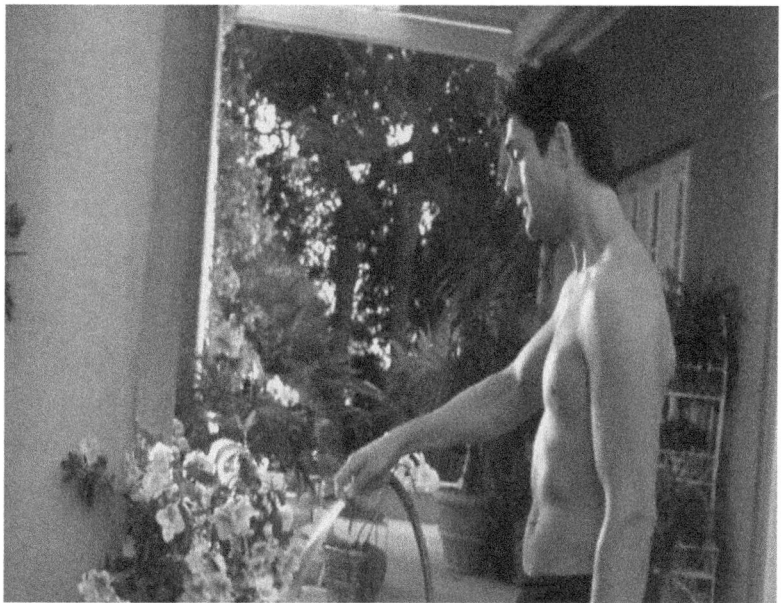

Figure 1.4 Safe spectacle in *The Next Best Thing*: the New Gay Man is always on the move

as healthy, robust and, most vitally, *active*. Working, gardening and boisterous parenting, among other domestic labours, are part of the work required to stave off the abject. Whether driving, designing, filming his son's birthday party or watering plants, Robert is constantly on the move, substituting activity for any homosexual libidinal energies that may threaten to contaminate the scene. During the July Fourth celebrations, for example, while Abbie sunbathes, Robert swims in the pool, spruces indoor plants and waters flowers (see Figure 1.4). The next day, after they have trashed Vernon and Ashby's house, Robert runs around frantically to get it back in order. These scenes create opportunities to admire Everett's beefcake physique, an erotic spectacle often mediated though Madonna's gaze, but in unselfconscious, seemingly un-posed activeness. That Robert is always on the move recalls the way in which refusing the abject requires constant, repetitive attention. The active gay body here literally *works* to counteract indolence and lethargy and their implications of degeneracy, illness, effeminacy and contamination.

If constant work is one of the central performative tropes of Gay Redemption, so too is the frequent exposure of Everett's body in these acts of labour. Everett has an athletic, muscular build, towering at 193cm. Like the gay male leads of other Hollywood buddy films, his body conforms to a type like that of the heterosexual male leads of romantic comedy: white, fit and handsome, often muscular and hairless. Until the introduction of Ben, Everett's body is the film's central object of scopophilic energy, far more central than Madonna's famously toned, yogic body. However, an active libido or even an indication of the character's awareness of his own sexual potency is completely disavowed by the costuming, acting and direction. It's a significant contrast to, for example, another of Everett's unclothed performances, as a languid, knowing, homoerotic Oberon in *A Midsummer Night's Dream* (1999), released the previous year. Here, the spectacle of a robust, attractive male form shows off a healthiness and manliness that is the visual antithesis to the sick, immobile, wasting body of the PWA.

This combination of musularity, clean-cut good looks, large proportions and the absence of sexual threat recalls the star body of Rock Hudson, the gentle beefcake of Sirkian melodrama. Rock's starbody, according to Richard Meyer, 'promised straight women a space of sexual safety – he would acquiesce to domesticity without insisting on male domination.'[84] In films and publicity stills, Rock often appeared shirtless, in 'quiet communion with the outdoors', in settings and poses that emphasised his largeness: 'Rock Hudson's was a body to fill, even to overflow, the enlarging screen of the 1950s'.[85] In the visual semiotics of Rock's star image, Meyer identifies a type of 'passivity' unlike that of Rock's contemporaries who did not 'acquiesce to this position of "to-be-looked-at-ness".'[86] That is, 'as the object of a desiring, *implicitly female* gaze, Hudson's masculinity is at once less aggressive and more eroticised than that of the conventional male hero of Hollywood film.'[87]

Ironically, the visual codes that frame Everett's body recall those that framed Rock Hudson's: codes of hygiene, domesticy, cleanliness and hetero-social communication. I say 'ironically' because, as Meyer recounts, in the 1980s Rock became the 'face of AIDS', a scan-dalous image of disease in which KS and wasting, the visual signifiers of AIDS-related illness, became evidence of the 'horrific opening of [Rock's] closet' to a public unfamiliar with the disease and previously unaware of Rock's homosexuality.[88]

Gay Redemption

In Everett's case, an out gay actor plays an out gay character, but the visual conventions are compellingly similar to Rock's at the height of his career. Like Rock, Everett is available as a safe erotic object sans the menace of phallic action. Likewise present are the 'gentle giant' conventions: Everett's height is exploited in numerous scenes where he seems to overfill doorways and in parenting scenes where, in contrast to his son, Sam, he appears to be huge.

Also recalling Rock, what Meyer calls a 'fantasy of sanitation' helps to code the body of the New Gay Man as a safe body, made wholesome and hygienic through its frequent proximity to water. As Meyer explains, 'Hudson's promise of self-restraint extended not just to his romantic relations on screen but to the very surface of his starbody.'[89] Fanzine images and publicity shots pictured Rock washing his car, fresh from a shower or lying in the bath, the watering and washing rituals signaling cleansing and purification, a 'somatic wholeness' without the threat of abject fluids or bodily functions. Rock's starbody, Meyer writes, is 'the consummate safe sex object'; any fluids 'were ones which had come from outside the body to cleanse it rather than his own bodily fluids which have leaked and were soiling the surface'; 'There were no layers of conflicted identity to be recovered beneath the surface of the starbody, no reason for it to break out into a sweat.'[90]

In scenes of swimming and plant watering, Robert/Everett's body is surrounded by similar iconographies of sanitisation. Most notably during his short-lived gay relationship – right at the moment when his body poses the greatest symbolic threat of contamination – we are privy to a scene of ritual cleansing. Abbie casually chats with Robert while he showers and prepares for a date with his lover. He dries himself vigorously, shaves quickly and applies deodorant – a simple, manly grooming routine, but evidence that Robert is disinfected and squeaky clean. All the while, the platonic couple discussing parenting issues establishes the bathroom as a sexless, mundane, domestic space. It's another opportunity to admire Everett's physique and yet, in this ritual of washing and grooming, the film works overtime to ensure that the gay body does not become a site of danger (see Figure 1.5). In case we aren't convinced, Robert breaks up with his cardiologist boyfriend in the next scene.

These rituals of sanitation produce a subject who is redeemed from dirt and the threat that it portends. It's a visual fantasy that recalls Mary

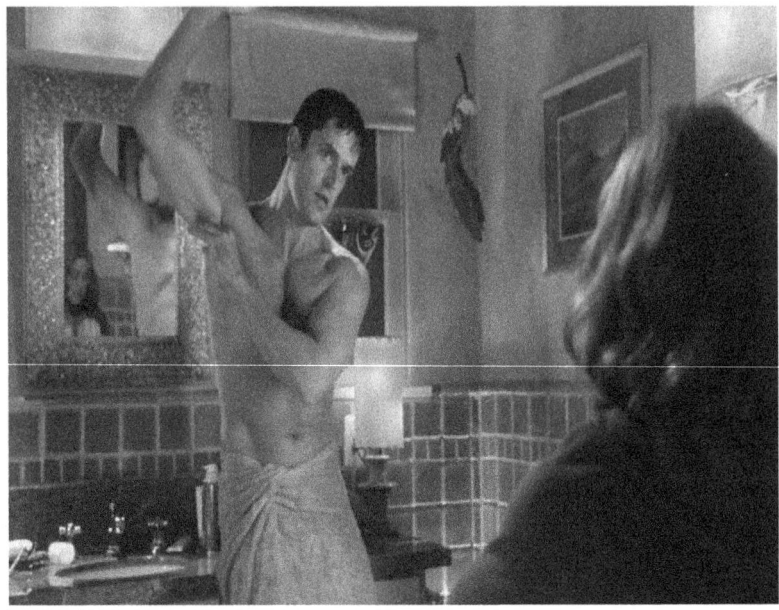

Figure 1.5 Sanitation fantasy in *The Next Best Thing*

Douglas's formulation on the social role of dirt in her classic work of symbolic anthropology, *Purity and Danger* (1966). Douglas argues that pollutants play a central role in maintaining social structures: we put objects into categories, and objects that don't fit are classifieded as dirty, polluting or disgusting and thrown away. The paradigmatic example is dirt, or, 'matter out of place', which plays a central role in the organisation and regulation of everyday life. Symbolically, dirt 'is essentially disorder',[91] and the removal of dirt is a way of controlling both bodies and the environment. For the film and for the New Gay Man, work and sanitation are part of the everyday routine of keeping the abject at bay. Kept both busy and clean, the New Gay Man is prevented from lapsing into a feminine idleness, or worse. Most importantly, the fruits of his labour aren't personal pleasure but are re-invested into the projects of family and futurity, at the heart of which are the fortunes of The Child.

Sadly, when we discover that Sam is actually someone else's son, Robert ends up like the Fab Five of *Queer Eye* who have toiled and preened in the service of heteronormative futures but are then excluded from them.

Much like the end of each episode of *Queer Eye*, with the Fab Five watching the rituals of heterosexual romance unfold, the final sequence of *The Next Best Thing* has Robert gazing longingly while Abbie and her new partner Ben collect Sam from school. In spite of all the vigorous activity, all the labour, Robert is retrenched from the role of parent and reduced to a mere spectator.

Look What Happened to Me

If fantasies of sanitation, work and a safe erotic spectacle are deployed here to disavow the spectres associated with AIDS, none are as effective at furthering the project of Gay Redemption as the severing of Robert from the corrupting influences of the queer world, and his juxtaposition to queer figures who are either stereotypically flamboyant, HIV positive or dead. This quarantines the New Gay Man from the abject qualities associated with these other types of queers: leaking sexualities, effeminacy, immaturity, anti-normative or anti-family sentiment, hedonism, narcissism, sickness, disease and abject meaninglessness. These characters provide a 'foil' for Robert, a generic device through which the New Gay Man is heterosexualised and masculinised; in the process of redeeming him, the foils are pathologised.

Vernon and Ashby (Jack Betts and William Mesnik), the retired, older couple whose garden Robert maintains and whose Hollywood home is the setting for a lot of the film's action, are the first instance of foil. The silk cravat-wearing, gin-martini-drinking couple spend their time on holiday, entertaining and floating torpidly in their pool (see Figures 1.6–1.7); they share a passion for catty humour, show tunes and musicals – the classic canon of gay fandom; they walk around in an 'alcoholic haze' and possess a vast collection of antique furniture and Hollywood memorabilia ('These people are maniacs about their stuff'). Vernon and Ashby are instantly recognisable as throwbacks to the Production Code Era's repertoire of homosexual stereotypes – aristocratic affect, sophisticated taste, effeminate mannerisms, camp and bitchy humour.[92] Robert may be something of an heir to their legacy – he benefits from their patronage, the use of their house and the freedoms of being an out gay man in a more progressive America than the one in which they've lived most of their lives. However,

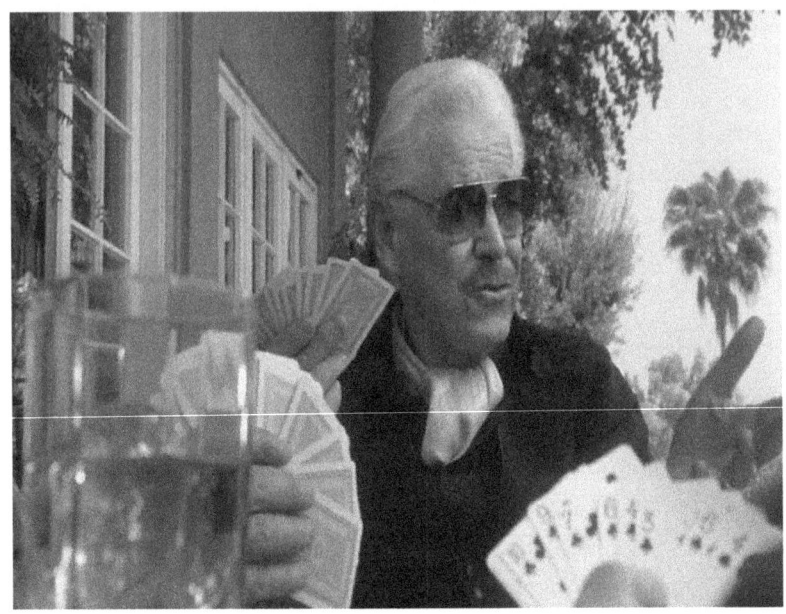

Figure 1.6 Vernon (Jack Betts) in *The Next Best Thing*

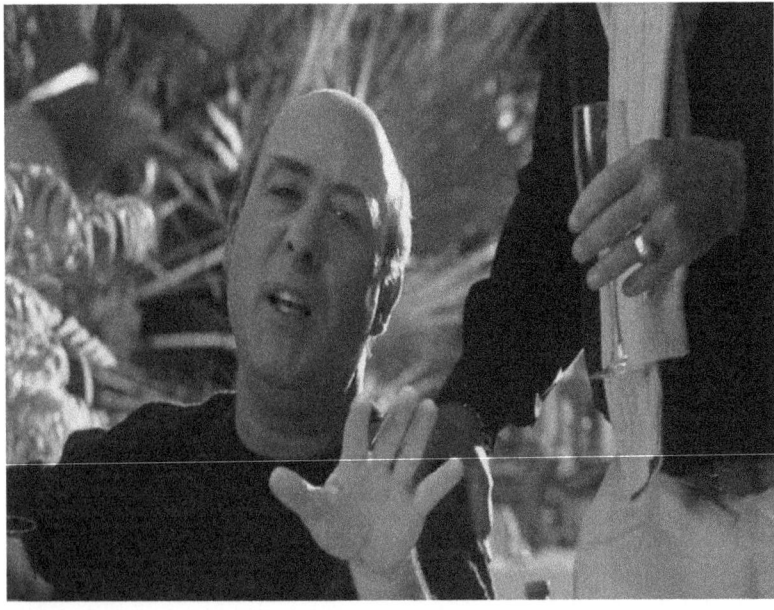

Figure 1.7 Ashby (William Mesnik) in *The Next Best Thing*

he disavows this lineage by dismissing them and their history as anachronistic. He calls them 'the most evil queens in Christendom', says they have been together 'since the Ice Age', and when they quiz him on Classical Hollywood trivia ('Oh, good, Robert's arrived, now we can settle this *Annie Get Your Gun* controversy once and for all'), he distances himself by saying 'Don't ask me, I'm afraid I flunked gay history'.

Though he sometimes performs campily himself, Robert here rejects camp and camp archives as anachronistic, as 'history'. The implied evaluation is that camp is no longer relevant in the affirmative gay present because of its association with self-mockery, self-loathing and therefore with more oppressive, homophobic cultural contexts. Here, camp becomes an example of what Heather Love calls a 'backwards feeling', a discourse with a consciousness of negativity and one that invokes a traumatic history. Many queer critics have discussed camp as a practice that emerged as a defence against homophobia, a mode of 'defensive offensiveness' or a reparative discourse. However, post gay liberation, camp has also often been viewed disparagingly as either or both a lack of gay pride and a supposedly immature unwillingness to embrace normative gender. The latter is significant here, for camp may be degraded for its strong association with gay male effeminacy. This is in spite of the fact that camp tends to ironise gender by caricaturing gender performance. Nonetheless, Robert distances himself from camp and its potential connotations – anachronism, self-loathing and abject effeminacy. Though Vernon and Ashby are sources of humour, they are not affectionately portrayed: they're sneering, selfish old queens who exist in a hermetic, outmoded world.

If this juxtaposition is at pains to distinguish Robert from recognisable gay stereotypes, it isn't nearly as central to the project of gay domestication as the film's ritual disavowal of the gay male PLHIV and the burial of the AIDS corpse. Early on, Robert and Abbie attend the funeral of a friend called Joe whom we learn has died from AIDS. At other moments later in the film, we catch up with Joe's boyfriend David (Neil Patrick Harris), giving us short glimpses of his miserable life as it has unfolded since Joe's death. This sub-plot provides the film with its most fully 'fleshed out' portrayal of gay life beyond Robert and Abbie's alternative family. It is a grim portrait indeed.

Joe's funeral presents us with a piteous vignette of gay life. Its bleakness, however, propels the narrative forward, motivating Robert to forge a family with Abbie. When Robert and Abbie arrive at the cemetery, David thanks them for coming, saying 'I'm so glad you guys are here. If it weren't for you, I'd feel like I was crashing my own boyfriend's funeral'. Accordingly, David and his entourage of grieving LA friends are outsiders, standing together on one side of Joe's grave, facing off against Joe's relatives who are on the other side looking conservative and accusatory. It's a pointed arrangement of the *mise en scène* to dramatise both the institutionalised exclusion of sexual nonconformists and the importance of friendship and community – families of choice – to the latter (see Figure 1.8). As David explains, Joe's family have hijacked the funeral arrangements: the pallbearers are 'a grab bag of Joe's relatives' who weren't part of his life, but would 'drive across three states to attend his funeral'; the death rites are contrary to his wishes ('Joe did not want all this Gothic hocus-pocus'; he wanted his ashes 'scattered to the wind with Don McClean's 'American Pie' playing really, really loud on a boom box'). 'I feel like I'm in *The Omen*',

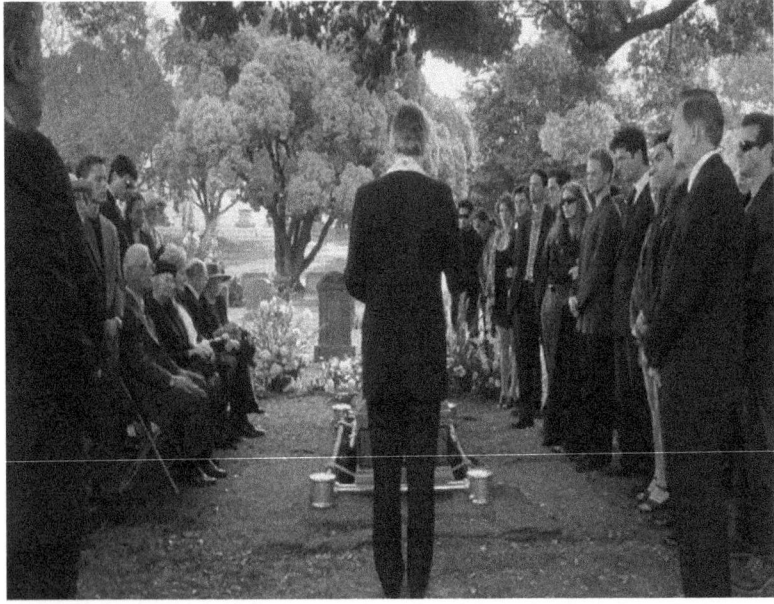

Figure 1.8 The straights v the gays at Joe's funeral in *The Next Best Thing*

Gay Redemption

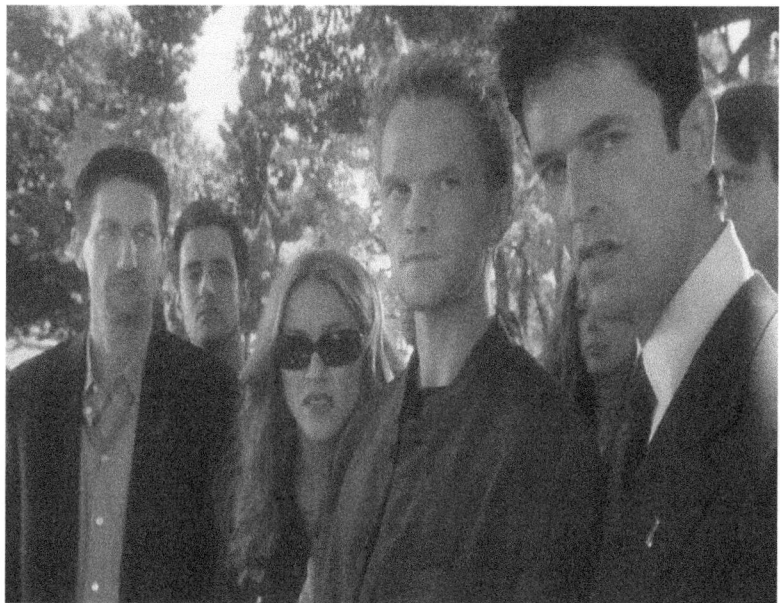

Figure 1.9 Abject dread: (from R-L) Robbie (Rupert Everett), David (Neil Patrick Harris), Abbie (Madonna) and other friends at Joe's funeral in *The Next Best Thing*

Robert says, and indeed, he wears an expression of outrage and abject horror throughout the scene (see Figure 1.9). In a clear dramatisation of HIV/AIDS stigma, the eulogising priest says that Joseph was 'struck down in his prime by pneumonia', a common euphemism for AIDS-related illness at funerals where the disease was unspeakable. Interestingly, HIV/AIDS isn't mentioned by name at all in *The Next Best Thing*, but Abbie, Robert, David and a number of their friends are wearing red ribbons, the universal signifier of HIV/AIDS awareness. Against all the gloom, Robert begins to sing the words to 'American Pie' as the eulogy trails off. In what may be cinema history's most cross-promotional moment of queer defiance (Madonna recorded a cover of Don McClean's song for the film's soundtrack that was also released as a single), Abbie and the rest of their entourage join in, proudly reclaiming the scene.

In its melodramatic dramatisation of homophobia and exclusion, the funeral scene advertises the extreme otherness of gay life – or rather, the abject spectacle of gay death – from which Robert's narrative will subsequently recoil. Afterward, Robert breaks down in tears and asks Abbie to stay the night, and the next day is the fateful Fourth of July when the accidental conception supposedly takes place. Although the latter is an ostensibly drunken mishap – a serendipitous 'accident' that becomes the premise for a quirky family melodrama – the funeral of the gay man, and the object lesson it portends is the turning point for the New Gay Man. After this harsh confrontation with gay mortality – with the corpse of his friend who has died from AIDS – Robert's narrative becomes oriented toward family and he becomes increasingly estranged from gay life. Robbie's literal burial of the AIDS corpse is a ritualistic burial of the (HIV/AIDS) past in order that the post-crisis present be constituted as one oriented toward a reproductive future.

The object lesson does not end there. Robert is juxtaposed to the increasingly pathetic David on three more occasions. First, they are pictured visiting Joe's gravesite. While David and a friend pour glasses of wine and make references to Joe being 'forever young and beautiful' and leaving 'the party too early', Robert plants a tree beside the grave, signifying his commitment to the nurture of new life. When he reminds David that the plant will need looking after, David can only respond with sarcasm: 'Doesn't perpetual care include sprinkler service?' Next, Robert helps David move his possessions into Vernon and Ashby's cabana where it is revealed that David's fortunes have worsened: he has been kicked out of his house by Joe's parents. These tragic circumstances aren't further elaborated, but they're a strong advertisement for the more homonormative life directions Robert is pursuing. In spite of his pitiable state, David asserts that he should be taking 'a stand' against 'this insane decision' that Robert has made to father a child:

> This is ridiculous. You're gonna be miserable. Have you thought about all the details, like your sex life? Are you even gonna have one?

In response, Robert explains his motivations. But first, he defends himself against David's sceptical judgement:

> Listen, if I was straight, and I turned gay, you'd be thrilled. But the fact that I'm having a baby with a woman – Uh! That's blowing your mind David. That's such a double standard.

And then:

> Actually, you know what? I'm just bored of it all. I'm bored of the parties; I'm bored of the drugs; I'm bored of the body obsession. I'm not in a relationship, I don't see one coming, and it happened. It's not a sacrifice, you know. It's an opportunity. I do love Abbie. I trust her. And here comes a baby that's gonna be part of our lives forever.

'And what happens when you do meet Mr Right?' David asks. 'I'll cross that bridge when I get to it,' says Robert. 'You'll burn that bridge when you get to it,' says David, foreshadowing Robert's abortive relationship with the cardiologist.

Although only a brief scene, this is central to understanding the disavowals at work here. David's criticism gives Robert the opportunity to voice a critique of queer culture, rehearsing the clichéd but powerfully pervasive perception of gay male culture as immature, superficial and obsessed with sex and surface. In his insistence that Robert consider his sex life, David is made to embody that culture's childish preoccupations. In Robert's patronising retort, he rejects this body and sex obsession and narcissism. This chimes with the advice that he has just received from his mother, who says 'I'll tell you one thing: having a child is the best thing in the world. It stops you from worrying about yourself.' In these exchanges, becoming a parent emerges as a method of repudiating the narcissism of gay culture ('the parties', 'the drugs', 'the body obsession') in exchange for something meaningful ('a baby that's gonna be part of our lives forever').

What makes this small conflict with David so instructive for thinking about the project of Gay Redemption, not only in this film but more broadly, is its insistence on the meaningfulness of parenting as opposed to the meaninglessness of other queer life narratives. Having a child may be an opportunity rather than a 'sacrifice', as Robert says to David, but within the conventions of Gay Redemption, it must involve certain renunciations – including pleasure and community, and most crucially, sex.

Edelman's argument in *No Future* is illuminating for understanding the significance of Robert's increasingly strained relationship with David. *No Future* highlights the 'antisocial bent of sexuality' – its resistance to normative social forms and institutions.[93] In *The Next Best Thing*, David comes to embody a symbolic queerness: the antisocial, the death drive and the dissolution of social meaningfulnses. Robert, on the other hand, makes an argument on behalf of 'good gay' citizens who are future-oriented, who insist on the project of normalisation via one of its central hallmarks: family-building. Edelman's comments on American writer and commentator Dan Savage, who spoke in the *New York Times Magazine* (1998) about 'the commitment to having a future' that childrearing entails, elaborates this opposition between queerness and reproductive futurity:

> Choose life, for life and the baby and meaning hang together in the balance, confronting the lethal counterweight of narcissism, AIDS, and death, all of which spring from the commitment to the meaningless eruptions of jouissance associated with the 'circuit parties' that gesture toward the circuit of the [death] drive.[94]

David – HIV positive, childlike, selfish, distanced from reproduction and committed to the antisocial energies of *jouissance* – embodies the radical negativity and meaninglessness of the 'queer'. He's a threat to the reproductive order.

Returning to Williamson, who identified the terror of HIV/AIDS as the terror of confronting meaninglessness,[95] Robert has a double motivation to repudiate his friend. The desire to parent here is the desire to be *redeemed from meaninglessness*. Explaining the impulse that structures the homonormative desire to reject and castigate the 'bad queer', Edelman writes:

> By denying our identification with the negativity of this drive, and hence our disidentification from the promise of futurity, those of us inhabiting the place of the queer may be able to cast off that queerness and enter the properly political sphere, but only by shifting the figural burden of queerness to someone else. The structural position of queerness, after all, and the need to fill it remain.[96]

HIV positive David is *The Next Best Thing*'s repository for this figural burden. In Robert's final encounter with him, the way in which the qualities associated with the queer that Robert seeks to repudiate fall together under The sign of 'HIV' becomes even more precise. The problems caused by the appearance of Ben in Abbie's life have reached a crisis point and what Robert doesn't know is that Abbie is about to elope with Ben and Sam, and the once best friends are on the brink of a bitter custody battle. Robert and David are sitting inside Vernon and Ashby's cabana on a grey, rainy day, contemplating the civil injustice of gay life. Here it is confirmed that David is HIV positive, and his trajectory just seems to have become more tragic:

DAVID: [*Struggling with a canister of pills*] I hate child-proof caps [*pauses*] I told you, Robert. I told you at the very beginning. You should have insisted upon getting married. Then you would have rights. Look what happened to me.

ROBERT: I have rights now. They're not going anywhere. Full stop. The end.

DAVID: You need to talk to an attorney. Just a consultation. A couple hundred bucks – know where you stand.

ROBERT: I know where I stand, David. Trust me. I'm not gonna see an attorney.

DAVID: I'll bet she is. [*pauses*]. Stupid pills. I can't even tell if they're working.

ROBERT: So stop taking them, and if you die, you'll know they work.

Robert patronises his friend with a sarcastic joke. As his own narrative moves more desperately towards outsiderdom, the need to distance himself from queerness, pathology and meaninglessness becomes more urgent. For his part, David has become such a hapless non-adult that he struggles even to unscrew the lids of his medication (see Figure 1.10). His partner is dead and he is homeless, lacking in legal or financial claim, living with a chronic illness that involves a (at that time) frustrating and complex regime of medications, and dependent on the support of friends for survival. David is socially unintelligible and powerless before the Law. It is a brief scene but a powerful object lesson, and one against which the New Gay Man must dis-identify. As the 'AIDS foil', David represents the unacceptable face of queerness that must be expurgated from the text. This is his final appearance in the flim.

Abject Lessons

Critics of *The Next Best Thing* were for the most part stumped by this HIV sub-plot. Nick Davis wrote that 'a gratuitous and unnecessary AIDS plot reminds us that Hollywood still prefers to represent homosexuality

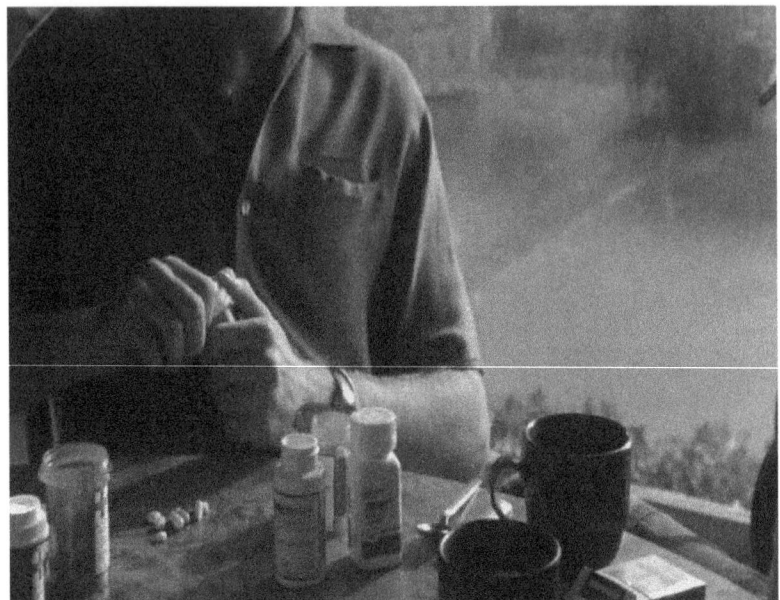

Figure 1.10 David (Neil Patrick Harris) struggling with his antiretrovirals in *The Next Best Thing*

as a garden path leading straight to death'.[97] Christopher Null wrote that 'no amount of Rupert Everett's delightful comedy and touching emotion can distract us from the hodge-podge of gay themes, one of which is the ever-looming AIDS. Instead of evoking sympathy, several scenes referring to AIDS only reinforce the idea that being gay means having AIDS'.[98] I would suggest that, rather than gratuitous, *The Next Best Thing*'s HIV/AIDS sub-plot is in fact *central* to the ideo-logic of the Gay Redemption narrative.

As we saw in the Introduction, 'The Big A' raises the fear of the meaninglessness of a virus and became in 90s 'positive images' a term invoking a powerful, terrifying association between sex and death. If these significations are frightening in themselves, the original association of AIDS with homosexual transmission conjures additional taboos: anality, with its significations of dirt, auto-eroticism, lack of gender-reference[99] and that most frightening reverie of crisis discourse – the 'intolerable image of a grown man, legs high in the air, unable to refuse the suicidal ecstasy of being a woman.'[100] In this phantasm, passive homosexuality, feminisation, prostitution and transmission are all invoked under the sign of promiscuity. If male homosexuality was to be publicised at this early moment in the era of post-crisis, it required the erasure of anything that could summon these spectres. Robert/Everett's embodiment of the New Gay Man works as a replacement for and a disavowal of the AIDS body of crisis discourse, the body of the person living with or dying from HIV/AIDS.

Redemption is not without its costs. The sympathetic portrayal of gay men in mainstream 1990s representation came at the expense of the expression of active homosexual desire, and since these men were virtually all white, educated, American and middle-class, it also came at the expense of other contaminating forms of class or racial difference. It's a trade off: for the family-values agenda to sustain itself, these characters need to work tirelessly toward rebuilding white, bourgeois, normative nuclear and reproductive structures by disavowing their dangerous desires and repudiating the perversity of gay culture. Across the landscape of post-crisis popular culture, versions of this figure are still prolific, participating in the same or similar trade offs: visibility and at least partial subjecthood in exchange for an investment in reproductive futurity. The New Gay Man, with his extremely marketable, palatable image, has become a pervasive figure across Anglo-American and global culture in the wake of AIDS crisis. Indeed, the successful integration of this figure into popular culture has provided a potent template for the types of ideal gay male citizenship that best represents the now widespread politics of homonormativity. Yet this 'rush to the mainstream', as Love describes it, 'is a betrayal of queer life and of those who still do not meet the criteria of legitimacy'.[101] The embrace of normativity always involves the disavowal of certain attributes and the queer persons that embody them.

In the dénouement to *The Next Best Thing*, the New Gay Man is swallowed up by the powers of the abject that he has striven so hard to keep at bay. Showing that homophobic systems have multiple means of disciplining sexual difference, the court battle reveals that Robert has no legal or biological paternity and therefore no claim to joint custody. The court will not recognise him as Sam's father but only as 'caregiver', publicly castrating the gay character and producing a space in which an eruption of that which the text has disavowed comes to consciousness. To everyone's horror, including Abbie's, her lawyer proceeds to demonise Robert on account of his homosexuality:

> 'In October of last year, did you go to a nightclub in Santa Monica called 'Sit and Spin?' / 'Did you notice drug use going on?' / 'Is it true that you are an active member in several militant gay organisations?' / 'Has Sam ever seen you have oral sex with another man?'

Robert loses all chance of custody and all access to the boy he has raised from infancy. Dropping his head onto the courtroom bench, he surrenders to the abject misery and injustice of it all (see Figure 1.11). Just prior to this, when the presiding judge asks if anyone has final statements to add, Robert makes a dramatic speech asserting that 'being a real parent takes more than DNA' and that 'Sam is my son… forever and always.' In a final comment that seems to refer partly to contested paternity (the institutional primacy of 'blood relations') and partly to concerns about HIV (a blood-borne virus), he says:

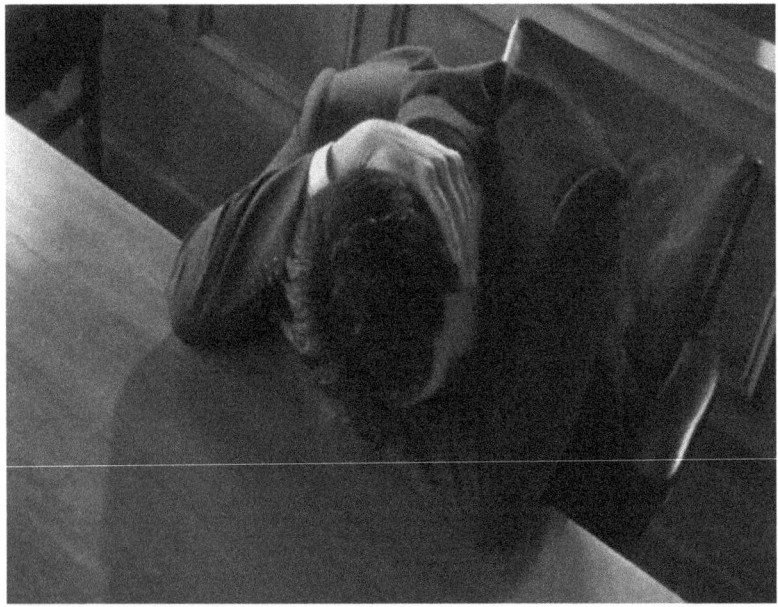

Figure 1.11 Robbie surrenders in abject defeat in *The Next Best Thing*

> Seems like I've spent my whole life thinking about blood. Worrying about blood. And blood… Well, it's just like shit. We're all full of it.

While the precise meaning of these statements remains ambiguous, they gesture to the universal battle with the abject, a conflict that emphatically underwrites this film.

The Next Best Thing and its unsatisfying engagement with the politics of queer families emerged from a broader cultural context in which questions about the relationship between queers and the institutions of 'normal life' were increasingly being posed. The fact that the film, when approached as an exploration of alternative family possibilities and queer kinship structures, provides such an unimaginative resolution is not necessarily a damning of the queer per se, but rather a negative appraisal of the potential for institutions like marriage and the family – and Hollywood cinema at this time – to accommodate queerness. It is for these reasons perhaps that *The Next Best Thing* – with its shambolic meshing of genres, its 'nasty' and 'highly revolting' characters, and its inability to imagine a future for them outside of social norms – was such an abjectly unsuccessful film.

In this instance of post-crisis representation, attempts are made to redeem the New Gay man via the expulsion of AIDS signification and its metaphorical conflation with radical queer negativity. And yet, paradoxically, he is still ultimately kept at a prophylactic distance from the sacred space of the family. In spite of this unsatisfying ending, the strategy of 'AIDS foil' among other visual and narrative conventions has attempted to resolve the problem of the conflation of AIDS and gayness in crisis discourse, which continues to haunt mass cultural images of gay men well into the era of post-crisis. The figural burden of queerness is shifted to the HIV positive gay man, who becomes a repository for the negativity and the antisociality of the sexual so that the New Gay Man may be redeemed – which is to say, made palatable and intelligible for the realm of the normative.

This, I would point out, demonstrates a proposition that I will explore further in the next chapter. That is, that the culture of post-crisis (of which this film is an early example) vacillates between a representation of both gayness and HIV/AIDS as both extraordinary and mundane. In this instance, the latter is made extraordinary so that the former may appear normal. In other words, HIV/AIDS is made to signify as an abject spectacle in order that new gayness may appear safe and redeemable. The New Gay Man is domesticated, while the PLHIV is left homeless.

The next chapter presents a case study in which the unresolvable tension between a spectacularised otherness and a mundane normativity exist together *within* the body of the PLHIV rather than as polar forces in the **diegetic universe**. In the significantly queerer world of *Queer as Folk*, in which HIV/AIDS is central rather than peripheral to the text, this tension between the extraordinary and the mundane still emerges. But, rather than relegated to the margins of the text (or the textual 'unconscious'), when this antagonism between the extraordinary and the mundane emerges it is exploited as a productive source of drama and narrative progress. Rather than an abject other from which the New Gay Man should recoil, here the body of the gay male PLHIV is enfolded in narratives and iconographies of the post-crisis everyday. The positive image here strains to *incorporate* HIV/ AIDS – to establish its normative place in the queer quotidian. However, this too involves symbolic and political conflict, compromise, and eventually dissavowal and irresolution.

2

Positive Men Are from Mars, Negative Men Are from Venus

Sero-Melodrama in Queer As Folk

'Sero-melodrama'

North American *Queer as Folk* (2000–5), the adapted and significantly extended version of the British TV show, was uniquely focused on HIV and post-crisis culture. Throughout its five series, the show consistently ploughed the terrain of the emerging, dynamic social landscape of post-antiretrovirals gay life for the matter of its drama, examining various issues including living with HIV, shifting generational attitudes to HIV, serodiscord in relationships, and the thrills and dangers of sexual risk-taking. These issues all emerged amidst the larger cultural re-scripting of HIV as a chronic manageable illness among gay male communities in the Global North after the advent of antiretrovirals around 1996. *Queer as Folk*, then, provides us with an opportunity to consider new, more complex and potentially more progressive representations of both HIV and gay male life from this period.

Queer as Folk was also extremely popular. It quickly became the most popular original program in cable TV company Showtime's history,[1] and in 2006 *The Advocate* identified is as a 'significantly important aspect of American readers' "LGBT experience".'[2] The shows's popularity was global: *Queer as Folk* screened on cable, free-to-air and gay TV stations throughout

Europe and the UK, in Latin America and parts of Asia. Internet and DVD editions, both authorised and bootlegged, have expanded the show's reach both geographically and temporally. Though it seems increasingly dated now that we are well entrenched in the era of sophisticated, quality, prestige and streaming TV, *Queer as Folk* became a cult TV show and one of the most popular, globally consumed representations of gay (predominantly male) life in the first decade of the twenty-first century. Its exploration of queer characters grappling with the ongoing HIV pandemic mark out the show as a landmark in post-crisis representation: it is one of extremely few popular Anglo-American TV dramas of the past two decades to consistently and meaningfully address HIV. No book claiming to consider HIV/AIDS and gay men in the popular culture of the post-ARVs world could ignore *Queer as Folk*. And, with the exception of a study of audience responses to certain HIV-focused plotlines undertaken by Kathleen Farrell (2006),[3] there is, to my knowledge, no sustained scholarly work addressing the representation of HIV in the series. As Farrell points out, the series deserves attention for, among other reasons, 'its departure from [earlier] patterns of televised AIDS stories.'[4]

Queer as Folk was indeed groundbreaking in some ways. During the 1990s, gay television characters became more commonplace, but by the time it arrived HIV-themed storylines and positive characters were, as Benjamin Ryan wrote for *HIVPlusMag* noted in 2004, 'woefully rare.'[5] HIV/AIDS had routinely featured in late 1980s and early 1990s American TV dramas like *ER*, *Life Goes On*, *Thirtysomething* and *The Real World*, and in made-for-TV movies like *An Early Frost* (1985), *The Ryan White Story* (1989) and *Something to Live For* (1992). But by the mid-'00s, HIV positive characters were 'so scarce that only the most dedicated couch potato [could] find them.' Ryan attributed this decline in visibility to the advent of ARVs and the dramatic decline in deaths from HIV/AIDS in the Global North. HIV has 'simply lost its status as a hot button issue', he wrote. 'After all, in the emotionally charged world of soaps, a relatively manageable disease provides far less dramatic fare than a ghastly fatal one.'[6] *Queer as Folk* bucked this trend with three HIV positive characters. It explored the new, transforming scene of HIV as a site of drama, even if *living with* HIV seemed less sensational than the sex/death narratives of the earlier, more spectacular moment of AIDS crisis.

Distinguishing itself from this earlier moment, *Queer as Folk* dramatised HIV differently to the AIDS movie-of-the-week, or the 'social issues' arc of TV soap opera. In the series' universe, HIV is integrated into the broader texture of the quotidian: to some extent, HIV is *made normal*. In narrative terms, HIV/AIDS does not appear as a singular disruption, not as a narrative *crisis*, but rather as a serial – that is, recurring – presence in the everyday (albeit one that can indeed present dramatic obstacles). Rather than a discrete or marginal event outside of everyday narratives, HIV becomes part of the complex, ongoing, tapestry of queer life.

Queer as Folk therefore provides strong examples of the interface between the spectacular and the mundane in post-crisis representations of gay life and HIV/AIDS that more broadly characterises the culture of post-crisis. Its stories about post-crisis life – including everyday living with HIV, HIV and relationships, changing and generational attitudes to safer sex, chemsex, negotiating safety, HIV medications, barebacking and bug chasing, fear of seroconversion – are frequently depicted as ordinary elements of queer life. However, at the same time, plots, characters and incidents relating to HIV are also offered as a site for the generation of interpersonal drama. If there is an unresolvable vacillation between the extraordinary and the mundane in post crisis culture's representations of gay male life, as *Positive Images* argues, then *Queer as Folk* absolutely exemplifies this tendency.

Beyond the representation of HIV, a broader dialectic of the extraordinary/mundane is enacted in *Queer as Folk* on a number of levels. In its meshing of formal, industrial and generic characteristics, the series inhabited the at-that-time groundbreaking category of 'quality TV' (edgy, novel) while also bearing the long-established hallmarks of TV soap opera (mundane, banal). Structurally, its combination of meandering, 'complex' narratives and the episodic/series format make it a combination of 'must-see', event television (spectacular, unique) and quotidian TV melodrama (conventional, associated with the everyday 'flow' of broadcast TV). Most importantly, *Queer as Folk*'s political dynamics veer from a sometimes radical representation of the lives of queer people to a more 'respectable' and homonormative vision of gay life. The next section of this chapter describes how these dialectics operate at the generic, aesthetic, narrative and political registers of *Queer as Folk* to produce an ambivalent, or 'hesitant', vision of contemporary queer persons, characters, aesthetics and life. A grasp of this context will help to explain the show's treatment of living with HIV and how the series depicts serodiscord. 'Serodiscordant' refers to a relationship in which one partner is HIV positive and the other is negative. Against the backdrop of quotidian queer life a drama unfolds around the dramatic obstacle of serodiscord in the relationship between central characters Michael Novotny (Hal Sparks) and Ben Bruckner (Robert Grant). This drama is organised around two narrative dilemmas: the problem of the HIV positive body and, subsequently, the more complex problem of relating across sero-difference.

Although Michael and Ben's relationship initially appears to work towards relating *across* difference rather than trying to obliterate it, as we shall see, to elaborate the 'problem' of serodiscord, *Queer as Folk* resorts to the well-trodden model of irreconcilable, gendered difference, or what Tamsin Wilton calls the logic of 'heteropolarity'.[7] Damien Riggs has shown how the biomedically-grounded discourse of 'HIV polarity' in public health discourses and elsewhere has encouraged us to understand serodiscord along this axes of gender difference, which, in turn, reinforces the perception that HIV status is both an essential trait of positive and negative bodies and an irreducible marker of difference.[8] This heteropolarisation of serodifference in *Queer as Folk* can be seen to collude with broader, neoliberal trends that have privatised the experience of living with HIV, and that have, more generally, enveloped gay life in the (narrative) conventions of the normative. Initially a seemingly insurmountable difference, serodiscord in fact becomes an ideal romantic obstacle. The body positive is enfolded into the domestic priorities of the Anglo-bourgeois couple, whose desire for monogamous, state-sanctioned marriage and family depends on the domestication and erasure of (sero) difference. Pressed into a model of gender difference, serodiscord then functions to reinforce Michael and Ben's marriage-like relationship so that in later series they can become a pop-culture example of what Jose Muñoz calls 'full-blown neoliberalism'.[9]

Queer as Folk's drama of serodiscord is one of several ways in which the show strikes me, as it has struck other critics, as 'not quite queer enough.'[10] Later series were increasingly aligned with a neoliberal, homoconservative gay politic, involving the re-enforcement of gay masculinity norms and marriage-like relationships, the privatisation of sexual culture and the repudiation of embarrassing and abject sexual elements and persons in the service of a 'pious idea of a respectable, dignified gay community.'[11] As part of this, living with HIV is assimilated to a vision of gay modernity that is homonormative. And so, in a cultural turn that will increasingly come to dominate the fictional (and, as we shall see, historical) narrative of post-crisis, HIV/AIDS is no longer an event that leads inevitably towards death, but, rather, a melodramatic event in a narrative straining towards *marriage*. Having overcome the melodramatic obstacle of serodiscord, Michael and Ben become poster boys for the marriage rights campaign that ultimately came to dominate the imagination of LGBTQI+ movements in the US, UK and Australia. Serodifference and HIV positivity are stripped of public, political and potentially radical significance in order that *Queer as Folk*'s characters can pursue a normative vision of gay life.

I use the neologism 'sero-melodrama' to describe this example of TV soap opera that trades in both the conventions of melodramatic romance narrative and the dramatisation of issues surrounding serostatus. As it has been theorised in recent scholarship, melodrama is a form that produces heightened drama from the quotidian and the ordinary; it draws 'exciting, excessive, parabolic story' from 'the banal stuff of reality.'[12] This makes it an ideal form for representing the paradoxes of post-crisis. As we shall see, the dramatic affordances of television seriality are especially important here. My term 'sero-melodrama' attempts to encapsulate both the mundane and the extraordinary status of HIV and gayness in the text.

How Queer is *Queer as Folk*?

'Quality TV' emerged from the brave new world of digital-global TV production, the period in which digital satellite's capacity to distribute transnationally generated new conditions of production, distribution and reception that have in turn influenced the styles, genres and production values of new TV products.[13] *Queer as Folk* is an early example of this turn, the late 1990s, a period of cable ascendancy and extremely competitive primetime network re-branding in response to pay TV's capturing of traditional broadcast audiences.[14]

Quality TV tends to feature outrageous predicaments, sprawling novelistic narratives, mythical structures and baroque generic compilations as part of its conventional stock and trade. Though it was less 'high concept' than some of its contemporaries, like *The Sopranos* (1999–2007), for example, *Queer as Folk* exhibits the five 'strategies' of quality TV identified by Trisha Dunleavy:

(1) inventive generic mixing;
(2) an emphasis on 'authorial' input;
(3) increased 'narrative complexity';
(4) the use of serial narrative to foster a 'must-see' allure; and
(5) the pursuit of a visual quality that further reduced aesthetic distinctions between TV and cinema.[15]

The series is a good example of what Robin Nelson calls the 'paratactic' character of TV in the digital-global era,[16] by which he means the ongoing juxtaposition of forms (e.g. the soap opera and the sitcom), of genres (drama and comedy) and of narrative styles (complex, conventional, meta-textual and hyper-textual).

Queer as Folk follows a group of predominantly queer friends with Michael at the centre. Michael is a sensitive, nerdy gay everyman in his early thirties with a long-harboured but unrequited infatuation with his best friend Brian Kinney (Gale Harold). Brian is a sharp, wealthy advertising executive: stylish, attractive, an insatiable consumer of clothes, cars, and men, a master seducer of prospective clients and sexual partners alike. Brian's income and success are superseded only by his exploits in the bedroom and the backroom; and, rather than tainted for being Pittsburgh's most notorious sex machine, Brian's promiscuity is a source of social capital, a fact that is central to *Queer as Folk*'s celebratory, sex-positive discourse. A new and more complex queer TV figure, drawing as much from the anti-heroes of the New Queer Cinema as the 'New Gay Man' paradigm discussed in the previous chapter, Brian was a kind of larger-than-life, homosexual superhero – an *überhomosexuell*. On the one hand, he's a hyper-consuming, hypersexual *fin de siècle* Anglo-American gay stereotype, but on the other, he's iconoclastic, angrily anti-homophobic and misanthropically anti-LGBTQI+ community. As Sally Munt describes the Stuart character from the UK version of the series on which Brian is based, he is 'a super-spunky vaguely Nietzschean hero.'[17]

Brian and Michael's entourage of friends also includes Ted Schmidt (Scott Lowell), a self-hating accountant who envies Brian's success with money and men, Emmett Honeycutt (Peter Paige), an unapologetically flaming queen from Mississippi, and Justin Taylor (Randy Harrison), a seventeen-year-old who becomes Brian's on-again-off-again lover. Completing the gang, albeit at a remove, are lesbian couple Melanie Marcus (Michelle Clunie) and Lindsay Peterson (Thea Gill), whose son is biologically fathered by Brian, Michael's flag-waving, gay rights–championing mother, Debbie Novotny (Sharon Gless), and Debbie's brother, Vic Grassi (Jack Wetherall), who is HIV positive.

In the globally competitive industrial context of quality TV, the demand for 'boundary-pushing', 'high-concept' television increased steadily. Premium cable companies like HBO and Showtime seduced viewers with novel or taboo subject matter, and frequently the drama produced in the spaces between the mundane and the unusual were what attracted eyeballs. For example, in the everyday life of a family of undertakers in *Six Feet Under* (HBO) viewers encounter a melodrama of the spectacular (death) and the quotidian (the workaday lives of those who administer the business of death). A dialectic of the extraordinary/mundane is inherent in the central conceit of *The Sopranos*, which concerns a New Jersey mobster seeking analytic therapy for a series of panic attacks he is suffering; likewise in *Breaking Bad* (2008–13), when a terminally ill high school chemistry teacher turns to the criminal production of methamphetamine. 'Edgy' content became a norm in the high-end television landscape, and *Queer as Folk* spearheaded this trend for Showtime with its frank depiction of everyday queer life alongside spectacularly explicit queer sex – 'spectacular' because such graphicness was groundbreaking on the American small screen. The first episode featured the very first sex scene between men *ever* screened on US television, and it included rimming, oral sex and anal sex. As we saw in the last chapter, mainstream images of homosexuality at this time tended to be anodyne and desexualised. Producers Ron Cowen and Daniel Lipman touted *Queer as Folk* as a direct antidote to those trends.[18]

Frequent, unapologetic sex between (mostly male) same-sex partners in hitherto unseen explicitness and sex positivity were two big reasons *Queer as Folk* has been called 'groundbreaking' time and again by critics.[19]

Fans applauded this sexual audaciousness. Walter Chow called it 'courageous in light of the open hostility still displayed towards homosexuals in the shockingly prudish United States'.[20] Andrew Holleran described it as 'frank and unexpurgated', the 'kind of show [that] is deeply welcome – the one gay people deserve, the one some of us have been waiting for – a long, long time'.[21] The predominantly queer cast of characters also broke new ground on TV, the medium 'widely fetishised as the ultimate conferrer of visibility, with the potential to "permanently [tear] the closet door off its hinges"'.[22] This queer-centric universe has been considered a form of 'counterpublic speech' or queer world-making by some observers.[23]

Owing somewhat to this exhilarated reception, scholarship on the series has been motivated by the question of whether *Queer as Folk* was indeed groundbreaking, and whether it qualifies for the designation 'queer' that it appropriates in its title. However, a distinction between 'groundbreaking' (unprecedented, novel or innovative) and 'queer' (reimagining or critiquing conventional sex-gender arrangements), has sometimes become blurry in these discussions. The reception of *Queer as Folk* as groundbreakingly *queer* was often emblematic of a reductive conflation of 'queerness' with a type of sexy, edgy media product that came to proliferate in entertainment culture at the time and ever since. This has led to the depoliticisation of the term 'queer' and its frequent use as a straightforward substitution for 'gay' or 'LGBTQI+'.[24]

So, how queer is *Queer as Folk*? There isn't a straightforward answer. While some have been quick to claim the series is either meaningfully progressive or slavishly conventional in its representation of sexualities and genders, other have remained undecided. In the latter, more ambivalent appraisal, *Queer as Folk*'s politics are considered both ideologically disruptive and reinscriptive.[25] Rebecca Beirne locates this political ambivalence in the show's 'embattled rhetorical conflict' between images, characters and stories that are sometimes pro-assimilation and sometimes radical and 'reminiscent of Queer nation'.[26] Similarly, Suzanne Fraser considers the show a 'boundary case' through which the distinction between public and counterpublic speech can be probed.[27] *Queer as Folk*'s political discourse emerges from these analyses as *paradoxical*: aware of the subordinate status of gay men in western culture, but also reproducing troubling universalisms and norms in its representation of them.

The clearest example of such norms is the fact that queer viewers who are not gay men may not extras are dominated by young, white, male cis-gendered middle-class Americans. As Noble writes, the show is a 'textbook case' of the five strategies of whitewashing identified by Allan Bérubé (2001) in his essay 'How Gay Stays White and What Kind of White it Stays'.[28] In addition, lesbianism is almost exclusively associated with stability, domesticity and parenting.[29] This isn't to say there are no viewing pleasures for lesbian-identified viewers or to imply that there aren't ruptures to a heteronormative visions of lesbian life,[30] but that queer viewers who are not gay men may not enjoy an easy fan-hood of *Queer as Folk*. Finally – but importantly for this chapter's analysis – sexual characterisation in the series consists exclusively of fixed top/bottom identities and positionings, reproducing a hetero-polarised, decisively fixed imagining of gay male desire.

A queer diegetic universe and the explicit depiction of sex are also signs of a TV product cashing in on a global market in queer aesthetics. As Davis wryly observes, 'almost every episode of the US remake contains at least one sex scene'.[31] At the time *Queer as Folk* started, as the previous chapter explained, queer content had an 'edgy' market appeal for certain audiences; racy queer sexual content appeared to be the means of courting them.

Indeed, *Queer as Folk* has become an iconic example of the 'hypercommodification' of queer aesthetics and representations, and the concomitant formation of a global gay modernity immersed in flows of consumption and burgeoning urban cosmopolitanisms. Alderson has charted the tangled histories of British *Queer as Folk* and the urban regeneration of Manchester in the 1990s, where the original series was set and produced. In this account, the LGBTQI+ community's role in the city's gentrification, including its 'licensed-carnival atmosphere',[32] is an example of the way in which queer spaces began to function in the 1990s both literally and figuratively as one among numerous key 'ethnic spaces' in international consumer culture that acted as an appealing 'marker of cosmopolitanism, tolerance and diversity for the urban tourist'.[33] North American *Queer as Folk* continued to deliver on these promises of queer consumption and the iconography of a global gay market. Its vision of gay modernity is of a highly developed material subculture, characterised almost exclusively by spaces of consumption (the nightclub, the gym, the café), homogenous identities and the atrophying of political and activist energies. This market in gay commodities is global, albeit with uneven economic and temporal flows and different implications in different locations. The consumption of *Queer as Folk* in Manilla in the early '00s, for example, became a key practice in the circulation of signs that compose the 'universalised, mediatised and commercialised' signs of 'gayness' in that city.[34] Both British and American iterations of the series and the practices of gay subjects' consumption across the globe are exemplary case studies of a gay modernity in which consumption is reconstituted as a form of citizenship.[35] Its participation and exploitation of a global gay commodity market is another way in which *Queer as Folk* has struck certain critics as 'not queer enough'.[36]

And yet, a text so widely circulated simply cannot sustain a singular or stable meaning over passages of place and time. While the series became an icon of an Americanised gay globality in many places, these signs are always modified – 'glocalised' – in geographically, economically and temporally specific ways. Benedicto defines 'gay globality' as

> an imaginative planetary geography built by the suturing together of other, distant city spaces and body spaces (e.g., clubs in ostensible "global" cities, international party circuits, celebrity DJ networks, the defined (white) torso, even fictional bars and characters).... [It is] a spatial imagination founded on claims and hegemonic representations driven by the market and sustained by a networking of (urban) scenes that separately, though similarly, depend on the erasure of othered gay men.[37]

Benedicto also describes the consumption of *Queer as Folk* as one of many glocalising strategies practised by Filipino queers in their reception of signs of gay globality. This is equally the case among different audiences. Noble's analysis of receptive anal passivity in *Queer as Folk*, for example, highlights the trans/queer potential of the series. Noble shows how the active labour of reception – a 'queering of the queer', or what he calls 'post-queer incoherence' – can lend itself to multiple 'libidinous cross-gendered identifications that defy both passive voyeurism and limited sexual taxonomies.'[38] A TV series will always accommodate a wide range of viewing pleasures and appropriations.

Positive Men Are from Mars, Negative Men Are from Venus

Textually speaking, there is a further political dialectic in the relations between characters. While some embody or articulate lifeworlds that are conformist and assimilative, other character's behaviours and attitudes disrupt hetero-social sex-gender norms. This seems to have been deliberate: *Queer as Folk* entered the fray of one of modern queer culture's most abiding conflicts: the tension between strategies of assimilation and strategies of subversion. Some protagonists seek recognition by embracing heteronormative respectability, sanctioned by legal and cultural institutions and the trajectories of the last two series moved 'progressively' towards 'responsible' marriage-like relationships for most of these characters. Others contested those lifeworlds.

The overall ambivalence about where the series sits *vis-à-vis* queer politics and the status of queer people in popular culture is apparent in the very title of the series, with its much-discussed paradoxical inference about the normality/strangeness of 'queer'. The phrase 'queer as folk' is derived from the traditional Yorkshire saying 'It's nought as queer as folk.' Here, 'folk' refers to everyday people and 'queer', as was historically the case in British vernaculars, means 'odd' or 'strange'. 'Queer', of course, also has a long history as a pejorative description for same-sex eroticism, and has been reclaimed, first by activists and academics and then by popular culture. So, if the traditional saying 'It's nought as queer as folk' implied that the average person is an odd creature, in its renewed context (which includes the shifting histories of the term 'queer'), the phrase now implies that the normal, everyday person is perhaps a bit queer. Peeren unpacks this 'discourse that is contrary'. As she explains, the original Yorkshire phrase is 're-signified to imply something like: "homosexuals are people in general... no longer incontrovertibly other, but... ordinary folk "'.[39] Queer people are, in other words, *both* a bit unusual and a bit mundane. Indeed, queer *ordinariness* may have ultimately been one of the most groundbreaking aspects of *Queer as Folk*: as Davis suggests, queer life is typically presumed to be 'interesting and engaging as a result of [its] liminal positioning', but it too is 'humdrum and ordinary'.[40] And yet, the detailed, unexpurgated representation of queer life at this historical moment was unusual, 'edgy' and spectacular.

If the phrase ('queer as folk') and the form (soap opera) make strong gestures to the everyday, they also can't help but gesture to the 'queer' in the older sense of the term: that is, the uncanny, the strange, precisely *not* mundane but, rather, extraordinary, spectacular, other. Melodrama, as it has been re-theorised is a form that negotiates this tension between the spectacular and the mundane, often filtering the former through the latter.[41] In melodrama, Brooks writes, 'states of being beyond the immediate context of the narrative [the "banal stuff of reality"], and in excess of it, have been brought to bear on it, to charge it with intense significances'. In other words, in melodrama the everyday becomes charged with excess, with 'queerness.'

By gesturing to all of these connotations of 'queer', the title *Queer as Folk* very emphatically sets the terms for an understanding of its cultural politics as fundamentally undecidable. The show is both queerly defiant *and* assimilative, both strange *and* everyday – all of which brings us directly back to the spectacular/mundane paradox that, as I have been arguing, lies at the heart of post-crisis representation. If the most productive way to read *Queer as Folk* is as an ambivalent or undecidable text on almost all registers (politically, culturally, industrially, aesthetically), then within this larger context of undecidability, the meanings surrounding HIV in the series also emerge dialectically. Life with HIV is in some ways ordinary – everyday, domestic, in a neat accordance with the priorities of the (homo) normal – but, in other ways, it remains radically other – melodramatic, a narrative crisis, a spectacle. As we shall see next, HIV becomes a privileged signifier of that which is both strange and everyday: the 'positive image', in other words, here becomes 'queer as folk'.

Perfect, Except for One Thing

Queer as Folk has three HIV positive characters. As an elder and a veteran of the epidemic, Michael's uncle Vic often acts as a source of wisdom and guidance. Hunter, a naïve young street hustler who is adopted by Ben and Michael in series three, acquired HIV through condomless street-based sex work. Both of these characters are worth closer consideration and certainly the relational dynamics between all three positive characters dramatises an interesting range of shifting 'generational' experiences of HIV. The attention of the analysis to follow, however, is on the relationship between Michael and Ben during Series Two and Three. Ben and

Michael's relationship was a highly visible HIV story in the circulation of signs that constitutes the global gay of the 2000s. It was a novel development in popular culture – one of very few depictions of serodifference in gay male relationships and surely the most widely circulated. Fans of *Queer as Folk* became very invested in this relationship and it became a key site for internet-based fan art and fan fiction.

The introduction of Ben in Series Two becomes a catalyst for a sequence of dramatic obstacles for both Michael and his close-knit circle. The drama of Ben and Michael's relationship can be divided into two overlapping problems: (1) the problem of the positive body; and (2) the problem of serodiscord. Both of these become obstacles to the consummation of a viable, long-term relationship. Our investment in the success of this relationship is stimulated along the way.

Ben's appearance in Michael's recently opened comic book shop appears as if it will finally settle the drama of Michael's unrequited love for Brian. Ben is a handsome, thirty-something college professor who specialises in gay literature and has published an autobiographical book on his experience of living with HIV – although we don't know that yet. Research on queer comic heroes brings him to the shop where, impressed by its proprietor's expansive knowledge, Ben invites Michael to deliver a lecture to his college class. This leads to a date. Yet, in spite of these promising beginnings, Michael and Ben soon break up, seemingly because Michael's friends and mother are anxious about Ben's HIV status, as is Michael himself. The troubling presence of the body positive is one of a series of early narrative obstacles that defer the consummation of the relationship.

In this initial phase, the gay male body positive is presented as a problematic and paradoxical space: ideal erotic object of the desiring (queer) gaze and simultaneously an object of (invisible) sexual danger. Also paradoxically: the HIV positive person, Ben, is both a subject with personal agency and narrative authority (literally the author of his own biography), while simultaneously the object of a verbally proclaimed stigma that attaches itself to his body, not in spite of but *because of* the invisibility of HIV. These paradoxes are neatly expressed through the oral and visual articulation of the trope 'perfect, except for one thing.'

From first appearance, Ben is presented as an object of intense erotic and romantic investment. Michael's uncle Vic encourages his nephew to approach the tall, good-looking stranger and, as we learn more about him, it becomes clear that he is indeed perfect in *almost* every conceivable way. The Showcase website (the cable channel that first aired *Queer as Folk* in Canada) described Ben thus:

> Hunky Buddhist Ben Bruckner is more than just eye candy for smitten comic store owner Michael. A professor of gay studies at Carnegie Mellon University, Ben is smart, sexy, funny and warm. He's the perfect mate for any eligible bachelor – as long as they are willing to overlook that he's HIV positive.

Something that must be 'overlooked', the presence of HIV is framed from the outset as an *obstacle to be overcome*. Ben discloses this single exception to his perfection at the end of the episode in which we meet him. The couple have been on their first date and are making out in Ben's apartment. Their shirts come off and it appears that the series' habitual trajectory towards easy sexual encounters will unfold. However, Ben interrupts proceedings to tell Michael that he is HIV positive. The disclosure of HIV bottlenecks the action, and the episode ends in a cliffhanger.

Importantly, this early revelation of Ben's HIV status characterises him as an ethical and altruistic sexual actor, modeling a particular public health ideal of the responsible disclosure of HIV.[42] Michael later recounts this to his friends ('I'm positive. It was the first thing out of his mouth') as an indication of appropriate sexual decorum (s2, e8 'Love for Sale'); it demonstrates to him and to the audience that Ben is rational, principled and sexually ethical.

The disclosure of serostatus is identified as a key rational behaviour in what Castel calls the 'hygienist utopia', an 'ideal society of risk avoiders, where personal conduct and public discourse converge to optimise health in the face of dangers to the self and for society.'[43] Somewhat didactically, then, *Queer as Folk* here implies two things: (1) that the self-regulatory practice of HIV disclosure is self-evidently good; and (2) that it is the responsibility of the HIV positive person. However, the issue of disclosure is more complex than this, and has shifted throughout the pandemic, alongside new technologies of HIV prevention, polarising international debates over the criminalisation of HIV transmission and HIV non-disclosure. These complex legal, technological and ethical issues aren't hinted at here. Rather, Ben's upfront disclosure naturalises the understanding that, as an HIV positive gay man, he has a 'moral duty to protect the health of sexual partners' in spite of the potential social and sexual risks that may come from disclosure.[44] In a telling double standard, there have literally been no instances of serostatus disclosure, either positive or negative, in *Queer as Folk*'s countless casual sex encounters up until that point. In spite of this, Ben's behaviour is configured as rational and responsible, as common sense sexual ethics, as right.

This rightness is indicative of a shift in perceptions of responsibility during the era of post-crisis where, as Race explains, 'the HIV-positive individual is located as the natural delegate of risk management.'[45] While earlier in the pandemic many education campaigns were invested in *non-*disclosure of serostatus (just use condoms with every partner every time) 'as a political strategy designed to combat the stigmatisation of those infected,' the ability to identify the HIV positive individual through antibody testing has helped bring about a model of governance where the responsibility for risk management is 'concentrated in the figure of the HIV-positive individual.'[46] In this disclosure and in later developments, *Queer as Folk* reflects and reiterates this augmented biopolitical investment of obligation in the HIV positive subject.

At the same time as Ben's serostatus becomes an obstacle to the development of Michael and Ben's relationship, Ben's body becomes a site of conflicted signification. In the episode after the disclosure cliffhanger, Ben returns to Michael's bookshop:

> I also wanted to see how you were, um, how you're doing after last night, after my big announcement. 'Hello, my name's Ben, I'm 33, Pisces, love the outdoors and I'm HIV positive'. Still haven't figured out a way to drop that bomb gracefully.

The inclusion of Ben's HIV status in a list of personal attributes is a nod to the way in which the statement of serostatus is a speech act with identity effects: the utterance of this form of health knowledge has become a statement of subjecthood that produces the (positive or negative) subject and positions them in a relationship of difference, of viral polarity.

The 'bomb' metaphor notwithstanding, Ben's revelation has not actually proved to be the climax promised by the cliffhanger. Michael doesn't mind: his liberal, sexually frank upbringing is offered as an explanation for his ostensible ease with the prospect of dating an HIV positive man. The relationship will continue.

The next hurdle is the judgement of others, and this is where the mixed significations of Ben's body are more powerfully foregrounded. Michael's friends become curious about the mysterious new man he is dating. 'Is there something wrong with him?' Ted asks, teasingly, to which Michael responds: 'There's something wrong with *you*. I would like this one to live before my best friends devour him' (s2, e7 'The Leper'). Michael's pun on the threat Ben's HIV status poses to his life and their relationship neatly articulates his (and the audience's) wish that their relationship will succeed in spite of the obstacle of HIV stigma. His response ('there's something wrong with you') also foreshadows the hostile reaction that will come from Ted in particular. We also soon discover that Michael's friends have already, figuratively speaking, 'devoured' Ben: Ted has read Ben's autobiography, while Brian hooked up with Ben at a dance party sometime in the distant past.

Despite his reticence, Michael's friends soon meet Ben in an extremely important and emblematic scene for the representation of the body positive in the image landscape of post-crisis. Here, *Queer as Folk* crystalises the idea that Ben's body is a space of paradoxical meanings: ideal, beautiful, healthy and even a locus of secular spirituality, but also infected and sexually dangerous at the same time. These mixed significations emerge both from dialogue and the adjudication of the camera's gaze.

Out on their second date, Ben explains to Michael that his outlook on life is strongly informed by Buddhism. 'Buddha', he says, 'teaches you to focus on the smallest details… the breeze against your cheek, the way your shirt falls against your body… It helps you realise that right now, this moment, is all there is' (s2, e7 'The Leper'). Michael is then pleasantly surprised when Ben takes him to Babylon, the gay nightclub that is one of the recurring locations in *Queer as Folk*. 'I thought when you said you wanted to "experience the now" you meant something spiritual?', Michael asks. 'I did', Ben replies, explaining: 'This tribe I visited in New Guinea would dance until they collapsed. That's how they freed themselves from… time. Looked just like them'. He gestures around to the men dancing in the club. 'Except for the light show. But they had shooting stars' (s2, e7 'The Leper'). On the dance floor, Ben takes his shirt off and both the camera work and

Positive Men Are from Mars, Negative Men Are from Venus

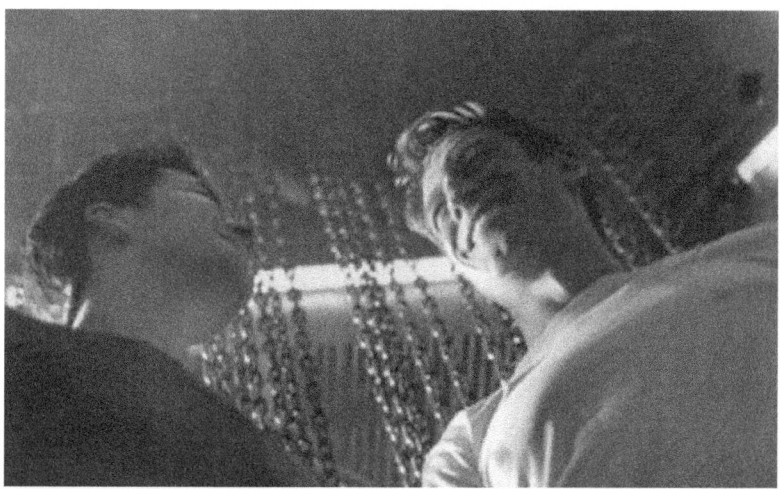

Figure 2.1 Michael (Hal Sparks) and Ben (Robert Grant) experiencing 'the now' in *Queer as Folk* (season 2, episode 7)

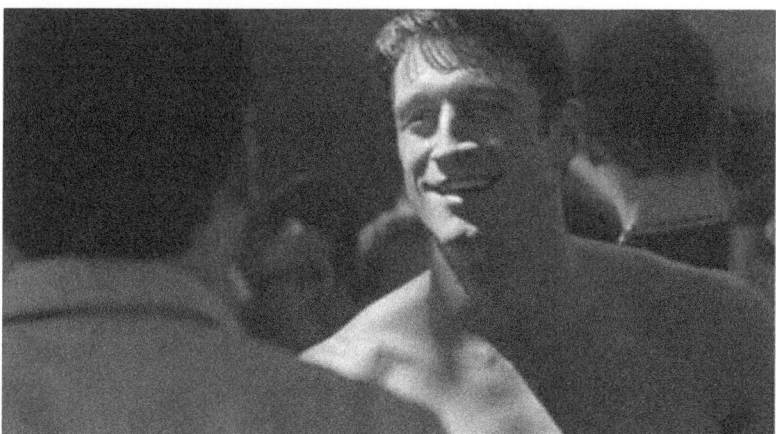

Figure 2.2 'Perfect except for one thing': Ben on the dance floor in *Queer as Folk* (season 2, episode 7)

mise en scène function to confirm what he has already suggested: for the HIV positive gay man the disco is a space of secular spirituality. The nightclub heavens gently shower silver leaf onto the dancing couple. They are shot from below, smiling, ecstatic, Michael admiring Ben's muscular body. They dance (see Figures 2.1–2.2).

As is often the case in representations of the disco in gay culture, this scene encourages us to view Babylon as a space of secular transcendence. The club has special resonance for Ben, and this meaningfulness is directly associated with his earlier comments about Buddhism's exhortation to register the sensual and haptic details of experience ('the breeze against your cheek'). It is strongly implied throughout this episode that Ben's HIV status has encouraged him to cultivate a thoughtful relationship with time, mortality and embodied experience. The importance of the disco becomes especially germane to the culture surrounding, and the experience of living, with HIV.

There is a tangled history of associations between HIV/AIDS, the disco, and the present-oriented secular–spiritual, communal experience. These associations were powerfully forged at the queer mega dance parties of the 1990s, many of which were HIV fundraisers. Especially before the advent of antiretroviral therapies, these parties occurred against a backdrop of 'a wide-scale experience and intuition of death – the death of hundreds of gay men a year,' a broadly felt awareness that contributed to 'a variously articulated practical philosophy of living for the moment.'[47] This nexus of associations between HIV, the dance party, and what Michael calls 'the now' is particular to a moment in the history of HIV/AIDS that has largely passed. Ironically, as Race points out, the advent of life-prolonging HIV drugs has contributed to the demise of a thriving queer dance party scene.[48]

While Race is particularly interested in the role of drugs – both 'licit' and 'illicit' – in the imagination and formation of community in the queer dance party scene, I want to emphasise the conjunction of the muscular gay male (positive) body and the idea of a secular sublimity that emerged from the context of these parties. An image of this particular, historically specific gay body is being offered in the Babylon nightclub scene. Recalling Ben's quasi-anthropological description of 'tribes in New Guinea', Bardella describes the circuit parties of the 1990s as a type of secular, postmodern pilgrimage, drawing on Victor Turner's formulation of the ritualised secular pilgrimage. Using the terms of ethnography, Bardella describes these parties as a communal custom of freedom and celebration – a key scene in the 'ritual repertoire' of the 'tribes' of an internationalised urban gay subculture that is intimately linked to the collective experience of AIDS.[49]

Though Ben and Michael are experiencing 'the now' in a latter, post-crisis moment, after the advent of ARVs drastically reduced the number of AIDS deaths, the memory of the former moment remains present. Curiously, it is the 'spiritualising' of the dancing gay body that helps us to assimilate Ben's wholesomeness with the figure of the disco queen. Ben is far from the image of unbridled hedonism, drug-taking and promiscuous sex often associated with party scenes, and yet he is still a potent image of 'experiencing the now'. How is this apparent paradox possible? As Race explains, the 'experience the now'–attitude of the queer dance party did not necessarily or only invoke excess, but also a thoughtful 'pursuit of intensified experientiality, in which the pleasures of the self are appreciably bound up in the nature and quality of relations with others – the practices of care, hope, memory, dance, excitement, and disclosure'.[50] The conjuring of some of these elevated experiences and affects enables us to imagine Ben's meaningful relationship with the space of the gay disco as something other than 'reckless', hedonistic, or 'meaningless' (as it is represented, for example, in *The Next Best Thing*). Through the orientalist sign of non-western spirituality ('Buddhism', 'tribes in New Guinea'), the gay disco is aligned with a present-focused (HIV) positive outlook that values health, life, responsibility, awareness, connection, and meaningfulness.

And yet, this becomes a scene of mixed significations: the idealised, mystico-spiritual mood is soon interrupted by the taint of stigma and sexual danger. Unbeknownst to Ben and Michael, Michael's friends are also hanging out at Babylon. The couple eventually bump into them and Ted, who recognises Ben from reading his autobiography, reveals to Justin and Brian that Michael's new boyfriend is HIV positive. As they're meeting this luminous new man, Ted, initially enthused, gushes to Ben about his book: 'It got rave reviews! It was so honest, so forthright, it was so, ah…' He pauses and an expression of misgiving comes across his face as he finishes the sentence: 'so *revealing*.' Ben responds to Ted's comment with a knowing pun on HIV disclosure: 'Yeah, well, that's what writers do, we just cut ourselves open and bleed all over the page.' After this awkward, loaded exchange, more shots of the ecstatic couple dancing and of Ben's perfect body are interspersed with another verbal revelation of HIV: 'He's hot', Justin says, looking on admiringly. 'He's OK', Brian qualifies. And then, in a foreboding tone, Ted says: 'Looks, brain, nice guy too. I'd say he's *perfect, except for one thing… He's positive.*' Justin looks to Brian for a reaction. Brian looks out to the joyful couple on the dance floor and again the episode ends with this dramatic, vaguely menacing moment of disclosure.

It is thus that *Queer as Folk* establishes the dilemma of the HIV positive body as an obstacle to the consummation of the romantic relationship – a dilemma centered around the paradoxes of visible/invisible and ideal/dangerous, and elaborated through these heightened moments of visual and verbal disclosure.

These strategies of revelation respond to the *invisibility* of HIV in the context of post-crisis. That is, in the absence of two cliffhanger-inducing verbal declarations, HIV would remain undetectable. This rehearses the investment in disclosure as the key articulation of the presence of HIV in the post-antiretrovirals universe, which Race dubs the 'undetectable crisis'. A riff on the aim of antiretroviral therapy to keep the level of virus in the blood at 'undetectable' levels, Race's phrase describes a socio-political climate in the places where HIV/AIDS has faded from the public arena into the anonymity of private lives.[51] 'Undetectable crisis' describes a shift in the pandemic from what was once an extremely visible, urgent public health crisis – evidenced in media coverage, activism and the politicising of AIDS deaths – to what is now considered a chronic manageable illness to be managed in private by affected individuals. This is the effect of a range of epidemiological and cultural transformations, at the forefront of which are the technologies of HIV antibody testing and ARVs. '[I]f antibody tests distributed and individuated the experience of HIV', Race explains, 'the presence of viral load testing allows the epidemic to be imagined as an aggregate of individuals with viruses capable of being managed by these individuals, "in partnership" with doctors.'[52] While this is neither a straightforwardly positive or negative set of developments, is has disciplinary effects. Key among Race's concerns is that alongside this 'withdrawal of HIV from public space and the "visible" ', there has been a 'privatisation' of the experience of HIV.[53] This privatising shift becomes an important part of *Queer as Folk*'s dramatisation of serodiscord as a personal issue to be managed within relationships, as we shall see shortly.

'Undetectable' may also refer to the fact that, for someone like Ben, there are no *visually detectable* signs of HIV infection, which is why *Queer as Folk* invents these elaborate dramatic disclosures. Prior to ARVs, images of people living with HIV/AIDS were culturally synonymous with Kaposi's sarcoma (KS) and wasting, 'the identifying and dreaded "signs" of AIDS'.[54] Now, when they are available and working effectively, ARVs have largely erased these signs. You cannot tell by looking at Ben that he has HIV. In Series Two he is hospitalised with acute pancreatitis, explained as a potential side-effect of his HIV regime (s3, e18 'Sick, Sick, Sick'). But even in hospital, Ben never appears sick. This presents a dilemma for visual culture in the era of effective treatments: if the 'dreaded signs' of AIDS are no longer detectable, how do you represent the body positive?[55]

Queer as Folk's solution to the invisibility of HIV is the motif, 'perfect, except for one [invisible] thing'. Announced first by Ted, this phrase is later repeated in Series Three when Lindsay and Melanie are discussing which of their gay male friends might father their second child. Running down a list, Lindsay suggests: 'Ben's brainy and brawny', to which Melanie responds: 'I'd say he's just about perfect, except for one thing'. 'Oh', says Lindsay, crossing Ben's name off (s3, e4 'Brat-Sitting'). Again, Lindsay and the audience need a verbal reminder of Ben's HIV status for otherwise there are no indications of HIV's presence. In the figure of Ben, popular culture has updated the wasting gay male PWA of crisis discourse – immediately identifiable as an image of HIV/AIDS – with a sexualised, athletic masculinity – the gay male person *living with* HIV. With this figure, the link between positive serostatus and potential illness (or death) is, in the absence of antibody test results, purely abstract, invisible and only available linguistically and or through clever subtextual and visual forms of signification. Paradoxically, HIV/AIDS becomes *separate from and yet coterminous with* the living, healthy, erotic body.

This paradox (dangerous but ideal erotic object; perfect except for one thing) may be further illuminated by what Sothern calls the 'spatial contradiction of the HIV+ body'.[56] As Matthew Sothern explains, the post-ARVs world has given rise to positive bodies with contradictory implications for representation. On the one hand, the PLHIV is the embodied site of HIV infection, a potential 'mechanism of the spatial diffusion of the virus' and thus in prevention discourse there has been a perceived requisite to represent the positive body as, a space that is 'inherently other', a 'space to be avoided (if only by latex).'[57] At the same time, we have also needed affirmative images of positive people as advocacy for the citizenship, justice, access and recognition of the positive community has become central to the agenda of ASOs. This creates a problem for representation, one that is ironically aggravated by improvements in medical technologies. The public image of the body positive in the era of post-crisis has been regenerated across a number of pop culture sites. For example, in American advertisements for ARVs, PLHIV have been represented as 'productive, useful and deserving of equal treatment and protection', as (sexually) active, an engaged member of the community, 'happy, healthy and normal, "just like everyone else".'[58] The paradox, as Sothern explains, is that 'people struggling with HIV/AIDS are productive and equal, they deserve justice and toleration and at the same time they are a threatening, diffusing, polluting other.'[59] The advent of PrEP and U=U has changed these meanings further. In *Queer as Folk*, this contradiction plays out in a melodrama of conflicting significations, with the desirable image of a shirtless, dancing Ben overlayed with an ambivalent, stigmatising verbal disclosure.

The mixed significations of Ben's body also recall discussions of the muscular gay body of the 1990s dance party and disco scene as a body that symbolically disavows sickness and death. In some commentaries, the 'circuit queen' was identified as a figure anxiously disavowing the wasting and sickness associated with AIDS through the accumulation of muscle. *Queer as Folk* draws on this idea in a later series, in a story arc involving Ben's use of steroids, as we shall see shortly. Arthur Evans has interpreted bodybuilding among gay men in the era of AIDS as, among other things, a means of masking the 'stigmatisation, isolation, loneliness, frustration and dependency processes triggered by the onset of illness.'[60] Lewis and Ross's qualitative study of the Australian gay dance party scene supported this hypothesis, concluding that 'one facet of the current fixation with the gay body-beautiful reveals deep anxieties about the epidemic.'[61] Andrew Sullivan expressed a similar reading of this body in his controversial *New York Times* essay 'When Plagues End':

> On the surface the parties could be taken for a mass of men in superb shape merely enjoying an opportunity to let off steam. But underneath, masked by the drugs, there is an air of strain, of sexual danger translated into sexual objectification, the unspoken withering of the human body transformed into a reassuring inflation of muscular body mass.[62]

In other words, the muscular gay body repudiates and replaces but can never entirely disavow the spectre of its anti-body: a diseased, wasting, feminised body, the 'AIDS body'. Is this alleged repudiation an individualised, psychic process? Or, is it a process of representation and collective cultural denial? Regardless of how well this account explains the body type that predominated in the circuit scene and other gay spaces in the 1990s, certainly the Babylon scene discussed above hints strongly at these mixed connotations. The muscle-bound disco queen exposes anxieties about the proximity between ideal objects of gay male desire and sexual risk that have been a particular problem for representation in the age of HIV/AIDS. The proximity of paragon and peril, of danger and desire, is deliberately exploited as a source of drama in the Babylon scene.

As we shall see next, *Queer as Folk* has other narrative uses for the built body in its dramatisation of serodiscord. In Series Three Ben develops an obsession with bodybuilding and starts using steroids. Across this story arc the problem of relating across serodifference emerges more emphatically. This drama is again manifest at the level of Ben's body, picking up and developing the associations between the fit, hard, disciplined, masculine body and the body positive first hinted at in the Babylon scene.

Positive Men Are from Mars, Negative Men Are from Venus

The drama of serodiscord emerges from a conflict around Ben's use of steroids. This story arc is precipitated by the death from HIV/AIDS of Ben's former lover. Ben hears this news at the gym:

MAN 1: Remember those five minutes in the 90s when everyone wanted to put on weight because it meant you weren't dying.
MAN 2: Didn't do Paul any good.
MAN 1: At least we don't have to go back to that goddamn hospice. Talk about depressing.

(s3, e4 'Brat-Sitting')

'Sorry, what was that about Paul?' Ben asks. One of the men turns to him and says 'Oh, didn't you hear? He died last night.' The details of Paul's death are kept very vague; it's somewhat strange that someone living with HIV would have died (from HIV-related illness) at this time, presuming they were diagnosed and treated, but the death remains an unexplained plot device.

Ben's reaction to the news is immediately articulated in relation to anxieties about health, diet and the body. He says to Michael:

> Why am I so goddamn angry at him right now? [Angry] for getting it, for giving it to me, and then not even bothering to take care of himself, or watch what he ate. I would tell him 'nutrition is essential' and 'exercise, you gotta exercise Paul, build up your muscle mass.' But it was as if once he knew he had it, he figured 'I'm gonna die anyway so what the hell difference is it gonna make?' (s3, e4 'Brat-Sitting').

Shortly after this news arrives, Melanie and Lindsay ask Michael to father their second child. Though Ben is nominally happy for Michael, he soon reveals deep feelings of loss: his serostatus excludes him from this bio-reproductive process, and having children, he says, 'was always a thought, but I never knew how much I wanted it until I couldn't' (s3, e4 'Brat-Sitting').[63] To cope with these feelings, Ben intensifies his training regime, redoubling his efforts at the gym and soon secretly injecting steroids. Over a number of episodes, his obsession with working out and the increasingly regular paroxysms of aggression anecdotally associated with steroid use or 'roid rage' lead to a relationship crisis (see Figure 2.3). Michael catches Ben in the act of injecting and though he initially agrees, albeit equivocally, to accept Ben's rationale that steroids are a 'preventative measure' against bodily wasting, he becomes worried (s3, e6 'One Ring'). These are the circumstances around which *Queer as Folk*'s drama of serodiscord develops.

As this drama unfolds, Michael and Ben begin to inhabit stereotypically gendered roles in their interpersonal dynamic with each another. Michael is anxious, upset, and sensitive to the changes in Ben; he wonders how to raise their issues and makes several attempts to communicate. The series goes to some lengths to establish his pensiveness and eventually he turns to best friend Brian for advice. Meanwhile, Ben is busily acting out his feelings, externalising them through the building of protective body mass; he denies that there is a problem, and he becomes angry and defensive when the subject is broached.

Positive Men Are from Mars, Negative Men Are from Venus

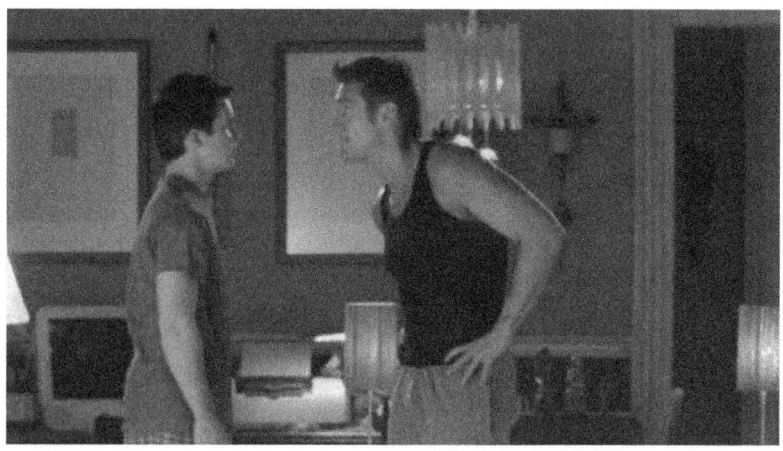

Figure 2.3 Ben has roid rage in *Queer as Folk* (season 3, episode 4)

As well as a potentially parodic or grotesque affront to conventional masculinity, the built gay body can also convey a disavowal of the feminine. The way Ben's anxieties unfold in *Queer as Folk* recalls both the commentaries on the muscular circuit queen discussed earlier and the laborious processes of disavowal enacted by the New Gay Man in the previous chapter. Marked as abnormal by virtue of its excess and its reliance on steroids – illicit drugs – Ben's bodybuilding is offered as an anxious practice of disciplining the flesh and as a means of psychic denial: denial of anxieties around HIV, denial of the spectre of the sick body – a *feminised* sick body. Bodybuilding has been theorised as a technology of masculinity enhancement through which femininity is 'evacuated'. The fantasy project of the bodybuilder, posits Marcia Ian, is the construction of a 'body-building' with 'no space left inside, because it has been transformed... into a thing made entirely of dense, hard muscle.'[64] Bodybuilding aims 'to substitute the "rock hard" for the soft, the monumental for the human, and the masculine for the feminine'[65]:

> One goes inside the gym to fill up, extirpate, or deny the inside... Femininity is unwelcome... [It] represents the spectacle, or the specter, of interiority, a reflection of oneself as penetrable and vulnerable with which the male body-builder does not wish to identify.... [Built] masculinity reassures itself that it is exactly what it appears to be: a body with no interior, and no aperture.[66]

Shredding and building muscle may be understood here as a figurative process through which an anxious evacuation of the feminine is enacted. In Ben's case, this evacuation is intimately linked to anxieties around HIV. The otherwise thoughtful, sensitive Ben becomes increasingly severed from emotional interiority, creating distance in his relationship with Michael.

At first glance it appears that *Queer as Folk* is running a straightforward anti-illicit drugs line, in spite of its earlier more permissive treatments of recreational drug use in gay male party scenes.[67] However, when Michael confronts Ben a more complex dynamic is explicitly revealed:

MICHAEL: It's fucking you up… It is and you don't even know it… You're acting crazy.

BEN: You don't understand anything.

MICHAEL: Understand what?

BEN: What it's like to wake up every morning and remember 'Oh yeah, I've got this thing,' because you *don't* have this thing. You never have to take a mouthful of meds, never knowing when they'll stop working, never knowing when a fucking cough or a fucking sniff will land you in a hospital, because to you, Michael, it is just a fucking cough, or a fucking sniff! And every time I go to kiss you, or suck you, or fuck you – even when we're protected, even then – there is still this shitty, nagging doubt that maybe, just maybe, you could get infected. Sometimes I just think…

MICHAEL: [*interrupting*] What? … Sometimes you just think what?

BEN: That it might just be easier being with someone who's positive.

(s3, e6 'One Ring') (see Figure 2.4)

Here the drama of relating across serodifference is explicitly announced.

'Serodiscordant' is a portmanteau term combining 'sero', the medical prefix relating to the diagnostic examination of blood serum (especially with regard to the response of immune system antibodies) and 'discordant', which implies incongruent, disagreeing or at odds. In HIV medical and prevention literatures, a 'serodiscordant relationship' describes a relationship comprised of one person who is HIV positive and one who is HIV negative. Because of its overtones of difference and conflict, alternatives to 'serodiscordant' have been offered, including 'magnetic',

Positive Men Are from Mars, Negative Men Are from Venus

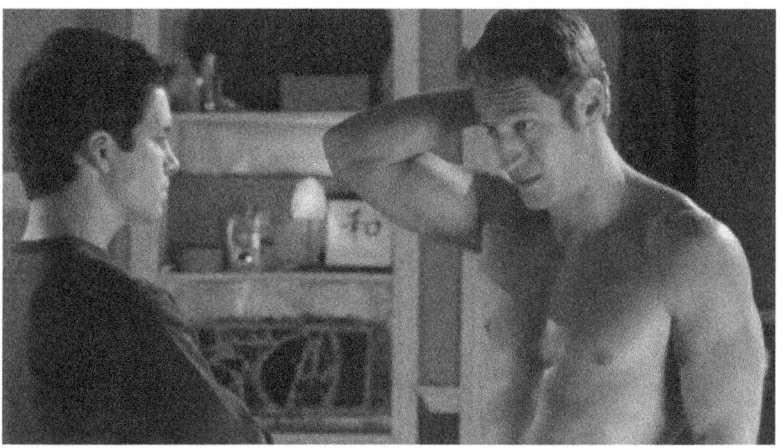

Figure 2.4 The drama of serodiscord in *Queer as Folk* (season 3, episode 6)

'sero-divergent', 'inter-viral', 'pos/neg' and 'mixed status'. ASOs and public health workers recognise that couples in serodiscordant relationships face specific issues surrounding the presence of HIV including: HIV prevention, adhering to treatment plans and other health issues, the effects of treatment or illness on sex and body image, care-giving responsibilities, disclosure and privacy, family and financial planning, potential rejection and abandonment. These issues have changed as medical and prevention technologies have developed, including the recent advent of PrEP. The deployment of PrEP and undetectable viral load make the risk of HIV transmission in serodiscordant couples virtually non-existent. At this time, however, the literature and peer education work of ASOs was focused on the need for communication and mutual responsibility for mutual health, care and safety in serodiscordant situations. In the quote from Ben above, some of these issues and the feelings they might raise are hinted at: isolation, anxiety, resentment and misunderstanding. In Ben's case, these feelings are organised around a generalised sense of being irreconcilably different and distanced from his partner, alienated and burdened in a way that Michael is not.

In HIV prevention and other discourses, a logic of serosame/serodifference has become part of the way that gay selves are conceptualised, and in this logic identity and relationality can seem polarised. Damien Riggs discusses this problem of the 'reification' of serostatus as a defining, biologised attribute of gay identity. He argues that:

> Whilst safer sex messages have been directed towards preventing infection, they have also promoted the ideas (a) that serostatus is a key aspect of gay men's identities, (b) that being HIV positive is something to be scared about, and (c) that being either negative or positive makes you incommensurably different from someone whose serostatus differs from your own.[68]

This idea of incommensurable, immutable difference may turn serostatus into a sort of defining, embodied 'nature', activating an essentialist understanding of identity and difference. Riggs calls this difference 'HIV polarity' and suggests the ways that, as a model, it borrows from and reiterates other commonly imagined role differences like butch/femme and top/bottom.[69] And, as is the case in *Queer as Folk*, serodifference has perhaps been most commonly expressed through the most ubiquitous model of difference in our culture: gender.

A gendered, or 'heteropolarised' vision of serodiscord plays out very clearly in Ben and Michael's relationship and the muscular body becomes a key symbol in this scripting of difference. HIV polarity is presented as a conflict between a hard, masculine Ben, working overtime to sublimate his fears of a diseased feminine interiority under a reassuring mass of muscle, and a softer, sensitive Michael, eager to communicate, trying to invent a means of overcoming these differences. Ben works out at the gym while Michael is pictured sitting, in thought and reflection, or talking to friends and family. From the beginning of their relationship Ben has been the top during sex, and Michael the bottom. Miscommunication and conflict are the consequences of these 'essential' heteropolarised (sero) differences. The effect of this gendered representation is to further entrench serostatus as a 'defining feature of gay men's identities', as 'central to gay men's modes of relationality and communities.'[70] Relationally, positive serostatus is associated with masculinity and negative serostatus with femininity. The articulation of serodiscord in this way comes to echo the hackneyed cultural script of a 'positive men are from Mars, negative men are from Venus'–type dichotomy.[71]

HIV polarity as a means of comprehending difference, Riggs suggest, may also become evident in the examples of barebacking and bugchasing

Positive Men Are from Mars, Negative Men Are from Venus

where 'HIV status is constructed through the categories of "haves" and "have nots", again privileging biomedical accounts of HIV.'[72] Indeed, once it emerges that serodifference is threatening their relationship, Michael daydreams his own deliberate seroconversion as a fantasy solution to the problem of HIV polarity. In Michael's dream, Ben is fucking him and the condom they are using breaks. Ben panics, but under Michael's insistence, they continue fucking in order that Michael may seroconvert. This seroconversion fantasy isn't offered as an actual or viable solution to their problem – it is presented as Michael's fanciful, irrational daydream (see Figure 2.5). As we'll see in the next chapter, seroconvertive discourses are complicated and can change dramatically with medical, scientific and somatechnological developments, and yet they may still be informed – sometimes – by our culture's time honoured, heavily naturalised ideological model of difference: masculine/feminine.

In the midst of this conflict, Michael's uncle Vic falls into a relationship with an HIV positive man called Rodney, a subplot that works to reinforce the notion of HIV polarity. Michael goes for dinner at his mother's house with the new couple. When he asks Rodney how he and Vic met, Rodney's story emphasises the idea that positive and negative men inhabit different universes. They met, Rodney says,

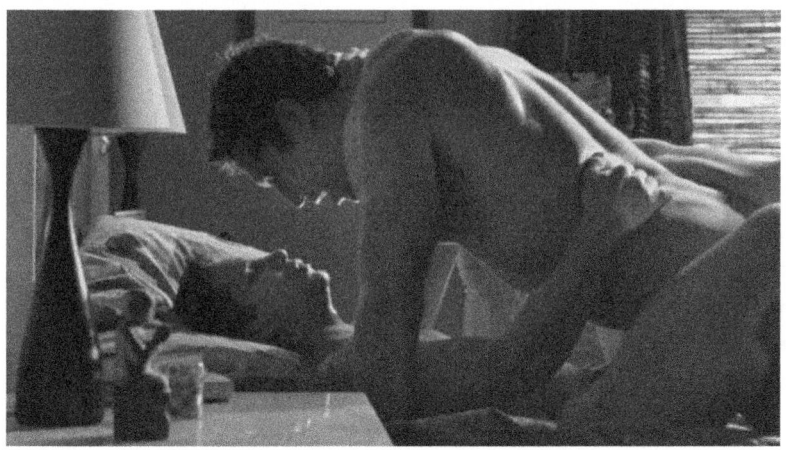

Figure 2.5 Michael's seroconversion fantasy in *Queer as Folk* (season 3, episode 6)

at a pos men's group. I didn't even want to go, but some friends of mine convinced me that I should meet some positive men. I'd been dating negative men for a while and it never really worked out. No matter how hard we tried they could never really understand what it was like living through this thing. And with Vic there's no need to explain. We already know what each other's going through. Instead of separating us, it brings us closer together. (s3, e7)

By this point, the series has gone to great lengths to suggest that positive and negative experiences are intractably at odds. In spite of grueling efforts to understand one another, there is a growing sense that this gulf may be ineluctable. For negative men, the experience of living with 'this thing', HIV, no matter how close you get to it, will forever remain incomprehensible. Like Michael, the audience is encouraged to wonder whether Michael and Ben's relationship will succeed. Will *Queer as Folk* overcome this obstacle to the success of Ben and Michael's relationship? All relationships may be a negotiation of difference, but can a relationship succeed between serodiscordant partners? Vic and Rodney's experience suggests not.

Later that evening, Ben returns from the gym to find Michael sitting alone in the dark in their apartment. He asks Michael what Vic's new boyfriend is like. 'They're so alike it's uncanny', Michael says dryly. 'Same interests, same temperament?' Ben asks. 'Same disease… They're both positive', Michael replies. Shock registers on Ben's face when he notices that Michael is holding a used steroid syringe. The confrontation that then unfolds is histrionic, bringing the conflict of HIV polarity to a decisive melodramatic climax. Alarmed, Ben asks Michael to put down the syringe.

MICHAEL: You know seeing Vic and his new boyfriend made me think. Y'know, maybe you're right, maybe you should be with a pos guy.
BEN: No, No… I was upset when I said that, I didn't mean that…
MICHAEL: Maybe that pos guy should be me? *[Gestures to inject himself]*.
BEN: *[Shouting]* Michael! Please!
MICHAEL: Please what? … All it would take is a quick jab in a vein and it'd be over in a flash. I'd hardly feel a thing and then I'd be just like you.
BEN: I don't want you to be like me.

MICHAEL: You said you wanted someone who knows what you're going through. Who wakes up every morning and suddenly remembers, 'Hey that's right, I've got this thing'. Who thinks every time he gets a cold, or the flu, 'This is it, this is the end.' Who's filled with resentment and anger 'cos he can never have kids… and who has to shoot himself up with *steroids* because his lover died… and he's scared shitless he's next and who has to *[starts shouting]* drive away the person he loves, and who *loves him*, because he doesn't understand. Well, now I will!

BEN: *[Shouting]* For god's sake, stop!

MICHAEL: *[Puts needle down and stands]* No *you* stop. Stop using this shit. Stop hurting yourself. And stop hurting us!

(s3, e7 'Stop Hurting Us').

The morning after this confrontation, Ben and Michael's conflict is somewhat magically resolved. Ben pledges to quit using steroids and insists that Michael come to Paul's funeral with him. 'But I don't belong there', Michael protests. 'You belong with me', Ben says. On the surface, the drama of serodiscord finds closure. Having offered itself as a sufficient but surmountable obstacle to their relationship, Michael and Ben now literally settle their (sero) differences.

However, the used syringe as an instrument through which Michael is able to 'put things into perspective' for Ben is a thorny, problematic signifier. The needle is intended to metaphorically and seemingly quite literally 'pinpoint' the difference between Michael and Ben, a difference that it could only take a tiny prick to overcome – trivial, not really a difference at all. Pos and neg are here offered as states of being that are merely an instant and a pinprick away from one another via the micro-event of seroconversion. But what makes this moment seem disingenuous is the polarising experience of serodiscord that the series has otherwise gone to such lengths to establish. Michael's syringe pantomine – his 'suicidal' threat – is a theatrical, manipulative gesture: it condenses Ben's experience of being positive (his grief for his dead ex-lover Paul; his anxiety about infecting Michael; his regimen of treatment and its side-effects; his concern for the future) into a disposable object; it trivialises Ben's experience of living with HIV. Threatening to inject himself, Michael reverts to a pre-post crisis discourse that spectacularises HIV and overdetermines transmission as a moment of suicide/murder. Michael's speech erases the legitimacy of Ben's emotional difficulties and prioritises the experience of the HIV negative man. Is it so unreasonable for Ben to feel sadness and resentment because he can't have children, or to sometimes be 'scared shitless' that he might die like his former lover? Beyond this erasure of his experience, the heightened melodrama of this scene scandalises the transmission of blood-borne viruses through intravenous drug use and the sharing of needles, reinforcing the heavily stigmatised associations with that practice.

But is silencing this crisis that has threatened the business of getting on with Ben and Michael's relationship a satisfying conclusion? Or, is this a soapy love-conquers-all palliative? If the syringe confrontation seems reductive or kitsch, perhaps this is because melodrama as a form tends to invest itself in 'cultural tensions, instabilities, and anxieties' that are, in many ways, *un*resolvable.[73] If *Queer as Folk*'s resolution to the drama of serodiscord seems insincere or unsatisfying, this is because melodrama often establishes problems it is unable to resolve. The syringe – a disposable object over-burdened with connotations of risk, blood transmission, criminality and addiction – is a melodramatic object that both condenses and heightens the stakes of the drama of serodifference into a single signifier, exposing it in all of its complexity and unresolvability; at the same time, it functions as a reductive agent of narrative resolution. The soap opera must attempt to present closure even when it cannot: with melodrama, the text opens up problems that it ultimately may not be able to resolve, that are instead 'laid open in their shameless contradictoriness'.[74]

Another disappointing aspect of this resolution is the missed opportunity to re-politicise the experience of living with HIV. With its erasure of the conflict that has preceded it, the syringe scene also erases the political history of the PLHIV, including decades of patient advocacy, medical activism, and efforts to view HIV/AIDS as a community responsibility. Despite its posturing against 'hurt', Michael's diatribe – which is then vindicated by the couple's resolution and Ben's promise to stop using steroids – erases AIDS activist history and reiterates the now prevalent model in which the onus is on Ben, on the HIV positive person, to manage HIV privately and quietly. While this 'resolution' facilitates a forward movement from the drama that has preceded it, it also reinforces the state of invisible crisis. If Michael's confrontation seems to trivialise Ben's experience and implies he needs to get over it for the sake of their relationship, it also implies that remaining quiet about the experience of living with HIV is somehow important for the future of the committed gay couple. The problem of serodiscord that has hitherto bedeviled the relationship gets dispensed with so that the couple can get on with other matters – like having their relationship recognised by the state, which becomes a key narrative preoccupation in later series. In this unsatisfying resolution to this dramatic arc, the series repudiates the contradictions of sero-melodrama in favour of a return to the polite, neoliberal quotidian. This privatising of serodiscord reflects the broader landscape of post-crisis culture where what was once an extremely public crisis inspiring collective action has shifted to one of a discreet, individualised health management exercise, a largely invisible one. The series characterises HIV as an intimate matter to be dealt with between couples, within families, and by individuals. Though *Queer as Folk*'s positive characters and its tackling of sero-melodrama suggest that we have come a long way from the sex-death narratives of AIDS crisis, the potential for HIV to inspire collective or 'counterpublic' action has disappeared. As Persson writes, the disease that 'was once an extremely public crisis inspiring collective action has largely become a discreet health management exercise on the part of individuals.'[75]

The key sites for the show's political investments in later series became the campaigns for legally recognised same-sex marriages. These issues come to the fore in Series Five with the introduction of a fictional political campaign called 'Proposition 14' that, like several real-life legislative proposals in US states since 2000, acted to prohibit same-sex marriage, adoption and other familial rights. The adverse implications of such legislative change for the lives of *Queer as Folk*'s characters are canvassed throughout this series, and Michael and Ben become active in the campaign against it. As a couple, they move into an equivalence with homonormativity. In a turn of attitudes and allegiances, Michael rejects his best friend Brian, who continues to embody unapologetic promiscuity and a cynicism towards homonormative life. More didactically, in a discrete narrative arc that confronts the then just budding issue of bug chasing, Ben rejects a young man who comes to him wishing to seroconvert (s3, e10). These are both instances where the politics of normal can be seen to cast 'shame on those who stand further down the ladder of respectability.'[76]

Melodrama, Narrative Complexity and Post-Crisis Ambivalence

Queer as Folk was the offspring of a TV landscape interested more than ever before in combining genres and forms. Like *Ally McBeal* (1997–2002), *Weeds* (2007–14), or more recently *Girls* (2012–17), it can be described as a 'dramedy', combining the soap opera and sitcom forms.[77] In its combination of accumulative, ongoing narratives and contained, episode-based stories, it combined 'complex narrative' with an episodic format. Complex narrative, with its rhizomatic plots and protracted character evolution, is a much-lauded characteristic of quality TV. As Michael Kackman explains, quality TV's 'extended back stories of plot and character' promote 'a particular kind of spectatorial pleasure in the mechanisms of narration itself'.[78] Critics who have lauded the viewing pleasures of complex narratives have, he argues, presumed that 'narrative complexity generates representational complexity; representational complexity offers the possibility of political and cultural complexity…. [and therefore] we're embracing the dream of a more complex world. Maybe, even, a more just one.'[79] What we need to remember, he insists, is that this move to celebrate complex narrative involves an embrace of that most denigrated of storytelling modes – melodrama:

> All of this [rhapsodising of complex narrative]… draws us ever closer to melodrama, as both narrative form and index of a kind of cultural longing. What's really key here is melodrama's investment in its immediate cultural environs, that is to say, not just its formal play, but its engagement of *cultural tensions, instabilities, and anxieties*. In fact, it's melodrama's *simultaneous invocation of, and inability to resolve, social tensions*, that makes it such a ripe form for serial narrativisation, and which makes it a central, and maybe even necessary, component of quality television.[80]

This critical reframing of quality TV 'as melodramatic complexity' suggests that the ir/resolution of *Queer as Folk*'s drama of serodiscord might be understood in terms of melodrama's capacity to thematise that which remains culturally unresolved, that which poses more questions than it answers. There is no doubt that *Queer as Folk*'s sero-melodrama is a more nuanced, progressive treatment of HIV than the coming-home-to-die and sex/death narratives of early Anglo-American AIDS movies and TV. And yet, even when the PLHIV is no longer an object of the horrified or sentimental gaze – a figure who must die for narrative closure – other aspects of difference too complex to find resolution to in this format are dispensed with, 'resolved'.

Although the trajectory of Ben and Michael's narrative starts with an emphasis on the importance of working through and beyond difference, in its unsatisfying closure, these experiential differences are trivialised. In the ideological universe of the show, serodifference as heteropolarity has been made central to our understanding of gay male subjectivities, and the sentimental closure of sero-disequilibria has reinstated the invisibilisation and the de-politicisation of HIV/AIDS. The articulation of this new, post-crisis cultural problem of serodiscord via the much older cultural logic of gender difference works to reify biomedically grounded conceptions of HIV polarity, reaffirming the idea that gay men's identities and relationships are structured fundamentally around serostatus. *Queer as Folk* illustrates the limitations of the quality TV dramedy format of its time, and its ability to imagine complex social issues, particularly ones that challenge notions of bourgeois personhood, embodiment, sexuality, and relationships under neoliberal conditions. Sero-melodrama, as I've identified it, dramatises the pressures of serodiscordant relationships on these structures. Ultimately, however, it though, releases those pressures in order to find resolution. In so doing, it reaffirms the primary unit of neoliberal gay politics – the monogamous, white, gay male couple. This hints strongly at the limitations of a neoliberal vision of queer life and what it does with HIV. A sentimental privileging of certain cherished structures of kinship and relationality forecloses the possibility of other more complex ones.

And yet, on the other hand, as Kackman says, 'complexity isn't just something we find in a text; it's something we *bring* to a text – and our recognition of certain characters as meaningfully conflicted, their narrative and moral dilemmas agonisingly or beguilingly puzzling, is a cultural identification.'[81] These agonising identifications speak powerfully to what Brooks calls 'the melodramatic imagination,'[82] in which closure is never certain, futures are always haunted by pasts and resolution always amounts to new questions. In the unsatisfying closure to *Queer as Folk*'s drama of sero-difference, new and important questions about the modes of relationality among gay men in the era of post-crisis are raised. What, for example, does it mean that sero-difference gets articulated through the scripts of heteropolarity? What are the implications of this? Is there an alternative way of thinking though the 'problem' of serodifference? And, could an alternative approach to this narrative of difference allow us, in the current moment of the pandemic, to think more imaginatively about the paradoxical space of the HIV infected but perfectly healthy body positive?

Michael's 'perfect, except for one thing' boyfriend, and their 'perfect, except for one thing' relationship are a key instance in post-crisis culture of the historically conditioned tension between the extraordinary and the mundane. Both the PLHIV and the romantic relationship with that person are sites of the narrative extraordinary, but both are ultimately subsumed into the neoliberal quotidian, and never more so than when they are recruited to the ideological priorities of the gay marriage narrative. This narrative demands both the privatisation of the individual's everyday management of HIV and the couple's quiet, domestic administration of the problem of serodiscord. These issues become invisible, personal, managed behind closed doors and drawn curtains where the contradictions of the positive body are politely and discreetly brokered.

In the next chapter I examine a more spectacular example of the extraordinary pole of the post-crisis dialectic: the sex panic surrounding condomless anal sex. In this site of post-crisis representation, the mundane is largely subsumed by spectacle as the subcultural practices of barebacking and chemsex are represented through the metaphors and images of a revivified – albeit somewhat re-invented – style of crisis discourse. In spite of the apparent normality of living with HIV in some quarters, the examples offered in the next chapter suggest that it is still impossible for popular culture not to get dragged back into the spectacular language and the high drama of AIDS panic. Chapter 3 also begins to more explicitly consider the ways in which a 'crisis logic' of gay history – a teleology from liberation to AIDS crisis to the present day – continues to underwrite post-crisis representation.

3

Crisis Re-Runs

Barebacking, Chemsex *and Post-Crisis Sex Panic*

Chemsex

VICE media's 2015 documentary *Chemsex* opens with an ominous image of London at night, then cuts to a full moon in a cloudy sky, then to a dark suburban streetscape, and then to the low-lit interior of an apartment with a close-up on a syringe balanced casually on top of a remote control. 'I'm gonna slam it in a minute,' a guy says. 'I'm pretty much slamming every day, four slams a day… About 400 pounds in a week.' The guy, the first of many 'automethnographers' in this controversial horror–documentary, fixes drugs. In the first of innumerable injecting close ups, we watch him tourniquet his bicep and inject slowly. He sits back into the couch, his eyes widening, his breath increasing. 'See, now all I wanna do it get fucked, have sex, it's crazy.' He starts playing with his crotch. 'Straight away?' asks a voice from off-screen. 'Uh-huh, yeah,' the guy nods, still fondling, 'just, like… cock cock cock cock cock…' He becomes silent, his eyes widen again and he stares vacantly into the camera. In the next cut he is on his mobile phone, using Grindr.

Released at film festivals and through various online streaming platforms internationally throughout 2015 and 2016, *Chemsex* brings audiences into intimate proximity with the 'Party and Play', or 'PnP', scene among gay men in the UK. Straight directors William Fairman and Max Gogarty assembled confessional interviews and actual footage of this 'underground' subculture where men have sex with each other in group or one-on-one settings using methamphetamine, mephedrone, gamma hydroxybutyrate (GHB) and other drugs. These drugs are used as aphrodisiacs, euphoriants, stamina-extending and pleasure-inducing stimulants; they have the potential to make sex feel better and last much longer.

One of the first things we are told in *Chemsex* is that if you start using the mobile hook-up app Grindr, 'within four conversations you are going to be introduced to chemsex, and within eight conversations you are going to get introduced to slamming' (injecting methamphetamine). This is a key premise of the documentary: that the expediency of mobile hook-up apps, combined with the dangers of illicit drug-taking, combined with 'risky' kinds of sex has created 'the perfect storm' for a 'hidden health emergency'. As the film unfolds, a more complex psycho-sociological explanation is developed alongside these technological and biological ones: lonely, alienated gay men, damaged by a culture of shame, homophobia and the relentless fear of HIV that continues to haunt the post-antiretrovirals era, turn to the disinhibition and disassociation induced by synthetic drugs to allay their sexual anxieties and find a sense of connection, community and intimacy. Drug use provides cognitive disengagement from homophobia, rejection, estrangement, bullying, sexual shame, illegality, the fear of and trauma surrounding HIV.

Although it promises to seriously contemplate these moods of shame and anxiety, such aversive feelings about sex and homosexual personhood are very likely also *Chemsex*'s effects. In a review titled 'Seriously Sobering', the *Telegraph* reported that

> many promiscuous gay men would prefer to know they have HIV than worry about getting it. Some even seek it out. This is a reckless strain on national health resources, of course, but should probably be looked at as a form of mental illness – a self-immolation in the most dangerous underground forms of sexual self-expression.[1]

A *news.com.au* article used the full-blown lingua of sex panic: 'hedonistic tempest'; 'reached fever-pitch'; 'a world that is as accessible as it is dangerous'; 'recklessness fuelled by drugs or even an extreme form of masochism';

Crisis Re-Runs: Barebacking, *Chemsex* and Post-Crisis Sex Panic

'the biggest crisis in the gay community in 30 years.'[2] This review exemplified the kind of outraged, distressed and moralistic reaction to the documentary and the colourful language of sex panic accompanying it, a hyperbolic script that is all too familiar to those who have witnessed eruptions of AIDS hysteria over more than three decades.

'Chemsex', 'PnP', 'WiredPlay' and the problematically named 'double epidemic' that links meth use to patterns of HIV notifications are all terms that describe practices in urban gay scenes internationally that have been the object of handwringing, debate and much clinical and sociological research and discussion in recent years. While the publicity surrounding *Chemsex*'s release has tended to confirm the documentary's assertion that this is a largely clandestine, furtive sex and drug subculture, in fact, there has been no shortage of discussions about sex and methamphetamine among gay men for at least the last fifteen years. *Chemsex*, I would suggest, is a fine example of a particular type of epidemic panic genre that has continued to crop up during the era of 'post-crisis', re-booting AIDS crisis anxieties about homosexuality and AIDS alongside other and newer forms of urban and sexual dis-ease.

Chemsex consists of roughly half talking-head confessions from men narrating personal meth stories and half in-situ recording from the chemsex 'underbelly' – footage supplied by participants at PnP parties, hook-ups and elsewhere. It's main editing principle is the montage, with repetitive images of parties, sex, injecting and more sex: blowjobs, buttfucking, group sex, sling sex, gags, collars, harnesses and hoods; dungeons, sex-on-premises venues, private homes and private parties; interviews with men in the midst of meth psychoses or the euphoric throes of having just injected mephedrone; elaborate pre-party planning, parties in full swing; the ritual and paraphernalia of drug use, smoking and snorting and countless close-ups of injecting. The unrestrained gaze, which is consistent with the style of other *VICE* documentary explorations of 'shocking' and 'uncharted' cultural terrain, gives *Chemsex* a licence to showcase more group sex among men than you would ever see outside of gay porn and more drug injecting than you would probably ever see onscreen anywhere.

This visual language bespeaks extreme excess through unprecedented, underground access. It is a kind of gonzo documentary style that deploys the patina of socially engaged and concerned ethnographic realism as a *modus operandi* for the spectacle of unexpurgated visibility. Paradoxically, what is initially framed as thus-far-unseen (the underground chemsex crisis) is revealed to the viewer through a kind of pornographic principle of maximum visibility. If chemsex, as it is implied, were indeed a stealth and un-exposed phenomenon occurring in dark backrooms, here it emerges into well-enough-lit, comprehensive visibility. Real sex and real drug taking are spectacularly documented as a means to circumnavigate what in other contexts might be categorised as 'obscene'. But, unlike porn, *Chemsex*'s voyeuristic titillations are glossed over on the grounds of the brutal seriousness of its subject. The visual conventions of ethnographic realism and the documentary's self-serious, worried mode of address means it may circumvent accusations of exploitative keyhole peering while continuing to deliver an endless spectacle of exceptional sex. This is part of a long history of the fascinated surveillance of modern homosexualities: the formerly 'hidden' practices of outlaw urban sexual subcultures are suddenly available for intense public scrutiny. This history of surveillance also goes somewhere towards accounting for the willingness of the subjects of *Chemsex* to speak openly and at length about their experiences to two straight men with a camera, largely without concealing their identities. As a demographic, gay men are well acquainted with having their curious sex lives scrutinised and surveyed, either informally, in media contexts, or by public health researchers, never more so since the rationale of sexual epidemic and public health have offered an alibi for ensuring these exotic sexual practices are examined, documented, analysed and publicly exposed.

Sex panics tend to involve what Stanley Cohen famously called 'folk devils' – protagonists of a sort; a group that pose a perceived threat to society and may be rendered inhuman in some way. Folk devils are 'social types' that serve as 'visible reminders of what we should not be'.[3] The meth-addled men of *Chemsex* are described by onlookers and participants as 'the walking dead,' an 'emotionless' community and 'possessed', all variations on the old idea of the homosexual as a self-destructive narcissist, rejecting the everyday social norms of work and family and health, pleasuring himself to death. One testimony from a gay sauna owner describes a couple who overdosed on GHB at his venue – one of them

Crisis Re-Runs: Barebacking, *Chemsex* and Post-Crisis Sex Panic

continued looking for sex while his partner was comatose, until he too fell unconscious. Another subject, 'Dick', recalls that his first experience with meth happened while he was tied-up for sex with two strange men he had hooked up with for the first time. Dick claims to have said no to the drugs, but was forcibly injected anyway while he was restrained. A voiceover reports that: 'you can find guys that will poz you up, that will give you HIV. For someone to be willing to give you HIV is such a brutal thing to do… a really extreme form of sadism, and just really extreme masochists will seek out those sadists'.

The chemsex underground is a bottomless pit of these depraved, dehumanised horror stories. Like the gay male PWAs we saw in Chapter 1, these monsters may be allowed to become objects of pity but only once they have dutifully and remorsefully confessed to their ruinous experiences, offering themselves as an object lesson to the spectator. Directors Goggarty and Fairman said of the interviews: 'When we were there listening to these men, they were like confessions, testimonials.'[4] These confessing talking heads describe loneliness and paranoia, struggling to get through the week before the next party, an increased inability to have sex without drugs. They speak of partaking in 'extreme' forms of sex that they would then crave more and more of. One of the subjects, Enrique, resorted to 'selling his body' to support his habit. Dick recounts the intimate disconnection of guys continuing to swipe through Grindr while they are penetrating other guys. Many of the autoethnographers report being diagnosed with HIV. Alongside their tales of bodies degraded, personal and professional lives ruined, risks taken and consequences paid, are the repetitive images of sex and syringe insertion.

Whatever experience you have with injecting, meth or adventurous sex, *Chemsex* is an orgy of emotional triggers. The problem with *Chemsex* is not that the sex itself is explicit or that there's so much of it. It's that the sex is depersonalised, risky, anonymous; it is sex with strangers, in slings, in dark underground places; it is sex combined with drugs and STIs; ruinous sex, sex that leads to more sex, sex that leads to addiction. The nebulous category of 'risky sex' is not really defined, having a kind of obfuscating effect on people's actual understandings and perceptions of risk; 'risky sex' becomes a euphemism for sex that is morally bad and to be avoided, or sex that inevitably leads to HIV seroconversion. The general brand of sex terror offered by *Chemsex* is the one in which sex will ruin your potential to have a normal, healthy body and a normal, healthy life. The documentary offers very little evidence of the way in which people who use hook-up apps to arrange sex and recreational drug users of all kinds may implement thoughtful and effective strategies to prepare themselves, care for themselves and one another, and protect themselves and others from risks of all kinds.[5] Conspicuously absent from *Chemsex* is any mention of PrEP or undetectable viral load, the highly efficacious uses of antiretrovirals as a preventative measure against transmitting HIV.

In spite of the changes wrought by antiretrovirals and other developments, the heady combination of drugs, epidemics and exceptional sex – group sex, anonymous sex, BDSM sex, sauna sex, anal sex – is a recipe for high-anxiety media, and is rarely handled with nuance or particularity in mainstream channels. Like much other media 'exposing' cultures of drug use and adventurous sex among gay men in the era of post-crisis, as we shall see throughout this chapter, *Chemsex* draws on the sensational genres of horror, social moralism and sex panic under the pretext of a generalised social or public 'concern'. The emotions stirred up by this genre are shock, disgust and unease. As we shall see in the rest of this chapter, when it comes to the treatment of gay sex in the contexts of HIV and within the landscape of post-crisis, this is an identifiable and recurrent pattern of representation.[6]

Déjà vu

Going back about a decade before the release of *Chemsex*, a very similar-seeming imperative to expose outré homosexual practices to the limelight of public scrutiny was emerging across mainstream and LGBTQI+ media in response to the controversial practice of deliberately having anal sex without condoms, or 'barebacking.' In Australia in 2007 'barebacking' and the sometimes conflated idea of 'bugchasing' made their first significant appearances in national news media in the coverage of a highly publicised criminal case of the alleged reckless infection of persons with HIV. Although discussions of barebacking had already been taking shape in the local gay community and among ASOs and there had been outbreaks of a global epidemic of barebacking anxiety for some years already, this was the first sustained account of an alleged subculture of men deliberately engaging in condomless anal sex that crossed over into the Australian news mainstream.[7] Unsurprisingly, it was not handled delicately.

At the nucleus of the controversy were the legal hearings of a Melbourne man, Michael John Neal, whom journalists nicknamed 'HIV man', and who was at that time alleged to have knowingly and recklessly attempted to infect at least sixteen men with HIV. The loaded terms, 'barebacking', 'bugchasing' and 'breeding' began cropping up in news reports, features and editorials across print and online media. Journalists correlated these new categories of sexual behaviour with both the heavily contested criminal category of the 'reckless infector' and with a reported twenty-five-year record high in HIV notifications in the Australian state of Victoria, where the Neal case took place. In summary, in the coverage of the Neal hearings the twin notions of reckless or deliberate HIV transmissions and escalating HIV epidemic were collapsed under the signs of 'bareback sex' and 'the barebacker' and delivered through the idiom of sex panic.

Moreover, the panic mobilised around the Neal case and the alleged epidemic of barebacking were controversies around which images from the archive of AIDS crisis discourse were reanimated. Like other chemsex and bareback panics across the Global North, the Australian case illustrates the ways in which earlier images of AIDS and AIDS-riddled homosexualities frequently get dredged up, re-worked and re-distributed in later, post-crisis moments. Much like the anxious images of the PnP 'epidemic' offered in *Chemsex*, the rhetorical inflations around barebacking in the Australian mainstreatm news re-booted the discourses of AIDS crisis, stimulating what I suggest we call a 're-crisis' – a recollection of the heightened feelings and spectacular images associated with AIDS crisis sex panic in aid of newer forms of neoliberal population management that are specific to the social and technological milieu of post-crisis. This involves familiar images that generate reliably familiar feelings, but not without some small but important shifts in representation, meaning and effect.

Researchers across the humanities and social sciences have been observing these phenomena of sex panic for several decades now. Both scholarship and popular commentaries tend to agree that shock, outrage and scandal are commonplace in everyday media.[8] In spite of the sensational, spectacular nature of the idiom, sex scandals, shock journalism and what Janice Irvine calls the 'dramaturgy' of sex panic[9] have become an almost banal, quotidian feature of the competitive news media landscape of twenty-first century life. Anxiety, outrage and disgust are routinely mobilised in response to a large range of phenomenon: paedophilia, pornification, the alleged mistreatment of women in Islamic countries and in demonised migrant communities, the booze-soaked endless spring break of teen hook-up culture, celebrity sex scandals, sex tourism, Tinder, Grindr and other mobile hook-up apps, to note just a handful of prominent and recurrent examples. Bareback and chemsex panics, with their links to epidemic disease, are an exemplary (but also particular) case of this, as we shall see in the remainder of this chapter.

Such eruptions of sex panic have become part of the management of bodies and practices in neoliberal times. HIV and homosexual panics are representative cultural scripts of post-crisis in their capacity to recruit an *extraordinary* set of images to a very *banal*, everyday form of ideological governance. Bareback panic, for example, can be understood as a key part of the system of biopolitical governmentality that Linda Singer calls 'the logic of epidemic',[10] an ideological model of the management of populations whose emergence is consistent with neoliberalism. As Singer's formulation suggests, the feelings (anxiety, repulsion, terror) roused by the rhetorical inflations of sex panic and the subsequent institutional interventions that respond to them (law reform, surveillance, criminalisation, mandatory reporting, quarantines) are disciplinary processes. In the journalism of sex panic, something – barebacking, chemsex and so on – is offered as a spectacular, outré practice and a danger to the community, calling for regulatory intervention. Extending Singer's model to apply to developments in the era of post-crisis, I suggest that we can understand the *recollection of AIDS crisis*, or 're-crisis' for short, as a new addition to this familiar ideological process. In other words, the legacy or memory of earlier representations of AIDS and the attendant feelings these memories arouse become an important part of the feelings mobilised in this new cultural moment. A 're-crisis' relies on memories and strategies of the past, revivifying old stories and images in the service of new cultural and biopolitical conditions – conditions that continue to reinforce the shift from public health models of managing HIV toward individualised, self-responsible, neoliberal ones: an 'increasing enthusiasm for criminal prosecution', 'escalating styles of social government' and the 'undermining of collective responsibility, social support and education.'[11]

In a broader cultural and media landscape where the sense of crisis around HIV/AIDS has well and truly waned, the potential for sudden eruptions of panic concentrated around 'viral sex'[12] suggests that the state of crisis originally associated with HIV/AIDS has, to some extent, become both quotidian and chronic. These extraordinary eruptions and their incorporation into the fabric of the everyday is a clear example of the dialectic of post-crisis culture that, as I have been arguing, underwrites the period after antiretrovirals: homosexuality and HIV/AIDS are signifiers whose functions are at once both extraordinary and mundane at the same time.

The remainder of this chapter focuses specifically on the example of the Neal hearings, happening as they did during a key moment in the eruption of bareback panic. In this example, sex panic scripts assembled a subculture of sexual outlaws or folk devils, siphoning off the once-illicit aspects of homosexuality into the new identities of 'barebacker', 'bugchaser' and 'breeder'. This reflects a broader, ongoing tendency in both mainstream and queer media to distinguish between responsible 'good' gay citizens and reckless 'bad' queers, a hierarchical distinction that is in part an effect of neoliberal styles of the management and representation of responsibility and safer sex and a legacy of the discourses of AIDS crisis. In this chapter's conclusion I will briefly consider the role that stories about the gay and AIDS past plays in these configurations, a consideration of how post-crisis culture narrates its history that I take up more seriously in the final two chapters of this book. Briefly, however, before we turn to the Neal case, some necessary background on the emergence of meanings and discussions associated with the post-crisis phenomenon of 'barebacking'.

What is Barebacking?

When used consistently and correctly, condoms are a highly effective means of preventing the transmission of HIV. Once discovered, this fact was at the heart of early HIV prevention efforts and it was game-changing: the effective dissemination of the 'condom code' helped to rapidly and dramatically reduce HIV notifications during the 1980s and early 1990s. Though condoms remain a mainstay of HIV prevention, they are now one among a growing list of prophylactic technologies including serosorting, strategic positioning, undetectable viral load, abstinence and recently pre-exposure prophylaxis (PrEP, often known by its drug name 'Truvada'), the success of which has rapidly altered the politics and practices of HIV prevention among gay men in the developed world.

Since the emergence of the latex paradigm and its swift naturalisation as a potentially *moral* as well as a behavioural norm within gay male communities, the practice – indeed, the very idea – of anal sex between men without condoms has been steeped in the semantics of scare. Though the meanings of an HIV diagnosis have shifted dramatically, from death sentence to manageable condition, the idea of seroconversion remains, as clinical psychoanalyst J. P. Cheuvront puts it, something that 'scare[s] up feelings of sadness, loss, anger, dread, guilt, and hopelessness.'[13] So, like chemsex, sex without condoms or 'barebacking', once named, quickly became the subject of the type of excited discussion and public anxiety that cultural historians and queer theorists call sex panic. What follows is a potted history of this term and its journey into a lexicon of sex panic. As well as a locus of anxiety, barebacking also became something of a generative entry point for investigating the meanings of HIV and male homosexuality in the period after antiretrovirals and thus became of particular interest to health and social science researchers and commentators. Moreover – and importantly – the languages, ritual and images that barebackers themselves have invented for thinking and talking about anal sex without latex include many positive, innovative and life-affirming signifiers of subculture, identity, intimacy, pleasure and fantasy.[14] As I discussed in the Introduction, anal eroticism among men is an entrenched sexual taboo. Already overburdened with a long cultural history of unspeakable, abject, identity-spoiling and identity-constituting meanings, in the age of HIV/AIDS, anal sex became an even more over-determined signifier of both sexual risk and sexual *jouissance*. Both the anxious and the affirmational representations of barebacking that have now emerged over the past two decades have only added to the complex repository of meanings surrounding this sexual practice.

Although men have doubtlessly had sex without condoms throughout the age of HIV, barebacking became a visible practice after the advent of

Crisis Re-Runs: Barebacking, *Chemsex* and Post-Crisis Sex Panic

antiretroviral treatments circa 1996, amidst the transformed perceptions of HIV infection they brought about. Anal sex taboos long predate HIV/AIDS, but the *frisson* of the term 'barebacking' is specific to the history of the pandemic, most particularly so to the period after antiretrovirals. It is the fusion of condomless anal sex with the twin notions of *wilful intention* and the potential risk of exposure to HIV that initially made the term meaningful (although, importantly, these meanings have again shifted with the introduction of PrEP). Despite this historically specific emergence of the term, the meaning of 'barebacking' has rarely been straightforward and there have been intricate debates surrounding its definition that themselves could fill several volumes. Although an encyclopedia would be needed to cover this literature, a brief overview of these discussions will help here to understand the misrepresentations that have emerged in the sex panics surrounding this sexual practice.

The term 'barebacking' comes from the equestrian world where barebacking refers to horseriding unsaddled, a practice associated with experienced horsemanship and an enhanced riding pleasure derived from the added thrill of an increased risk of injury. The added sexual proficiency implied by the term is a point not often mentioned: barebackers are better, more experienced riders. The equine context of the term also has potent masculine overtones. The horse as an image of male sexual potency is an old symbol in western culture and remains pervasive in the vernaculars used to describe masculine sexualities: 'stud', 'stallion', 'hung like a horse'. 'Bareback' also dips into the repository of masculine images and archetypes associated with horse handling: herdsmen, cowboys and rodeo riders. This is especially so in the US context from which the term first emerged, where such images are part of a broader national iconography. As the pioneering bareback porn director Paul Morris of Treasure Island Media has explained, 'the term itself, with its horsey allusion links to the same American mythic construct that, say, the Marlboro man is meant to connect with and exploit.[15] In his 'risk manifesto', 'No Limits', delivered at the world pornography congress in 1998, Morris identified a strain of adventurousness and risk-taking among US men involved in barebacking subcultures that he suggested might be connected to a 'national character' of experimentation and thrill-seeking.[16] These connotations give the emergence of the term a particularly American cultural slant – and likewise, they indicate why in other parts of the world, the term has sometimes had different connotations.[17]

Defining what is and what isn't barebacking has been fraught and rarely free of moral adjudications. Although we may start, as Mark J. Blechner writes, with a definition of barebacking as referring to 'unprotected anal intercourse between gay men, in a context in which there is some danger of HIV-infection', definitions have rarely been so straightforward. The variety of situations in which anal sex without condoms occurs are situations where the risk of HIV exposure varies from significant to fractional to non-existent. Nonetheless, as Blechner elaborates, 'in the near-panic atmosphere that has surrounded the AIDS epidemic, it has not always been specified precisely when anal intercourse without a condom is most dangerous and when it is most safe.'[18]

In aid of a more nuanced discussion, Benjamin Junge[19] proposed six axes around which variations of the term bareback can play out. These axes include: *intention* (i.e. does barebacking denote any anal sex without condoms or does it only describe the conscious discarding of them?); *consensus* among partners (did they all agree to condomless sex?); the *serostatus* of the partners (are they all negative? both positive? sero-discordant?); the distinction between *fantasy and practice*[20]; and, the distinction or lack of distinction between sexual *practices* and sexual *identities*. The latter draws attention to the tendency to slip between talking about bareback*ing* to talking about bareback*ers*, a problematic slippage that bedevils these discussions in spite of decades of efforts by HIV educators to transform representations of sexual risk from a characterological model ('risky persons' or 'groups') to a behavioural model ('risky practices'). The elusive categories of behaviour and affect render the task of defining barebacking even more complex, as Donna M. Orange has argued. Risk-taking, she writes, is not a 'behaviour' at all but the 'property of a relational system'.[21] Risk-taking isn't a discrete 'conceptual atom' available for isolated empirical analysis, but rather the upshot and the agent of dynamic historical, technological and interpersonal contexts.

A revealing example of when this terminology becomes subject to moral adjudications is, as Race points out, when behaviour labeled 'barebacking' is in fact (or also) 'serosorting.'[22] Serosorting describes a practice in which individuals pursue sex with partners who are of the same known

Crisis Re-Runs: Barebacking, *Chemsex* and Post-Crisis Sex Panic

HIV status as themselves, and it is widely recognised as an effective mode of HIV risk reduction. But, both 'serosorting' and 'barebacking' may be sex acts that deliberately eschew condoms. The significantly different connotations of the terms are telling. As Race explains, 'the valorisation of serosorting… rests on the ultimate erasure of gay anal sex as well as an invocation of matrimonial norms.'[23] For the serosorted (and perhaps even monogamous) sexual couple, not using condoms may be a mundane, normative 'safe' sex practice; in other contexts, 'barebacking' is considered a dangerous scandal. The semiotic distinction here reminds us that labels and categories have affective and material implications, and often work to distinguish between types of sexual personae and practices positioned on a hierarchical spectrum of risk, normativity and responsibility. In other words, labels have reality effects, and the prudent conjugal couple are almost always positioned at the centre of the 'charmed circle'[24] of sexual respectability.

Why do they do it? Just as quickly as the scandalised public reactions to barebacking emerged, the sexual riddle thrown up around the question of why healthy, informed men would knowingly risk exposing themselves and their partners to HIV, drove researchers across the social sciences, public health and HIV fraternities into the field in search of answers. This is partly because, as a topic for researchers, barebacking offers various titillations: it is provocative, sexy and troubling all at once; it presents thorny moral, ideological and methodological questions[25] that arise both from a long history of moral, medical, scientific, ethnographic and sexological inquiries into the 'strange' sexual practices of homosexuals and other deviant minorities alongside specific somatechnical issues that have developed in response to advances in HIV prevention and other technologies including the universe of digital communication. The vast literature of accounts seeking to *explain* barebacking, including research, policy and practical interventions, is itself something of a 'viral' phenomenon.

Within this discursive field, some material could be considered a kind of neo-sexology – a contemporary iteration of the nineteenth century scientific 'sex talk' identified by Foucault in *The History of Sexuality*.[26] The taxonomising, pathologising approaches of classical nineteenth century sexology was one of the key disciplines Foucault identified in the '*scientia sexualis*', 'the machinery of power' underwriting the modern system of sex. Classical sexology was particularly focused on 'dysfunctions' and 'variations' of sexual behaviour, bringing aberrance into increased visibility and specificity. Though contemporary sex researchers may offer more nuanced and considered accounts than, say, sex panic journalism, we are all implicated in the burgeoning definitions and understandings of sexuality that emerge from its discussion – and, concomitantly, the ways the sexual body is disciplined and managed. The scientific and media fascination with barebacking is a good example of the way in which, as Adam writes, 'AIDS has ushered in a further development of sexual speech which cannot but partake of the larger twentieth century "obsession" with sexuality and its colonising by the professions, the media and the state.'[27] This professional, socio-scientific engagement can also contribute to the pathologisation of homosexuality. As Gregory Tomso has pointed out, accounts of barebacking from pop journalism to qualitative social research have conventionally been organised around the question 'What makes them do it?'[28] Why do men who are aware of the potential risks they may be exposed to continue to fuck without condoms? While answers to this question are as manifold as the definitions of 'bareback' are varied, the epistemological framing of the question remains the same: asking 'why do they do it?' begins from the presumption that barebacking is a problem or a mystery in need of resolving. The question, Dean argues, 'proceeds from the assumption that if we can understand the forces prompting such risky behaviour, then we might be able to curtail it; in other words, it is assumed from the outset that barebacking is pathological.'[29] Wherever condomless anal sex is approached as an epidemiological, cultural or psychological riddle to be solved, the imprimatur of sexology is discernible.

Some studies of barebacking have been remarkably pathologising. For example, Moskowitz and Roloff reported 'the results of a study that casts bug chasing as symptomatic of sexual addiction';[30] they found that 'bug chasers are suffering at the most severe level.'[31] Similarly, Tewksbury, in the journal *Deviant Behaviour*, claimed to have provided 'the most complete profile of bug givers and bug chasers to date.'[32] The function of such profiling remains questionable, although it does illustrate an enduring scientific desire to code and organise aberrant bodies and behaviours.

However, beyond such studies, which arguably codify certain sex practices as aberrant, there is a genuinely diverse range of accounts of barebacking, many of which offer larger insights into gay men's history and sexual culture in the wake of HIV/AIDS. I will briefly consider a small selection of key themes operating across these accounts.

First, there are epidemiological and technological accounts of barebacking – post-crisis era developments in the management, treatment and perception of HIV/AIDS that are factors often called upon to explain a decrease in the use of condoms. The 'protease disinhibition hypothesis' was one of the first of such explanations, linking the advent of ARVs to the recorded increase in condomless sex. The idea here is that a new rationale for abandoning condoms may lie in the presumption that HIV, if acquired, is a 'manageable condition.'[33] Sociological research has backed this up, though in more nuanced ways: ARVs have indeed 'provided the conditions of emergence of a *partial* revaluation of risk among some gay men.'[34] Also from early on in these discussions, there emerged the notions of 'complacency' and a 'safe sex fatigue' that was somehow inevitable with the passing of time, and health promoters and ASOs were charged with failing to anticipate this and adapt accordingly. It was alleged by some that these agencies continued to flog a dogmatic condom code that increasingly appeared simplistic, patronising and absolutist, and that had lost its ability to account for the myriad sexual possibilities described above in which condoms may or may not necessarily figure. It is worth noting that a knee-jerk tendency to blame some group or agency is a common feature of sex panic and, in addition to gay men themselves, health, community and government agencies are not immune to such charges of culpability.

Increasingly, researchers have also considered the central role played by digital technologies alongside prophylactic and pharmaceutical ones. Mowlabocus, for one, argues that to bareback is to 'tacitly acknowledge the central role digital media technologies play with the pursuit, negotiation and performance of this kind of sex.'[35] As he argues, barebacking is to some extent unimaginable outside of the digital technologies that facilitate and sustain contemporary sexual sociality among men who have sex with men.

Alongside these techno-epidemiological explanations, there are a number of psycho-social accounts that explain the disregarding of condoms as the effect of a 'mangled social identity.' For example, US clinical psychologist Walt Odets argues that the media's oscillation between hysteria and silence over anal sex is the effect of a broader homophobic, sexnegative culture, and that barebacking in casual scenarios is a symptom of the internalisation of that culture's values.[36] Similar to the explanations offered for meth use in the *Chemsex* documentary, in these accounts barebacking is seen as a symptom of gay men's problematic socialisation in a homophobic society alongside the historical trauma of HIV/AIDS. Eric Rofes exemplifies this explanation with a cultural and historical argument that contemporary gay male lives need to be understood in the context of cumulative historical trauma, equating AIDS to the holocaust and the bombings of Nagasaki and Hiroshima.[37]

Such accounts might also be seen as examples of a school of thought that views anal sex without condoms as a form of symbolic cultural and/or psychic resistance to social and sexual norms, a form of conscious or unconscious sexual transgression. As Oliver Davis writes, barebacking 'evidently marks a certain distance from socially entrenched heteronormative ways of understanding futurity and kinship'.[38] Taking this line more explicitly, Crossley has argued that wilfully disregarding condoms is a transgression of mainstream culture's sexual mores, including the dominance of safer sex as a presumed norm of gay male sexual practice. Such transgressions have a history for queer people, and Crossley, drawing on French sociologist Pierre Bourdieu's concept of the 'habitus' (embodied practices functioning below the threshold of consciousness),[39] traces what she calls a 'transgressive habitus' back to the sexual values of gay liberation. Gay men as a social group, she argues, have historically forged identities tied to sexual transgression and these are core identarian practices. In other words, these practices are so entrenched in gay male identity that we are unable to let go of them, even when ours or someone else's health may be at risk. More broadly, if 'health' has a moral and ideological character because of its ties to 'good', 'correct' and 'responsible' personhood, the 'flip side' of this is that certain 'values and meanings' may become attached to '"unhealthy" and "risky" behaviours'; '"[o]pposing behaviours", like non-exercise, unsafe sex, eating junk food, drinking heavily, smoking, using drugs... may take on a certain *cachet* and value of their own.'[40] Individuals may not even be conscious of the 'latent emotional, social, cultural and value-laden meanings' of risky behaviours,[41] and their capacity to stir a 'psychological "feeling" of rebellion against dominant social values, which, in turn creates a sense of freedom, independence and protest.'[42] For gay men, since the period of gay liberation, sexual transgression has apparently become a key practice in a repertoire of identity practices and so the rejection of condoms is 'just one contemporary manifestation of such "habitual embodied" resistance.'[43]

I would call accounts such as Crossley's a 'resistance hypothesis'. In such an explanation, barebacking offers feelings of resistance to moral personhood, ideological good and the wholesome mainstreaming of safer sex. Sheon and Plant provided a useful early summary of the resistance hypothesis:

> Ironically the attention focused on anal sex as a risk activity has given it *even more symbolic meaning* as an act of *profound intimacy* or even *rebellion*. *This problem* is only compounded when the target population is one that *already sees its identity as a community tied to a recently acquired sexual liberation*.... This experimentation has always existed under the threat of sanction from powerful institutions such as the police, the church, schools, and the family. Barebacking can thus be seen as merely the latest in a long line of challenges by gay men to the sexual status quo and the institutions which support it. Attempts to 'manage desire', whether they originate from within or without the gay community, tend to produce 'transgressive desire', a fetishising of certain acts because they are dangerous, stigmatised, and emotionally charged.[44]

I have quoted Sheon and Plant at length because this early account of a resistance hypothesis highlights four key elements that have underpinned discussions of barebacking:

(1) it foregrounds the increased cultural fascination with – and overdetermination of – the meanings of anal sex since the advent of HIV/AIDS, which strengthened the association between anality and death, but also, paradoxically, stirred up a further politicisation of anality;
(2) it identifies the charged exchange of bodily fluids, namely semen, as another symbolically inflected sexual act;
(3) it identifies gay men as a marginalised community with a legacy of resistance to conventional (hetero)normative (sexual) cultures; and
(4) it highlights a 'recently acquired sexual liberation' as a key historical development in this heritage.

Ideas about the role of history are important here: a somewhat fixed idea of gay liberation as a watershed moment for key sexual practices is offered, albeit within a longer history ('a long line of challenges') of resisting 'the status quo and the institutions which support it.'[45]

While I recognise the importance of considering history and culture in these accounts, a psycho-social and historical account of sexual transgression is still at risk of trading in the logic of pathology, albeit a less medicalised version of that logic. If practices like meth use and deliberate exposure to HIV are considered 'coping mechanisms'[46] or identity practices in the context of societal homophobia, the norms of dominant culture (including dominant gay culture) and AIDS trauma, then barebacking may be viewed as a sort of historically and culturally derived sickness. While historical approaches indeed have their fruitful implications, especially in their turn to the subjective meanings in gay men's accounts of their own sex lives, the resistance model is also in danger of using history to *diagnose* barebacking as the most recent manifestation of a trans-historical 'habitus' of rebellion among gay men. The idea of a 'barebacking backlash' comes to look very much like the return of a repressed gay male psychopathology, but rendered in narrative and historical terms, with the trope of inexorable return as its organising logic. Homosexuality still tends to emerge from this analysis as pathologically transgressional ('it is subconscious'; 'they cannot control themselves').

In the discourse of sex panic around barebacking, gay liberation and AIDS Crisis histories return to haunt the post-crisis present like a pop psychology version of Freud's return of the repressed. Crossley's idea of 'transgressional habitus', for example, understands history as the chronicle of a pendulum swinging between the pleasure principle and a moral, rational sexual ethics. To quote her at more length:

> During the 'pre-AIDS' era, responding to threats imposed by dominant prejudices relating to homosexuality, 'promiscuous sex and sexuality' were advocated… as 'all good' with no space for criticism. During the AIDS era, existing in death infused environments, many gay men swung to the other side of the pendulum, experiencing a devastating lack of safety and loss of a sexual identity…. And then, 'post-AIDS', as a response to the depression and internalised stigmatisation of the AIDS era, a

renewed vigour is experienced, as activists… reinvoke a commitment to the 'pleasure principle' and the valued 'good' of a previous era. Here, it is possible to see the paranoid-schizoid pendulum swing back once more.[47]

For Crossley, the culture at the core of the problem is not a broader homophobic or heteronormative culture, but the already degraded, impersonal sociality of gay culture, engendered particularly by the sexual practices attributed to liberation (bathhouses, beats, unbridled sex, multiple partners and open relationships). This perverse history, congealed as a 'sexual habitus', has incubated a class of gay men acting out unconsciously anarchic, rebellious behaviour, a refusal of ethical sexual responsibility in favour of a culture of impersonal promiscuity and dangerous stranger sociality. Barebacking becomes, in Shernoff's brief but cogent summary of Crossley's work, 'a current manifestation of gay men's need to hold onto the transgressional aspects of their outlaw sexuality.'[48] History becomes the paradigm through which a negative evaluation of contemporary sexual 'problems' takes place. History is used to account for the meanings of certain sexual practices, and that history itself is tainted with irrationality and pathology.

A more complex, queer analysis of barebacking-as-sexual-resistance would expand the purview from a narrow perspective on an allegedly transgressive subculture to a more universal context that includes heterosexuality and heterosexual masculinities.[49] Adam, for one, positions dominant and mainstream ideologies centrally when he argues that the languages used by barebackers in in-depth interviews 'adapt some of the major tenets of neoliberal ideology by combining notions of informed consent, contractual interaction, free market choice, and responsibility in new ways.'[50] Other researchers have focused on masculinity norms. Alex Carballo-Diéguez, for example, reported that barebackers described condomless anal sex as 'the essence of masculine, aggressive, hot wonderful sex' and the only kind of sex 'real men' have.[51] Michael Graydon's study of online bugchasing and giftgiving discourses found giftgivers portrayed as 'masculine, powerful and giving', and bugchasers as 'feminised, voracious and needy.'[52] Ridge found that individuals' accounts tended to be 'brimming with masculinised meanings': 'experimentation, initiation… not being a "sissy", "letting go", the smell of sweat, "rough" sex play, wrestling, and muscles grinding'.[53] Barebacking sociology has thus been a productive site for examining gendered and sexual signifying systems among MSM. Dowsett et al.'s work found a complex recalibration of masculinities and endless possibilities for 'doing gay' in the online world of popular bareback sites.[54] They call for a rethinking of 'how gender and sexuality intersect' based on the variety of gendered orientations their research uncovered – orientations that include the (re)construction of gay men's subjectivity in terms of the desiring anus, models of relationality that are not 'easily mapped onto heteronormative expectations', and the decentering of the penis.[55] Byron Lee's analysis of bareback pornographies argues for a similar kind of reconstruction of gender, in which recognisable forms of masculinity are 'queerly articulated' and a 'queer erotics' are developed through the conventional frames of normative masculinity.[56]

Radical theoretical interpretations of barebacking have also been offered from queer, psychoanalytic and biopolitical perspectives, where barebacking has become a complex topos for a rejuvenated exploration of theories of sexuality and sexual relationality. With or without the presence of HIV, anal sex without condoms emerges from these readings as a life-oriented and meaning-saturated practice: a survival mechanism; a key ritual in the reproduction of gay male subcultures through viral consanguinity;[57] part of the queer psychological work of abjection;[58] a recalibration of masculinities;[59] and a resistance to the dominant meanings of life itself in neoliberal society.[60]

As something of a 'topic du jour' in health and social sciences, queer masculinity studies and sexuality studies, barebacking has inspired an extremely broad range of accounts. The quantity and variety of interpretations themselves are, as I noted earlier, something of a viral phenomenon – another epidemic of signification and knowledge production. Much has been productive about these conversations, however, at the same time, these research-based and analytical discussions can't be entirely separated from the emergence of sex panic. The two are coterminous, as Adam writes: the emergence of barebacking sex in the media as a scandal is partly what has 'sent researchers into the field in search of new impairments and pathologies to explain this ostensibly irrational behavior.'[61] These socio-sexological and research accounts aren't part of the purview of popular culture, which is the primary focus of this book's interest, but I have diverged into an overview of them here because they are in dialogue with sex panic discourses in interesting and important ways, as we shall now see.

The Neal Hearings

In Australia in March 2007, 48-year-old Michael John Neal went before the Victorian magistrate's court facing charges of attempting to infect at least sixteen men with HIV between 2000 and 2006 while he was subject to Department of Human Services orders not to engage in unprotected sex or attend any public places where men have sex with men.[62] Neal was charged with attempting to infect a person with a serious disease, intentionally infecting a person, rape, reckless conduct and possession of child pornography.[63] He allegedly had unprotected sex with 200 men in one year.[64] Journalists covering the hearings also noted that increases in HIV notifications were at a 20-year record high in the state of Victoria. In one article, the 17 per cent increase from the previous year was mentioned just after a witnesses' testimony at the hearing that Neal had targeted teenage boys in toilet blocks in order to 'breed' them.[65] Such was the logic throughout the coverage: reckless infection and Victoria's escalation in HIV notifications were repeatedly connected,[66] establishing a cause-and-effect logic in which deliberate condomless sex was responsible for increasing rates of HIV.[67] But this was not all.

Barebacking and breeding were also associated with the idea of recruitment. At the first committal hearing, prosecutor Mark Rochford reportedly said that 'in conversations and other material Mr. Neal has demonstrated an intention to infect people with HIV'; ' "He indicated", the Prosecutor continued, "that his reasons for doing that is for more people [to be] introduced to a particular group of HIV-infected persons actively participating in unprotected, or "bareback"… sex.' Neal allegedly held 'conversion parties' where he offered methamphetamine to HIV-negative men who were 'targeted for deliberate sero-conversion.'[68] 'Deadly Party Game' reported that 'an HIV positive man organised sex orgies known as "conversion parties" where gay men would be recruited and deliberately infected with the deadly disease'; 'Mr. Neal also bragged about "making 75 people pos" and referred to one lover as "Daddy's little pos boy".' Neither of these reports explained that HIV is not 'deadly'. Using the online name 'filth pig Melbourne', Neal 'lured men on gay websites', he 'was a regular at several Melbourne gay "sex-on-site" venues [...] and was involved in a lifestyle of sexual deviance, rampant drug use and sexual maliciousness.'[69] The coverage reported a witness' testimony that Neal had hosted a conversion party at which 'a 15-year-old boy was injected with crystal methamphetamine and then "bred" by about fifteen HIV-positive men'.[70]

This mainstream public debut of the concept of barebacking associated it closely with the concept of 'breeding' (deliberately transmitting HIV) and 'bug chasing' (deliberately exposing oneself to potential HIV infection). The *Herald Sun*, one of Australia's then most widely circulated tabloid newspapers, ran the testimony of a former of Neal's lovers that presented the first 'bugchaser' as a speaking, confessing subject. 'HIV Infection Fantasies' reported that

> a gay man has admitted in court [to] harbouring fantasies about becoming HIV positive, years before he was diagnosed with the virus... '[T]he fantasy) was intermittent. Most of the time I had a rational approach to remaining (HIV) negative and at other times I had other inclinations,' the man told the court....
> 'I didn't set out to become HIV positive but my will to remain (HIV) negative had lapsed on some occasions.'[71]

The man admitted to having unprotected sex with Neal in moments of 'passion and intoxication' but didn't blame Neal for exposing him to HIV, saying 'anything I did with the defendant at any time was consensual'. He added that there were HIV negative men in the gay community dubbed 'bug chasers' who actively set out to become infected 'so they could indulge in sex with other infected men without fear of catching the virus.'[72] Another of Neal's male lovers testified that 'Neal looked triumphant when he asked him how it felt to "take a big pos load" when they had unprotected sex in 2000'; '"There was absolutely nothing arousing or erotic about what he said. It was more a statement of violence", the witness said.'[73] In week two of the hearings, another of Neal's partners testified that he had been registered with the local council as a dog as a sign of commitment in their master-slave relationship. The man reported being tricked by Neal who assured him he couldn't transmit HIV because of his low viral load levels.[74]

During the hearings the court also heard that Neal used ropes, slings, snooker and golf balls and pegs during sex.[75] He allegedly wore a 'genital meat grinder' – a large penis piercing – in order to damage his partners' tissue and thus increase the likelihood of HIV transmission when they had sex.[76] Neal admitted to possessing child pornography, saying it reminded him of his days in an orphanage.[77] A tendered report from a psychiatrist testified that Neal was 'the most evil man' he had seen 'in 20 years'.[78] The court heard that Neal himself contracted HIV deliberately by having sex on the altar of a Catholic Church with two men he knew were HIV positive.[79]

By the end of March 2007, magistrate Peter Reardon ruled that there was sufficient evidence for a jury to possibly convict Neal of 106 charges and he was committed to stand trial in the Victorian county court in June 2008. When Neal was brought to trial in June/July 2008, the jury found him guilty on fifteen counts, including nine of attempting to infect a person with HIV, two of rape, three of reckless conduct endangering a person and one of procuring sex by fraud. In October 2008, Neal was sentenced to eighteen years and nine months jail with a non-parole period of thirteen years.

'HIV Man'

The portrait of the man that emerged from the coverage of the hearings was lurid indeed. Michael Neal materialised as a kind of monstrous, hybrid type of sex offender – a polymorphous composite of other deviant and criminal personae including drug addict and supplier, paedophile, rapist, S/M practitioner and reckless infector. Because Neal was identified as a father and grandfather, and because of the recurring trope of youth recruitment, there was a strong whiff of intergenerational sex surrounding the case. Bisexuality as a vector of disease (its 'crossing over' from the homosexual to the heterosexual community) has a potent history in AIDS discourses. While it is not clear whether Neal identified as bisexual, the intimation of bisexuality and intergenerational desire made Neal seem omnivorous and a contaminating threat beyond the homosexual community. The coverage also presented someone insidiously mobile: Neal had two houses, attended nightclubs and sex-on-premises venues and prowled the viral, impossible-to-police realms of the internet. His Gaydar profile photo (see Figure 3.1)

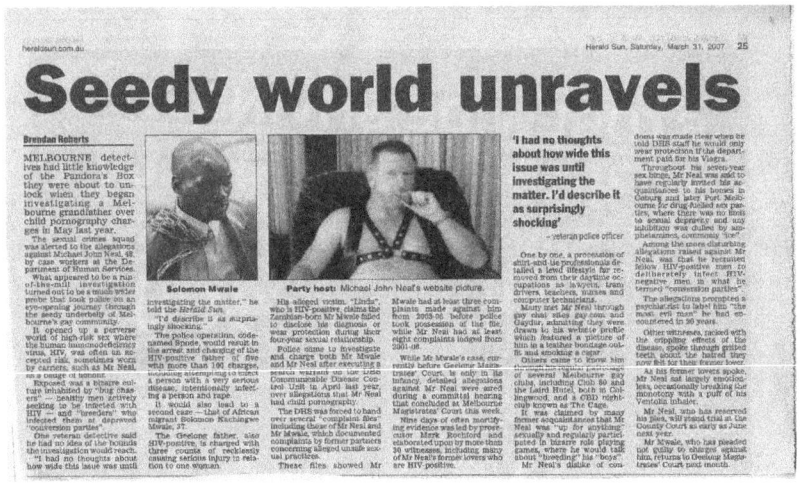

Figure 3.1 'Seedy World Unravels', *Herald Sun*, 31 March 2007

functioned in the coverage as a kind of self-produced mug shot, like an illustrative image from colonial anthropology or criminology.

Organising these disparate deviant and criminal tropes and types into a semi-unified whole is the category of the 'AIDS Monster', a spectacular figure who has moved beyond the pale of 'quotidian sex crime' into the exceptional cultural space reserved for monstrosity. Neal's much-fixated upon ability to have sex with hundreds of partners and to seduce men into subordinate roles in BDSM relationships suggests a charismatic, almost mind-controlling power. The recurring use of the moniker 'HIV man' throughout the coverage gestures to the desire to personify HIV – attach it to a single person or type. This of course recalls the story of 'Patient Zero', the original reckless, deliberate 'superspreader' of AIDS popularised by Randy Shilts' 1987 book *And the Band Played On*, as discussed in the Introduction. In journalistic and fictional crime genres, abstract monikers are often used to describe serial killers, child abductors, sex criminals and other menaces to society. Origin stories and superspreader mythologies are common in cultural storytelling around epidemic disease.[80] In some cases, like organised crime, sex and drug epidemics, an individual genius or sociopath is imagined to be the central architect of social dis-ease, despite the fact that these phenomena can never be reduced to the machinations of a single individual. This 'supervillain' fantasy is evident in the psychiatrist's description of Neal as the 'most evil' man he had seen 'in 20 years' and an *Age* article that expressed the desire for a straightforward resolution to the problem of sexually transmitted disease implied by this fantasy: 'Lock him up'.

In *Notorious H.I.V* (2004), Thomas Shevory examines the media of moral panic surrounding the 1997 case of African American man Nushawn Williams who allegedly perpetrated reckless transmissions of HIV in heterosexual encounters. In contrast to the Neal coverage – in which Neal's whiteness remained uncommented on – the Williams case demonstrates the extent to which epidemic sex panics are produced through racialised frames. Beyond this key difference, the Williams case sheds some useful light on the production of the 'AIDS predator'[81] in the Neal case: the transformation of a 'real life' alleged criminal into an imagined monster. The exaggerations and distortions that riddled the coverage of the Williams case, Shevory argues, served the political purposes of producing representations that helped to foster the passage of HIV-transmission statutes, criminalising what had been previously handled as an issue of public health. Shevory's analysis demonstrates how the media transformation of an alleged criminal like Williams into an 'AIDS Monster' de-humanises the individual in order to enhance the atmosphere of anxiety and threat surrounding the case.

How and why does the alleged reckless infector cross over into the special realm of monstrosity, and what role does HIV/AIDS play in that transformation? As we saw in the Introduction, early AIDS representations borrowed from Gothic literary conventions, *fin-de-siècle* monsters and vampires of the Decadent novel. Images of gay male PWA, as they were called at that time, drew from a historical archive that included the decadent anti-hero of Oscar Wilde's *The Picture of Dorian Gray* and the portrayal of Neal recalls these 'Dorianesque' characteristics: drugs narratives, violence, perverse sex and other identity-spoiling vice; an unfixed gender-of-object-choice; intergenerational sexual relations; super-human promiscuity; irresistible powers of seduction; and a complete abandonment of the moral self to the pleasure principle in spite of the potentially homicidal effects of that recklessness. Neal's lovers' testimonies invoke the seductive, lascivious vampire, a figure with the capacity to blur the paradigm of criminal/victim by refiguring the latter as unable or unwilling to resist (Neal's partners exposed themselves to him/HIV consensually). Indeed, much like the *Chemsex* documentary, the Neal media spectacle recalls Hanson's critique of AIDS crisis media as a discourse peopled with 'spectacular images of the abject' and a 'late Victorian vampirism': gay men represented as 'sexually exotic, alien, unnatural, oral, anal, compulsive, violent, polymorphic, polysemous, invisible, soulless, superhumanly mobile, infectious, murderous [and] suicidal.'[82] Not only does Neal move between places, persons, generations and sexual categories, but because of the advent of ARVs, *he does not die*. The extended temporal horizon of HIV brought about by medical technologies helps to revive the vampire metaphor – the idea of death inhabiting life.

As a type of folk devil, then, the AIDS Monster has also undergone important historical shifts, which offer telling revelations about the scene of post-crisis. Between Patient Zero/Gaëtan Dugas and HIV Man/Michael Neal there are significant differences. While Dugas had only limited knowledge of the 'gay cancer' he, according to myth, was deliberately spreading, the conversion-party hosting, methamphetamine-pushing, genital meat grinder-wearing Neal is fully aware of HIV and how to enhance the chances of its potential transmission, innovating opportunities to expose his partners to it. The coverage presents him as a sort of HIV 'mastermind', confusing his lovers with the then emergent concept of undetectable viral levels. There is also something of a subtle masculinisation in the comparison of Dugas and Neal: Neal is resolutely HIV *man* rather than the feminised 'patient' of Patient Zero.

Perhaps even more significantly, the knowledge that many of Neal's partners consented to condomless sex in full awareness of his HIV status, and with an understanding of HIV (as opposed to the ignorance of many men who were exposed in the very early days of HIV/AIDS), enhances the sense that gay men are inherent masochists, lusting for self-annihilation. While the crisis-era concept of 'AIDS victims' rendered PLWHA as objects available for the pity of onlookers (passive and lacking in agency), today these gay men who had consensual relations with Neal and other HIV positive men are no longer 'victims' in the crimino-legal and epidemiologic sense. In other words, we cannot pity them when they should be responsible, informed sexual actors. The coverage of the Neal hearings resurrected images from the AIDS crisis archive, but in ways that are a more specifically instructional object lesson for gay men: barebackers and breeders – intentional transmitters – are criminals as well as pathetic victims.

The AIDS monster has an entourage of deviants. The coverage of the Neal hearings gave way to the discussion of a seedy underworld, a subculture of reckless barebackers, suicidal bugchasers, murderous gift-givers, and risky sex-addicted, drug-addled gay men – bolstering the idea of an organised subculture. The terms 'barebacking' and 'bug chasing' emerged from the coverage as signifiers of a criminal and pathological (homo)sexuality that connects HIV/AIDS, risk and perverse sexuality in a chain of metonymy. As Hallas writes, 'since the virulent pathologisation of gay men's lives that defined the initial media reporting of AIDS in the United States during the early 1980s, several further waves of gay moralism have resuscitated figures from the archive of pathology and abjection.'[83] The case of the Neal hearings very distinctly recalled AIDS crisis media from the 1980s and 1990s. It suggests that the 'dirty little story of gay male promiscuity and irresponsibility'[84] has remained both resonant and marketable in the era of post-crisis, and that the rhetorical and emotional force of certain styles of sex panic remain useful for the governance of populations in this new milieu. However, at the same time, this post-crisis sex panic reflected changing technologies and sexual identities. In particular, the earlier depiction of gay men as AIDS victims – as *infected* – was re-calibrated to gay men as *infectors*.

'Re-Crisis'

Unsurprisingly, bug chasing became especially fertile territory for the heightened language of sex panic. An article called 'Seedy world unravels' (Figure 3.1) reported that:

> Melbourne detectives had little knowledge of the Pandora's Box they were about to unlock when they began investigating a Melbourne grandfather over child pornography charges in May [....] What appeared to be a run-of the-mill investigation turned out to be a much wider probe that took police on an eye-opening journey through the seedy underbelly of Melbourne's

gay community. [...] It opened up a perverse world of high-risk sex where the Human Immunodeficiency Virus, HIV, was often an accepted risk, sometimes worn by carriers, such as Mr Neal, as a badge of honour. [...] Exposed was a bizarre culture inhabited by 'bug chasers' – healthy men actively seeking to be infected with HIV – and 'breeders' who infected them at depraved 'conversion parties' [....] One by one, a procession of shirt-and-tie professionals detailed a lewd lifestyle far removed from their daytime occupations as lawyers, tram drivers, teachers, nurses and computer technicians.[85]

Here, anal puns like 'wider probe' and 'opened up' places the scandalous but unmentionable image of sodomy centrally in the reader's mind. The Pandora reference invokes the exotic, 'bizarre' nature of these sexual practices, as does the portrayal of an organised, underground culture ('seedy world'; 'seedy underbelly'; 'perverse world'), an only partially visible spectacle, rendered more titillating through this mode of 'Peeping-Tomism'.[86] The seedy underworld is positioned in stark opposition ('far removed') to the daytime respectability of 'shirt-and-tie' professionalism – the benign, quotidian occupations of the witnesses. In a familiar line-up of risky personae, Neal's photo was published beside an image of Solomon Mwale, a Zambian-born migrant who was then also facing charges of reckless infection. Another story of HIV and boundary trespassing (African migration to Australia), the coverage of the Mwale case symbolically linked criminal sexualities with criminal migration, creating another gendered, racialised and geopolitically specific AIDS Monster.

The breakout quote from a 'veteran police officer' is indicative of the expected shock response from readers: 'I had no thoughts about how wide this issue was until investigating the matter. I'd describe it as surprisingly shocking'. The tautology, 'surprisingly shocking', is an almost comic breakdown in language's capacity to register the sexual phenomenon under discussion – a quite literal crisis of linguistic representation. Characteristic of the language of sex panic, what the actual phenomenon is remains opaque: is 'this issue' that has spread so 'wide' the culture of men engaging in condomless anal sex? The seedy gay underground more broadly? Or the HIV pandemic? There are slippages here with the descent into the corrupting spaces of a gay underworld conflated with the mysterious, abject space of the anus. The reader is called upon to consume the image of anal sex between men, the 'black hole' of AIDS discourse,'[87] in the mode of what Laura Mulvey calls 'sadistic spectatorship': the gaze is surveillant, voyeuristic and homophobic; curious, prurient and thoroughly moralising.[88]

'Seedy world unravels' paints a portrait of a 'perverse world': a clandestine, unregulated, underground, urban sexual universe whose capacity to nurture epidemics is based on the 'cesspit' metaphor, the idea that people's sexualities are shaped by the environments in which they dwell. Audiences may be familiar with such imagery from popular culture: from William Friedkin's notorious homosexual serial killer film, *Cruising* (1980), released amidst much controversy right before the beginning of the AIDS crisis, to more recent examples from Gaspar Noe's Hades-style sex club 'The Rectum' in French rape-revenge film *Irreversible* (2003), to the *Chemsex* documentary. These depict 'deeply unpleasant sensory images' through what William Miller (1998) calls 'the idiom of disgust.'[89] In the Neal case (as in *Cruising*), we are privy to them via the gaze of law enforcers. Davidson calls this the 'expose-like mode' of 'ghetto noir.'[90] The point of identification is an everyman law enforcer encountering the criminal underworld firsthand. Simultaneously ethnographic and hardboiled investigation, the generic qualities of 'ghetto' or 'homosexual noir' work to 'extract a substantial frisson quotient from their revelatory strategies.'[91] Not entirely unlike some forms of sexology, they are prompted by and contribute to the increased 'visibility of urban gay culture.'[92]

The coverage of the Neal hearings invokes anxiety and outrage, key emotions in what Irvine calls the 'dramaturgy of sex panic.'[93] As she explains, 'sex panic scripts rely heavily on tales about sexual groups or issues that use distortion, hyperbole, or outright fabrication' and 'evocative sexual language and imagery.'[94] Barebackers, bug chasers, reckless infectors, black heterosexual migrants, HIV positive gay and bisexual men appear here as a cast of folk devils in this dramaturgy – minority sexualities that are demonised via their association with stigmatised sexual practices and the spectacle of sex itself. But in addition to the aversive feelings of disgust and anxiety is a 'palpable frisson of pleasure.' Foucault described this as 'the pleasure that comes of exercising a power that questions, monitors, watches, spies, searches out, palpates, brings to light'[95], and Irvine considers it key to the machinations of sex panic. Emotions 'not only attract individuals to moral conflicts such as sex panics', she writes, 'they may perpetuate them' through the pleasures of augmented sociality, the 'passionate emotional arousal' and the sense of righteousness promoted by moral sentiments.[96]

In the Neal coverage, the moralising thrust of sex panic scripts also developed over a series of editorials in which authors drew generalisations about 'barebackers' in the context of rising HIV infections. An investigative article ran on the front of *The Age's* Saturday 'Insight' supplement called 'Dance with Death' with an ominous, paternalistic article summary: 'AIDS: Recent criminal charges over the alleged deliberate spreading of HIV have called public safety into question and exposed a worrying subculture within the gay community'.[97] The article was typeset around the image of a fraying HIV awareness ribbon dangling from the scythe of the Grim Reaper, combining Australia's two most recognisable AIDS images (Figure 3.2).[98] Though the image is anachronistic it remains potent in its capacity to remind Australian readers of a terrifying public campaign from a moment when AIDS was a far more pervasive source of sexual terror. Reminding readers of a historical moment of fear, it is an almost literal instance of what I have been calling 're-crisis'.

Let's consider the 'Dance with Death' feature in more detail. This exposé is drawn primarily from the testimonies of one anonymous gay man and one anonymous HIV worker. The anonymous HIV worker claims that probably at least 50 per cent of HIV positive gay men will not disclose their HIV status before having sex with someone. Despite the fact that this does not mean the partners of these non-disclosers are being exposed to HIV (they may be using condoms; they may have negotiated other practices that don't involve disclosure but nonetheless prevent HIV), this unverifiable statistic leads to another unverifiable assertion: 'The majority of people that I have known have all been recklessly infected'. The alarming generalisation offered here is that sexually active HIV positive men are reckless liars. Though this charge is then contradicted or qualified by several quoted and *named* experts in the HIV sector, the anonymous worker accounts for this contradiction by claiming that ASOs propagate a public relations line that denies the existence of the bugchasing culture. The implication here is that corruption is so endemic to the gay community that it has infected the institutions charged with 'managing' HIV.

Crisis Re-Runs: Barebacking, *Chemsex* and Post-Crisis Sex Panic

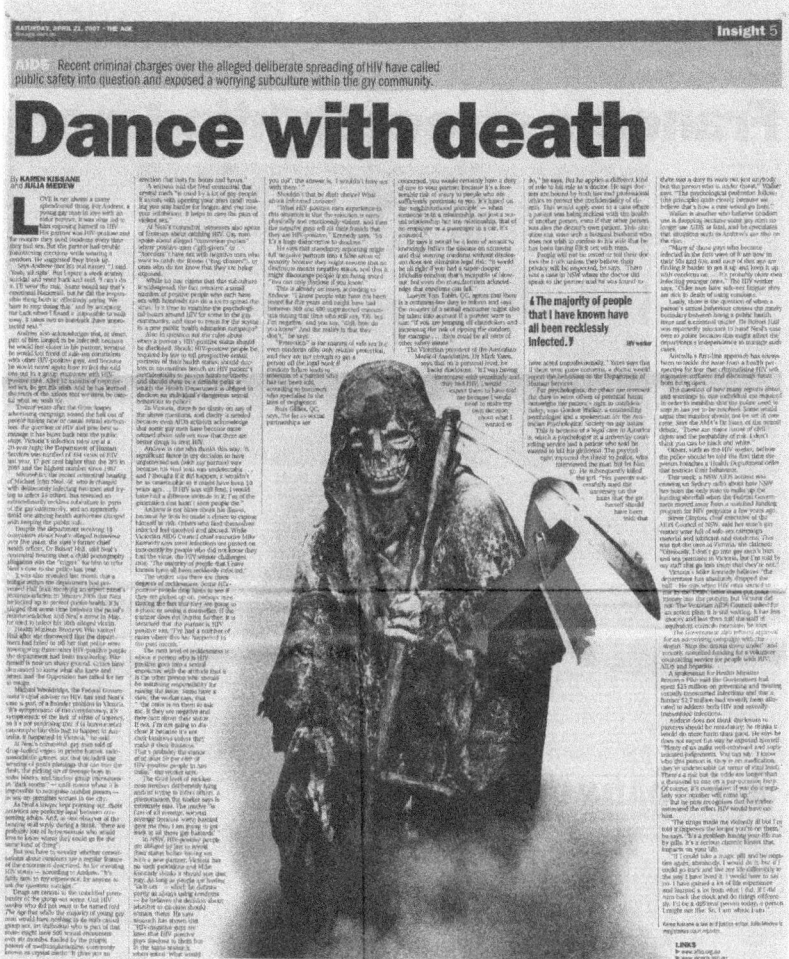

Figure 3.2 'Dance with Death', *The Age*, 21 April 2007

It also implies that the oft-celebrated, effective Australian policy of the HIV affected community managing the epidemic 'in partnership' with government[99] is itself in crisis. The article later describes the infamous sexual heroics of gay men, 'jumping off chandeliers' and having '500 sexual encounters over six months fuelled by the priapic powers of methamphetamine which gives you an erection that lasts for hours and hours and assists with opening your anus.' As if every available shock trope of

AIDS crisis discourse hadn't already been trawled out, it also mentions the hypothetical 'bisexual husband' who hides the 'illicit sex he has with men' from his wife, and brings HIV into the 'wider population.' These examples of 're-crisis' are utterly reminiscent of the framing, images and logics of earlier AIDS discourses that created a division between the 'general population' and 'risk groups', a fantasy underpinned by the wish to quarantine the self from the contaminating other. Perhaps the most inflationary aspect of 'Dance with Death' is its unqualified conflation of the rise in HIV seroconversions with the alleged recklessness of gay men. Like *Chemsex* and numerous other examples of epidemic sex panic, the insistence that the increase in HIV notifications is the direct result of deliberate or reckless exposures might at first seem logical, it entirely overlooks the complex range of scenarios mentioned above in which people may have anal sex without condoms – many (if not most) of which are scenarios with little or no risk of exposure to HIV.

The dramaturgy of sex panic is aimed at the production of spectacle at the expense of analytical complexity. Then it paves the way for less equivocal declarations of blame. An editorial in national news broadsheet *The Australian* asserted that 'someone has to take the blame for this outrageously long-lived, unbelievably reviving, preventable epidemic.'[100] This article called for 'accountability' and 'a proper sense of personal and collective shame':

> It is time to state that a reasonably well-educated, western gay man who contracts HIV in 2006 because of sex is at least a reckless fool, and if he deliberately brings it upon himself, at best a suicidal sociopath.
>
> Yes, believe it or not, there is a whole gay subculture that rests upon 'bug-chasing', or the despicable sport of actively seeking out or passing on HIV infection for the satisfaction of sexual or other perverse fantasies.

Here the lurid coverage of the Neal case slides into the wholesale blaming of gay men for the continuation of HIV.

These unpleasant images and rhetorical inflations contribute to the production of 'an affect of paranoid dis-ease'[101] and an atmosphere of 'generalised emotional combustibility',[102] the first effects of a sex panic. Then, they may also become part of some more official, disciplinary, legislative intervention or apparatus. Though it can be brushed off as a form of excess, panic merchantry may in fact incite increased forms of surveillance and the disciplining of bodies in the name of 'public welfare'.

Neoliberal Biopolitics and the Logic of Epidemic

Sex panic studies have considered the ways in which the mobilisation of negative in a sex panic emotions has a connection to the way in which sexuality is regulated. The panic metaphor has been used by a number of researchers, including Gayle Rubin, Lisa Duggan, Jeffrey Weeks and Michael Warner among others, as a means to explore 'political conflict, sexual regulation, and public volatility about sex.'[103] In the heightened moments of sex panic there is, as Irvine explains, a 'transmogrification of moral values into political action.'[104] 'Collective emotion, evoked discursively', she writes, 'brings publics into being, organising diffuse, sometimes inchoate beliefs and moralities in political action.'[105] More recent work in sex panic studies has honed in on the role of emotions as both the function and effect of panic, and as a force implicated in structures of sexual regulation. Ahmed (2004) and Cvetkovich (2003) have been influential in this 'affective turn' in sex panic studies, exploring, respectively, how affect shapes public culture, and how emotions function in the governance of the self. Sex panics theorists have also worked against the traditional dichotomy that views the 'private sphere' as emotional, and the public sphere as the space of rational discourse.[106] Instead, they have shown how the so-called 'rational' public sphere is in fact riddled with emotional politics and how affect saturates all forms of civic life.

AIDS panic, like sex crime panic and sex panic more generally, has been a key site for the expression of late twentieth-century and post-millennial social anxieties, and the transformation of these anxieties into forms of population governance. The sex panic model is useful for thinking about the vexed, emotional discussions of barebacking in the mainstream Australian media context, and the implications these discussions have had for policy and official intervention. The bareback panic surrounding the Neal case in Australian can be understood as part of a model of biopolitical governmentality that Singer called 'the Logic of Epidemic', a model that draws on existing studies of sex panic. In Singer's formulation, an epidemic is 'a phenomenon that in its very representation calls for, indeed seems to demand some form of managerial response, some mobilised effort of control.'[107] An epidemic, she argues is 'a situation that is figured as out of control, hence at least indirectly a recognition of the limits of existing responses, hence a call for new ones.'[108] As the 'Dance with Death' feature anxiously asserts, certain practices in the gay community, most notably sex without condoms, 'have called public safety into question and exposed a worrying subculture in the gay community.' Such a 'threat to the very order of things' demands a response. Singer explains that 'because the destabilisation effect is also represented as a threat… epidemic conditions tend to evoke a kind of panic logic which seeks immediate and dramatic responses to the situation at hand.'[109]

Singer's model helps illuminate events in Australian HIV policy that unfolded after the Neal hearings. In the wake of the coverage of the Mwale and Neal cases, the conservative prime minister John Howard announced that new government policies could see HIV-positive migrants banned from entering Australia, and that, if admitted, their movements would be tracked.[110] The Victorian state health minister Bronwyn Pike recommended that the federal government introduce a mandatory HIV test for refugees [111] and called on limitations to the immigration of HIV positive persons. To distract attention from what the coverage of the Neal hearings had exposed as a potentially inadequate system for preventing and/or disciplining potential reckless infectors, HIV positive migrants were scapegoated.[112] In turn, the federal health minister recommended a further form of surveillance: the introduction of mandatory reporting by doctors of 'risky' HIV patients to state health authorities.[113] At the same time, a research team was established at Victoria's Monash University to 'scrutinise national clusters of infections' in order to 'track down what groups or behaviours are responsible for the increasing rate of HIV infections over the past three years.'[114]

Once created, anxiety must be allayed through strategies that appear to address the problems so named. The relationship of the bareback panic that circulated around the Neal case to these federal and state policy assertions exemplifies Singer's logic of epidemic. Under epidemic circumstances, the production of sexual anxiety is conducive to official interventions – law reform, surveillance, criminalisation, mandatory reporting, quarantines.

Crisis Re-Runs: Barebacking, *Chemsex* and Post-Crisis Sex Panic

These regulatory apparati appear to address or compensate for the sense of 'crisis' stirred up by the anxious sex panic talk. Scandalised proclamations and inflated feelings in media coverage create a type of fertile atmosphere for the sorts of law enforcement, legislative and policy interventions that, internationally, have surrounded the criminalisation of HIV transmission.[115] It warrants noting here that the threatened Australian ban on HIV positive migrants was a racialised response and wasn't focused on gay migrants per se. The extent to which media and policy debate beyond the Neal case was targeted at gay men exclusively should not be overestimated – much of it had nationalist and racist overtones.

Discussion of the legal issues surrounding so-called reckless infection is best left to legal researchers and theorists, however, we can draw on the theories of sex panic and the logic of epidemic to speculate on this figure's *symbolic* function in the landscape of post-crisis. In the episode of re-crisis described above, the reckless infector emerges as a high-visibility sexual persona who can transition from 'everyday' sexual criminal to AIDS monster. In this transformation, his utility is at least threefold:

(1) As a criminal spectacle, he reinforces the myth of the nuclear family as the optimum social and sexual space, and, by contrast, all alternatives are correlated with danger and risk;
(2) He helps to manufacture highly marketable forms of storytelling. Sex crime is excellent business for tabloid and online media; and
(3) He becomes a template for the creation of a criminal class that 'justifies the mobilisation of various disciplinary and even militaristic forces'.

Criminality is troped as disease and disease is figured as criminal. So-named 'high-risk sexualities' are conflated with contagion and HIV becomes the associative link between them. In sex panics, the spectacularisation of sexual types and subcultures as monstrous or criminal is part of a more diffuse model of social governance through which good sexual citizens are encouraged to recognise themselves in relation to or against figures of public menace, like barebackers. As the Neal case suggests, sexual spectacle may function alongside public health responses in which good (gay) citizens are those that prioritise the maximisation of health, and the 'evil irresponsible barebacker… embodies the transgressive pleasure of unprotected sex.'[116]

Ambivalent Afterlives

> Although from one perspective fucking without condoms represents sex at its most mundane, from another perspective the history of AIDS has made gay sex without condoms extraordinary, endowing bareback sex with enormous significance.
>
> Tim Dean[117]

The Neal case suggests that AIDS crisis discourses have had afterlives – an ongoing albeit transformed currency in the political, cultural and epidemiological scene of post-crisis. The popular fascination with 'gay sex as an erotics of suicide and murder'[118] remains a key theme. And, while such sex scandals may seem a banal and recurrent part of our mediatised quotidian, the rhetorical inflations they stir up can (re)create emotions that in turn create the potential for states of exceptionality. This paradoxical alliance of the exceptional and the mundane is part of the ongoing apparatus of representing and managing HIV under neoliberal conditions. Rather than episodic, crisis has become chronic. The Neal hearings, in which the logic of epidemic was revived via both generic homosexual and epidemic sex panic scripts and new developments in HIV and subcutural sexual practices, reflects the simultaneously spectacular and mundane status of both HIV and homosexuality that defines 'post-crisis' culture. In the quotation that opens this book, the late William Haver described this state of affairs eloquently when he wrote that we 'have erected… structures of intelligibility and comprehensibility on and around the pandemic, structures that themselves render AIDS normative and routine: the business of AIDS, constructed and carried on around an impossible object, has become – like genocide, nuclear terror, racism, misogyny, and heteronormativity… business as usual.'[119]

If barebacking emerged into public discussion as a spectacularly bad sexual signifier – an outré sexual practice, dangerous, irrational, a source of anxiety and a behaviour calling for intervention – it has also accrued many alternative meanings. The history of AIDS has given anal sex without condoms a special status, but on the other hand, as the quote from Tim Dean above suggests, sex without condoms could not be more ordinary. As I mentioned earlier, condomless anal sex between 'serosorted' men may for many be a very mundane, quotidian sex act.

Moreover, barebacking representations and cultures have in some quarters amplified the positive revaluation of anality, especially receptive anality, and have thus taken their place among 'arse-sex-positive' expressions of gay sexuality.[120] As Dean observed of bareback culture, a special masculine status 'accrues to the man who assumes what used to be thought of as the female role in homosexual relations. The more men by whom one is penetrated, the more of a man he becomes.'[121] This masculinisation of bottoming in barebacking culture can be seen, he argues, 'as a compensatory response to modern society's feminisation of male homosexuality – a response, that is, to the gender-inversion model of same-sex desire.'[122] Dean argues that these cultures have re-signified the meaning of being penetrated, so that bottoming becomes 'a matter of "taking it like a man", enduring without complaint any discomfort or temporary loss of status, to prove one's masculinity.'[123]

Across a spectrum of sites, then, from panic to porn, barebacking is a paradigmatic example of the logic of post-crisis culture: vacillating between the extraordinary and the mundane, and ambivalently inhabiting both of those meaning spaces simultaneously. When my investigation into the Neal hearings began in the early 2000s, most commercial gay porn producers were committed to the condom code.[124] Early examples of gay porn sans condoms like that infamously produced by Treasure Island Media were the subject of derision and alarm among industry players, commentators and gay community media alike.[125] Since then there has been a large-scale, digitally enabled and seemingly rapid *banalisation* of barebacking in ubiquitously circulating gay male pornographies that increasingly incorporate anal sex without condoms into their routine repertoires of representation. Now, barebacking has journeyed from the margins to the centre.[126] As this has unfolded, other spheres, like ASOs and health promoters have begun to address barebacking in a tone that acknowledges the reality of its myriad manifestations, rather than treating it like an aberration or an outlaw practice. Condomless anal sex is much less fussed over than it was ten or even five years ago, demonstrating the ways in which shifts in the language and understanding of epidemic sex can happen rapidly. The advent of PrEP, U=U and other new technologies of HIV prevention have and will continue to contribute to these transformations. In the years since these initial eruptions of bareback panic, barebacking has become something of a routine – perhaps even *normal* – part of the cultural landscape of gay male sexual representation.

In the final two chapters of *Positive Images* I turn to the history of the AIDS Crisis, or, rather, to the increasingly popular re-envisioning of that history in recent film, documentary and TV. How is this past being depicted? Why this turn to the AIDS past now? What are the implications of telling AIDS histories in certain ways for how we understand and live with HIV/AIDS in the present? These investigations may seem somewhat removed from the contexts of nouveau sexology and media sex panics discussed in this chapter, and yet, as we have seen, certain understandings of gay and AIDS history have emerged in accounts of both barebacking and chemsex, suggesting that our understandings of sexual practices, communities and identities today are informed by how our histories are told. As we shall see, the 'pre-AIDS/AIDS crisis/post-crisis' historical narrative has often been narrated in either fatalistic or moralistic terms, where a reductive image of liberation (as a carnival of naïve, promiscuous recklessness) gives way to AIDS crisis as a dire historical punishment or 'lesson' that sets the stage for the (neoliberal) post-crisis present as the mature and logical solution to the turbulence of earlier eras. Crossley's appraisal of the post-crisis landscape in terms of *déjà vu* is a clear instance of this kind of narrative logic. Similarly, in the vision of bareback offered in mainstream journalism, both liberation and the AIDS crisis return to haunt post-crisis representation in powerful ways. The lessons of this history are implied in Heard's call for accountability cited earlier in this chapter: 'someone has to take the blame for this outrageously long-lived, unbelievably reviving, preventable epidemic.'[127] Here we have the deployment of historical narrative as moralistic object lesson: AIDS is positioned as something from the past – an anachronism, but one that can resurface to invade and discipline the post-crisis present. Despite the passing of time, the homosexual and his behaviour remains essentially the same: driven inexorably to transgress the prevailing sexual orthodoxy.

The next chapter charts the first of two turns to AIDS memory and the ambivalent feelings and complex negotiations that post-crisis culture has with the complexities of gay history and AIDS history. It examines the construction of an Anglophone 'AIDS heritage' in BBC2's adaptation of *The Line of Beauty*, a text that looks back to the moment of British AIDS crisis through the lens of a complex crossover of national and queer historical gazes. Rather than a punitive trajectory from chaos to common sense, from sexual carnival to prudent politics, the narrative line drawn by this example of AIDS heritage is a more nuanced historical trajectory from innocence to experience, presided over by the ambivalent influences of Henry James and the generic conventions of heritage cinema.

4

AIDS Heritage in *The Line of Beauty*

> It's glittering, but it's deadly at the same time. It doesn't want you to survive it. It's totally negative.
> Catherine Fedden to Nick Guest, *The Line of Beauty* episode 1

While 'HIV/AIDS' has often been associated with the concept of 'crisis' – exigency, urgency, states associated with the here-and-now – 'heritage' conjures history, tradition, cultures of preservation and recreation. Before ARVs, the literature and cinema of AIDS tended to invoke a finite or apocalyptic sense of time. In heritage culture, time is supposedly frozen. While HIV researchers, prevention efforts and AIDS service organisations strive to maintain a sense of urgency and dynamism in response to rapidly and constantly changing circumstances, the archival, curatorial and artifactual work of producing 'AIDS heritage', with its backward-looking orientation, may seem like the antithesis to their aims.

In 2011 the HIV/AIDS pandemic turned 30, and in 2012 it seemed as if an official decision had been made to collectively look back on 'The Plague Years'. After the widespread absence of large-scale, popular or mainstream representations of AIDS, a critical mass of crisis era and ACT UP documentaries emerged in 2012. These were followed by a number of narrative cinema and quality TV recreations of that historical period, including

AIDS Heritage in *The Line of Beauty*

Dallas Buyers Club (2014) and *The Normal Heart* (2014), which I discuss in the next chapter. More broadly, in archival, historical and retrospective projects, HIV/AIDS has become a properly historical object. It appears to have become the case that in the popular culture of the developed world, the 'nowness' once associated with HIV/AIDS has increasingly transformed into an association with the past.

This is the first of two chapters reflecting on the recent 'boom' in screen memories of the AIDS crisis. While the next chapter considers the emerging narrative of AIDS history in recent film and TV more widely, this chapter returns to a forerunner of this retrospective turn, BBC2's miniseries adaptation of *The Line of Beauty* (2006). My inquiry in both chapters is motivated by questions about the significance of these 'retrovisions' in the contemporary, post-ARVs, post-crisis era. What does the way we write the history of AIDS mean for how we understand HIV and queer life today? How does this history reflect or react to the dynamics of post-crisis culture identified in the previous chapters of this book?

In spite of the apparent tension between 'AIDS' and 'heritage', these categories came together in BBC2's serialised adaptation of Alan Hollinghurst's Booker award–winning novel, *The Line of Beauty* (2004). Hollinghurst's novel follows the coming-of-age of Nicholas Guest, a middle-class gay man from Barwick, as he progresses through the world of Britain's rich and powerful Tory elite during the boom period of the 1980s. Befitting his name, Guest becomes a lodger in the Notting Hill house of wealthy Tory MP Gerald Fedden and his family. In this milieu he rubs shoulders with Britain's rich and powerful and becomes privy to the goings-on of the inner sanctums of the Thatcher-era political elite. Reghina Dascăl describes the novel as a comedy of class that turns to 'the dark underside of, and the profound lack of compassion that characterised Margaret Thatcher's 1980s London.'[1] Simon During has declared it a 'masterpiece' of 'the anti-Thatcher fiction sub-genre' that emerged from intellectual and literary antipathies to British conservatism from the 1980s onwards.[2]

Thatcher-era political culture is often recalled for its traditionalism and conservative family values. This included an unapologetically homophobic public policy and currents of legal moralism, as exemplified in the notorious Section 28 clause of the Local Government Act of May 1988. Section 28 stated that 'a local authority shall not (a) intentionally promote homosexuality or publish material with the intention of promoting homosexuality; and (b) promote the teaching in any maintained school of the acceptability of homosexuality as a pretended family relationship.' The clause was passed amidst widespread AIDS panic and an 'increased pathologisation of homosexuality associating it with promiscuity, disease and a risk to both public health and morality.'[3] A particularly violent effect of the Act was its stipulation that no public activity could be taken to positively value or 'promote' homo-sexuality, which stifled the matter-of-fact discussions of sex required urgent community efforts at AIDS education, stigma reduction and prevention.

The heritage film cycle that emerged in this era was widely regarded as reflective of and implicated in this sex negative, homophobic, retrograde political culture. Early heritage films were attacked by critics for their alleged nationalism, their 'conservative recreations of a fossilised past in the context of Thatcherite traditionalism and new liberalism'[4] and their prim, neo-Victorian sexual politics.[5] Critics argued that the rearward heritage gaze fostered the type of reactionary, nostalgic political moods that displaced and neglected contemporary social issues, of which HIV/AIDS was a particularly urgent example. It may therefore seem odd or ironic that *The Line of Beauty* – this early vision of AIDS history – should be housed in the signature genre of that conservative strain of British culture that it in turn examines. However, I want to suggest that heritage style, including its detailed period *mise en scène*, functions here to produce a deeply critical form of social history. Rather than a merely 'pictorialist' space – an artful tableau for gazing at the attractions of English past – the loving historical re-creation of 1980s Britain in *The Line of Beauty* exposes the darkness of this period, highlighting the complicity of the rich elite in a scandalous national policy of indifference to AIDS. While preserving the novel's elegiac qualities and drawing out the capacity of heritage screen conventions to evoke longing and nostalgia, BBC2's adaptation remains faithful to the novel's dim view of 1980s social politics and, in fact, magnifies its scathing critique of the official response to AIDS.

The 1980s were the best of times and the worst of times. Cartmell, Hunter, and Whelehan use the term 'retrovision' to describe screen representations with a mixed, ambivalent perspective on that past – images that 'demythologise', gazing back sometimes with horror at violence and oppression, and sometimes with 'nostalgia for lost innocence and style.'[6] 'Retrovision' nicely accounts for *The Line of Beauty*'s mixed relationship with the Thatcher era – its combination of requiem for what has been lost with its sentiments of disgust towards cruelty and tragedy.

As I have been arguing throughout *Positive Images*, images of gay men and HIV in post-crisis popular culture tend to express paradoxical meanings. The memory culture of this era is no different: AIDS retrovisions contend with a fraught legacy that is at once both painful and commemorative. AIDS memory, as we shall see both here and in the next chapter, is a category of cultural memory that is fraught with grief and epic narratives of suffering. But, on the other hand, it is an archive filled with affirming, defiant nostalgia for experiences of collectivism, visibility, groundbreaking activism, artistic flourishing and loud counterpublic demands for recognition. The nostalgic recollection of AIDS community activism may constitute what Lucas Hilderbrand calls 'subcultural utopian nostalgia', a feeling that counterbalances the trauma of AIDS history with affirmative and potentially galvanising feelings of 'historical fascination, of imagining… [of] drawing from history.'[7] As an example of 'AIDS heritage', *The Line of Beauty* is similarly reflective of post-crisis culture's complex, divided disposition towards the AIDS past.

This mixed orientation towards a past that is simultaneously both painful and stirring may also be seen as an example of what Heather Love calls 'feeling backwards'. In *Feeling Backward: Loss and the Politics of Queer History* (2007), Love takes the 'progress narrative of queer history' as a focal point for critique. She argues that the reclamation of shame and stigma in dominant LGBTQI+ politics and culture has been beholden to the logic of a positively-inflected reverse discourse, requiring that suffering and stigma be always transformed into positive feelings, a transformation of 'social abjection into… political agency.'[8] Returning wilfully to the 'unhappy archive' of queer literature, instead Love refuses to 'rescue' the 'troubled figures' of the queer literary past and to thereby reverse the threat they pose to a progress narrative of LGBTQI+ history. Instead, she asks, 'what if the threat of "queer damage" could be enabling in the present?'[9] For Love, the haste with which queer thought seeks to 'refunction' the unhappy and tragic experiences of the past results in the failure to 'adequately reckon [...] with their powerful legacies.'[10] As we shall see, the complex and paradoxical meanings of heritage conventions enables *The Line of Beauty* to do some reckoning with the unbearable but powerful legacy of AIDS history.

Queer High Pop Heritage

Prestige adaptations of literary classics and bestsellers have risen exponentially on TV and cinema screens since the early 1990s and show very little sign of abating in their popularity. These are usually marketed to a broad, crossover audience and they draw hybridly from serialised soap opera, historical costume drama, family melodrama and the 'movie-of-the-week', among other genres.[11] These 'blockbuster adaptations' combine 'the romance of authorship [and] the commercial bond of personality and popularity' in the adaptation of recognised literary material, the most 'popular, reliable, and profitable sources for the movies.'[12] It is a trend that Jim Collins called 'high pop', spearheaded variously by Miramax, Austenmania, and the transnational blockbuster adaptations of the 1980s and 90s, and it has settled in as a permanent feature of globally popular culture. As Collins explains, 'high pop' is the fourth phase in the relationship between mass culture and high art: if the third phase involved the de-sacrilisation of culture, epitomised most iconically by the Wharhol soup can – Pop Art's self-conscious dragging of the popular into the realm of the rarefied – 'high pop' is the reverse: in high pop, capital C 'culture' is transformed and spun into forms of mass entertainment.[13]

In its trajectory from Booker award-winning novel to BBC series, *The Line of Beauty* exemplifies elements of the high-pop trend. The BBC itself has long been associated with literary tradition, heritage culture and quality TV. In addition to its commercial imperatives, the BBC maintains a civic designation as Britain's national broadcaster, 'a learning resource for the nation' with a pedagogical vocation 'in [it's] bloodstream.'[14] BBC2 is its second major channel, specialising in 'intelligent' yet popular programming, and with a founding ethos of public improvement and education.

Alan Hollinghurst is also canonical. An award-winning British writer who foregrounds Britishness, British queerness, and a dialogue with canonical British writers like Henry James, Evelyn Waugh, and Ronald

AIDS Heritage in *The Line of Beauty*

Firbank, his novels are about 'the Comedy of Being English.'[15] The coveted Booker prize, traditionally awarded to the best original full-length English language novel by a citizen of the Commonwealth or Ireland (but open to American writers since 2014) catapulted him into a more global canon. Hollinghurst is now considered 'the most important gay novelist in Great Britain since E. M. Forster.'[16]

And finally, Andrew Davies, *The Line of Beauty*'s adaptor, is another English household name. The Emmy award-winning writer of screenplays and TV series is the national doyenne of literary adaptations. Like the authorial brand Merchant Ivory, Davies is firmly associated with prestige literary adaptations and heritage cinema. But rather than the simmering corseted eroticism traditionally associated with the genre, Davies has been a trailblazer of the 'bodice ripper.' He was most (in)famously the man behind Mr Darcy's iconic wet shirt in the BBC's 1995 *Pride and Prejudice*, which turned Colin Firth into a costume drama sex symbol and helped reignite international Austenmania. His work is characterised by playfulness, irreverence and departures from classic heritage conventions, social critique, 'gothic heritage' and meta-heritage.[17] Given the varied but all 'quintessentially' English status of Hollinghurst, Davies, the Booker, the BBC and Anglo-American heritage cinema, *The Line of Beauty* is very much a nationally significant *English* text, authored and authorised by authenticated English cultural institutions.

Although *The Line of Beauty* trades in various generic modes, including melodrama and social realism, here I am most interested in its use of the conventions of heritage, a genre closely associated with English national culture. In order to unpack the functions of heritage style in the series, it will be necessary to take a brief tour through the heritage debates of the 1990s and beyond. These discussions show how the emergence of revisionist and hybrid forms of heritage cinema have developed the genre so that by the time we reach *The Line of Beauty*, heritage has reached its 'baroque' stage. In Thomas Schatz's influential taxonomy of genre evolution, the 'baroque' follows from the experimental, classical and refinement stages of a genre, offering its core conventions but in revisions, inversions, parody or ridicule; the baroque involves a high degree of formal self-consciousness and reflexivity.[18] BBC2's adaptation is a good example of baroque heritage – while it revels in the pleasures of pictorialist cinematography and the so-called 'museum aesthetic', it is also a strong example of revisionist 'post-heritage' and self-conscious 'meta-heritage', working reflexively against a fixed and glorified reification of the nation's past.

The Heritage Debates

'Heritage' initially described a small group of film and TV dramas including *Brideshead Revisited* (1981), *A Passage to India* (1984) and *A Room with a View* (1986). Though most of these were actually British–American co-productions, heritage brought about a 'renaissance' in the then flagging British film industry.[19] Primarily, these films were recognisable by their use of a well-known literary source and/or historical event and 'a museum or antiques aesthetic' – settings and costumes 'based upon meticulous research, presented in pristine condition, brightly or artfully lit.'[20] The genre grew in concurrence with the British heritage industry: the marketing and commodification of the past and British museum culture as part of the new enterprise culture of the Thatcher era.[21]

Andrew Higson's influential (and since-revised) critique positioned heritage cinema against the backdrops of Thatcherism, Toryism, emergent neoliberal enterprise culture and neo-Victorian family values. His evaluation quickly congealed into a critical orthodoxy that surpassed scholarly discussion and moved well into popular discourse. In this Leftist reading, heritage culture is considered to be bad nostalgia: it celebrates elite, conservative traditions and mythologised versions of the national past. Heritage has an ideological agenda: it solicits nostalgia for the white British Imperium by fetishising the lives of its *haute bourgeoisie*, forgiving the rich and privileged their sins and distracting viewers from the social problems of the present. 'Heritage cinema' became critical shorthand for reactionary, easily digested fantasies of a supposedly 'authentic' British past.

This account zoomed in on the use of period spectacle in heritage – meticulously reproduced sets, elegant costumes, authentic rituals, manners and iconography that deliver the past as 'a museum of sounds and images, and iconographic display.'[22] In the heritage gaze, culture is put on display, frozen; 'heritage culture', Higson argued, 'appears petrified, frozen in moments that virtually fall out of the narrative.'[23] 'Heritage space', he continued, is produced for the display of heritage properties that become attractions in and of themselves, rather than as 'narrative space' for the enactment of drama.[24] As such, the camera work is dominated by long takes and a deep focus, long and medium shots rather than close-ups and rapid cutting; its movement is languid, 'dictated less by a desire to follow the movement of characters than by a desire to offer the spectator a more aesthetic angle on the period setting.'[25] The use of framing devices (figures flanked by others; persons standing in doorways), and the editorial method of 'string[ing] together single shots like beads', produces a visual rhetoric like that of the still life painting; this camera work has hence been called 'pictorialist'.[26] Hipsky described this particular variety of cinematic spectacle 'circumambience'. A 'Baudrillardian simulacr[um] of the traditionally defined locales of "high culture,"' circumambience administers an overdose of historical and cultural allusion and iconography.[27] Moreover, one must possess the requisite cultural and educative investments – cultural capital, in other words – to appreciate them. A lucrative transnational film export product, 'Anglophil(m)ia', as Hipsky cleverly dubbed the genre, profits from aspirational, class-based cultural appeal. Educated audiences 'want their increasingly expensive college educations to pay some cultural dividends.'[28]

The problem with all of this for these critics is that in heritage cinema, history and literary culture is co-opted by a nationalist, neo-imperialist agenda. The genre's distinctive visual pleasures solicit nostalgia in the viewer for the imperial homeland, for luxury and for the privileged bourgeois spaces of the past. At the heart of the genre's scopophilic energies is the heritage house, an emblem of property ownership, landed aristocracy; this is the genre's most persistent, recurrent image. The English country house set in a picturesque, verdant landscape is the key icon of inherited value, conspicuous consumption, and the psychic yearning for the lost home.[29] Affectively speaking, the genre's appeal lies in the fundamental desires to find a home – the pleasures (and anxieties) of belonging and identification. As we shall see, this desire for the (lost) home is aroused and deeply interrogated in *The Line of Beauty*.

After this first wave critique of heritage cinema, other critics, particularly feminist and queer scholars, began to defend the genre for its revisionist approach to minority histories and its liberal viewing pleasures. Since the 90s, the critical and political consensus on heritage's supposed inherent conservatism has shifted. Cook and Gaines et al turned their attention to costume as a site of feminist histories and flexible gender performance, drawing from Butler's work on masquerade and performativity. Other critics have identified examples of the genre with anti-imperial, post-colonial and critical race and class-conscious agendas. Dyer, for example, catalogued the great hospitality of heritage to homosexual representation, listing literally hundreds of examples of queer themes, characters and proto-gay identities, 'clearly inspired by a gay or sexually liberal political agenda.'[30] Monk saw the genre as opening up historical and textual spaces in which genders and sexualities are 'shifting, fluid and heterogenous'.[31] For these defenders of the genre, heritage cinematic space may indeed be 'pictorialist' but it may also be understood as 'semantically charged'.[32] Rather than a 'separate discourse of scenic display, in conflict with the narrative… [and functioning] as spokespersons for the heritage industry', settings, props and costumes can be regarded, rather, as 'symbolic indications of the inner life of the characters.'[33]

Heritage defenders have also often sought to rescue the category of nostalgia from its pejorative associations. Nostalgia has long been the poor cousin of history and memory because of its aura of inauthenticity. Nostalgia gets associated with a retreat into fantasy and the desire for something lost, never had or irretrievable: as Ben Gook puts it, a 'longing for the past which buffs away at rough edges, a kind of soft-focus history…. [A]t best, diversionary and pleasant; at worst, wrongheaded and dangerous.'[34] Presided over by Frederic Jameson's influential critique in 'Postmodernism, or the Cultural Logic of Late Capitalism' (1984), the prevailing critical approach has been to view postmodern nostalgia culture as a negative, reactionary mode, a flattening or stereotyping of the past largely in the interests of commercial cultures.[35] But, since the 1980s, numerous critics have worked at reclaiming nostalgia,[36] arguing that the Jamesonian view foreclosed the *productive* possibilities of nostalgia: its affective pleasures, its self-conscious engagements with the past, and its potentially progressive political investments. Cook, for example, argues that 'rather than being seen as a reactionary, regressive condition imbued with sentimentality', nostalgia 'can be perceived as a way of coming to terms with the past, as enabling it to be exorcised in order that society and individuals can move on.'[37] In particular, what she calls 'memory films', like

The Line of Beauty, engage critically with the construction of history: they explore the limitations of dominant histories, interrogate traditional modes of representation and self-consciously highlight the relationship between past and present.

Although the nostalgia debates are too wide-ranging to dissect in detail, I want to note two further elements of this reconsideration of nostalgia that I think are important to understanding the recent turn to AIDS heritage. First: nostalgia is a feeling that is constituted by its *awareness of the irreversibility of the past*. As Jason Goldman explains, nostalgia 'implies a rupture between the present and some bygone era.' The nostalgic knows they can never return. The rupture cannot be undone. The intensity of the desire to return to the past inherent in nostalgic feeling is countervailed by an acknowledgement of the 'absolute foreclosure of the past.'[38] Second: Svetlana Boym draws a useful distinction between 'restorative' and 'reflective' forms of nostalgia. The former is invested in ideals of truth and tradition and tends to 'reconstruct emblems and rituals of home and homeland in an attempt to conquer and spatialise time.'[39] Reflective nostalgia, however, is a more creative and ambivalent approach to the past: rather than seeking to reconstruct a lost home, reflective nostalgia places critical pressure on the very states of longing and belonging, and the hierarchical organisations of culture that prop these systems up, even as it often revels in the pleasures of the past. In the case of *The Line of Beauty*, the question of 'belonging' (to the family, to the nation) is deeply interrogated.

Since the 1980s, heritage has significantly diversified. In the 1990s, for example, arthouse feminist auteurs Sally Potter and Jane Campion, in films like *Orlando* (1992) and *The Portrait of a Lady* (1996), experimented with and extended the genre's gendered, affective and erotic dimensions. Queer filmmakers, like Derek Jarman in *The Last of England* (1987) and Todd Haynes in *Far From Heaven* (2002) and *Carol* (2015) have played with heritage formalisms to draw out queer narratives and themes. These types of films, dubbed 'post-heritage' by Monk, tend to ironise the class-bound culture of Old England and to foreground gender and sexuality, anti-Imperial, anti-canonical, revisionist or minority histories.[40] Heritage is a genre with 'porous boundaries' that has developed in multiple directions in the new millennium.[41]

In the analysis to follow, my key interest is in the gay bachelor's difficult relationship with the 'semantically charged' spaces of elite culture. Initially, Nick Guest is welcomed into these spaces, but when scandal, economic downturn and epidemic disease threaten to invade, the elite culture of Thatcherite England can no longer abide nor afford his presence. In a state of ignominy, Nick is discharged from the house of privilege and symbolically expelled from the house of the nation.

In this shrewd observation of the position of outsiders – *guests* – in the sanctified spaces of British culture, *The Line of Beauty* can be read as an allegory for the limits of tolerance as well as a narrative about the fortunes of homosexuality in the moment of epidemic panic. In these early moments of the AIDS crisis, with the media and the government colluding in homophobic hatred, Nick's status shifts from privileged guest to what Giorgio Agamben calls *'homo sacer'* ('bare life'), from the Latin term for 'the accursed man' who is banned and may be killed by anybody, the most radical form of human alterity.[42] The degenerate homosexual, the repository of AIDS scandal and abjection, is banished from the heritage house, the symbolic space of national belonging.

And yet, at the same time, a queer presence has inhabited both the heritage house, and the classic cast of heritage genre aesthetics. This is *baroque* heritage; the genre has been 'queered'. Among various generic diversifications, critics have identified 'post heritage', 'alternative heritage', 'revisionist heritage', 'gothic heritage', and 'meta heritage'. To this taxonomy we can add the category of 'AIDS heritage.'

AIDS heritage may incline either way: towards restorative or reflective forms of nostalgia. As this chapter will hopefully show, in the complex turn back to an unhappy historical archive, the practice of reflective nostalgia may be a particularly queer sort of memory practice: queer because of its deliberate turn towards histories of pain, trauma, shame, and other 'ugly feelings';[43] and queer also because the ritual of sharing these feelings calls into being what Warner calls 'a special kind of sociability' in queer culture.[44] A shared consciousness in the present of a history of shared abjection, as Crimp argues, may be a basis for articulating 'collectivities of the shamed'.[45] As we shall see, the rearward gaze of AIDS heritage in *The Line of Beauty* reaches backwards to the homophobic past not only to acknowledge that past but to acknowledge what is still of that past in the present. In its historical 'account of the corporeal and psychic costs of homophobia',⁴⁶ the backwards feeling text, as Love describes it, can 'serve as an index to the ruined state of the [contemporary] social world... [it can] indicate continuities between the bad gay past and the present; and show up the inadequacy of queer narratives of progress.'⁴⁷ In BBC2's *The Line of Beauty*, Hollinghurst's merciless critique of the birth of neoconservative neoliberalism hints more than strongly at a critique of the neoliberal present, and therefore, perhaps, helps us to re-imagine the future.

Heritage Ga(y)ze

How does the re-genrification of heritage play out in *The Line of Beauty*? On the one hand, the formal and aesthetic conventions of classic heritage are all in place – set pieces, soft focus, long takes and middle-distance shots, party sequences, drawing rooms and establishing shots of houses. The production design is steeped in 'authentifying' period settings and lavish, correct costuming. Describing the goal of making the sets look 'convincingly 80s', production designer Mellanie Allen said, 'we just montaged loads and loads of references, so we knew exactly what would have been used in the 80s, the shapes of milk bottles, the cars, the graphics.' And yet, from the moment the pink cursive titles appear on-screen, it is clear that this will be a vision of the 80s through queer eyes, even if that view is itself limited or distorted.

The series begins in 1983 with 20-year-old Nick (Dan Stevens) arriving in London to start working on a PhD on Henry James. He's brought by his Oxford mate Toby Fedden (Oliver Coleman) to stay in the Fedden family mansion in Notting Hill. Toby's father, Gerald Fedden (Tim McInnerny), is an MP in Thatcher's recently re-elected government which had a strong majority. Nick lusts after Toby but finds close comradery with Toby's sister, Catherine (Hayley Atwell), and begins to emulate the detached, aristocratic bearing of Gerald's wife, Rachel (Alice Kridge).

The opening sequence frames the series via Nick's point-of-view, but also complicates identification with it, placing the viewer in a paradoxical relationship with the visual seductions of the heritage gaze. Inside Toby's car, Nick emerges from the shadow of a bridge into glittering sunshine; he gazes admiringly through the car window, his view of the tree-lined streets reflected back onto his face (see Figures 4.1–4.2). These three adjustments of viewpoint – low angle, vitrification, and character's point-of-view – flag a distortion of perspective, alerting us from the very beginning that Nick's impression isn't entirely reliable. Nick's emergence from shadows suggests that he himself is a shady character and although we're encouraged to sympathise and identify with him, he will at times

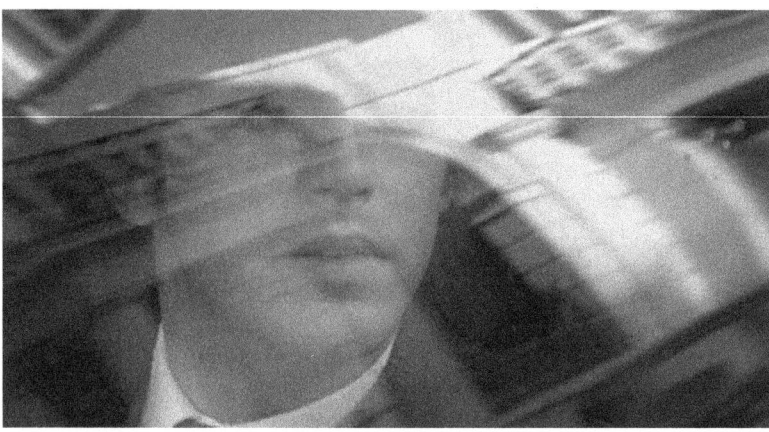

Figure 4.1 Distortions of perspective: Nick Guest (Dan Stevens) emerges from the shadows in *The Line of Beauty*, episode 1

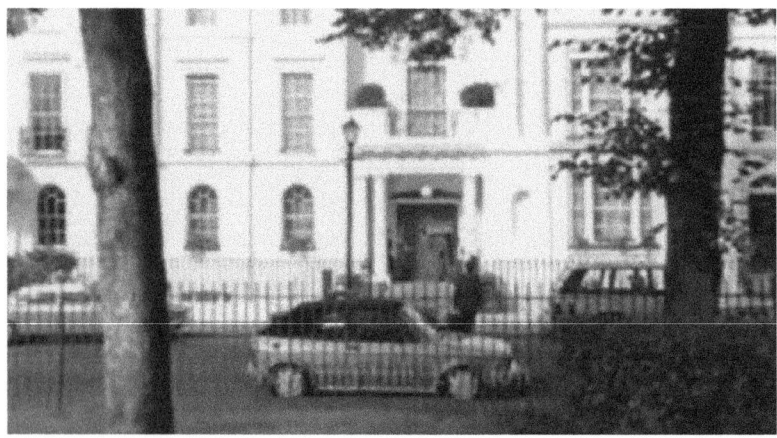

Figure 4.2 Toby and Nick are dwarfed by the Feddens' mansion in *The Line of Beauty* (episode 1)

AIDS Heritage in *The Line of Beauty*

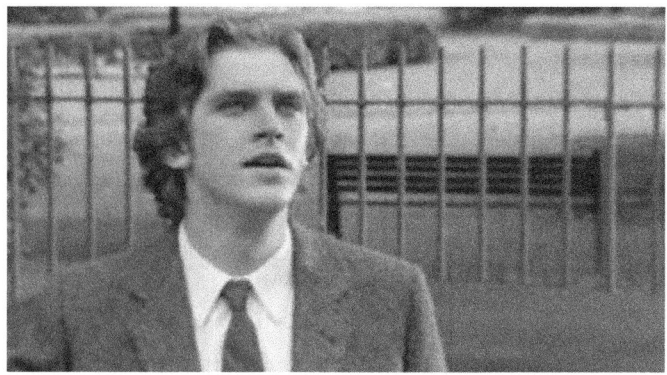

Figure 4.3 'Is this really where you live?' Nick gawks at the house in *The Line of Beauty* (episode 1)

conceal or misrepresent, knowingly or unconsciously, to others or to himself.

The Feddens' house is the central narrative space and the most semantically charged feature of the *mise en scène*. It is the site at which both the romantic seductions and hostile exclusions of privileged life take place. Its significance becomes apparent in an establishing shot in the opening sequence in which Nick and Toby are literally dwarfed by the house (Figure 4.2). Nick looks on reverentially (Figure 4.3), but the audience is privy to a more daunting perspective, with Martin Phipps's brooding, portentous theme on the soundtrack suggesting there are mysteries, if not dangers, present. From the very outset, then, *The Line of Beauty* puts its viewers at a subtle but discernable (queer) slant in relation to the seductions of period, luxury and property, positioning us ironically, ambivalently or at a distance from the luscious heritage spectacle.

'Nick Guest' is of course a deliberate naming. 'Nick' alludes to other literary Nicks, including Nick Carraway, the paradigmatic modernist narrator of F. Scott Fitzgerald's *The Great Gatsby* (1925), neither an insider nor entirely an outsider, complicit with the culture he observes. He also recalls Charles Ryder, the narrator of Evelyn Waugh's *Brideshead Revisited* (1945), another outsider–observer who has a fascination with the aristocratic life and with real estate. Like Guest, Ryder is 'politic, adaptable, and mild-mannered', and 'ingratiat[es] himself' into high society whilst 'leading a very different life outside it, or alongside it.'[48] And of course 'Guest' foregrounds this young man's complicated relationship to his surroundings, a relationship of both privilege and obligation, as we shall see.

Nick is cheerfully absorbed into the Fedden *ménage*, although his role there is subject to some brokerage and it is clear that he must discharge certain oblique functions beyond his ostensible status of friend and guest. Toby and his parents depart for Europe, leaving Nick to 'look after the Cat' (Catherine) and act as custodian of the house. As well as a keeper of the house, Nick becomes a keeper of secrets: while her parents are away, Nick discovers Catherine cutting herself and, on her request, agrees to withhold the incident from them. When they return and invite him to stay on, his guest status is again qualified and re-framed as an exchange that involves obligations on his part. He thanks the Feddens for their generosity but Gerald rebuffs this gratitude, saying 'Nonsense, you'll be doing us a favour. Subbing for Toby sort-of-thing, surrogate son of the house'. Gerald then pointedly thanks Elena (Carmen du Sautoy), the housekeeper, for preparing their evening meal, reminding us that these aristocratic types manage their domestics with an air of congeniality that smudges the line between friendship and employment.

Nick is a sexual and class outsider who is able to participate on account of the human capital he offers as a scholar, aesthete and confidence man. His father is a provincial antiques dealer, and Nick's schooling in art and furniture are his calling card in the Feddens' milieu. When Nick arrives at Hawkeswood, the country castle owned by Rachel's brother, Lord Kessler, his appraisal of the furniture is observed by the Lord and appraised in turn: 'What a beautiful writing desk. It must be about 1770?' 'Very good', says the Lord. Like other Jamesian aesthetes, Nick is an avid voyeur of houses and their contents. He's the heir to a long lineage of modern queer figures whose homosexuality is concealed by, articulated through, and inextricably twinned with an appreciation of aesthetic forms; his class-based knowledge and cultural capital is what makes him both intelligible and a source of value in the world of old money and New Right politcs. Like gay men in popular culture including the antiques appraisers on *Antiques Roadshow* and the 'lifestyle specialists' of *Queer Eye for the Straight Guy* – avatars of design, lifestyle and consumer culture knowledge and know-how – Nick

AIDS Heritage in *The Line of Beauty*

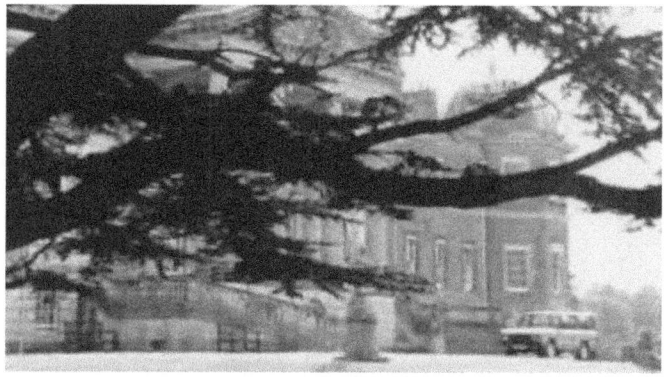

Figure 4.4 Gothic Heritage: Hawkeswood in *The Line of Beauty* (episode 1)

cultivates an aestheticised homosexuality as a key resource of self-entrepreneurship and advancement in Thatcherite neoliberal society.

Hawkeswood, where the Feddens throw a lavish twenty-first birthday party for Toby, is an iconic country estate of heritage cinema – powerful and brooding like the Pemberleys of *Pride and Prejudice* adaptations. Nick is instantly seduced by it, but the viewer is offered a portentous long shot of the castle, obscured by the branches of a huge Norfolk pine blowing about in the wind. It's a Gothic image: more Manderley than Pemberley – beautiful, awe-inspiring, but foreboding and full of dangerous secrets (Figure 4.4). This ambivalent framing of the house originates in Hollinghurst's novel: Nick admires the 'sheer presence' of the place, but it gives him 'a hilarious sense of his own social displacement.'[49] Hawkeswood is 'a complex climax', a 'strange and seductive fusion of an art museum and a luxury hotel.'[50]

The party sequence that unfolds at the castle showcases the series in its most baroque inhabitation of heritage. The genre's classic stylings are here in abundance: slow panning, circular-shots, set pieces, costume and pomp. As Held writes, the lavish society scene is 'the essential ingredient in the heritage formula'[51] (see Figures 4.5–4.6). However, the pleasures of gazing at this spectacle of British aristocratic display are called into question by a series of striking reminders that looking can be exploitative and or dangerous. Before the party Lord Kessler declares that 'there are umpteen beds

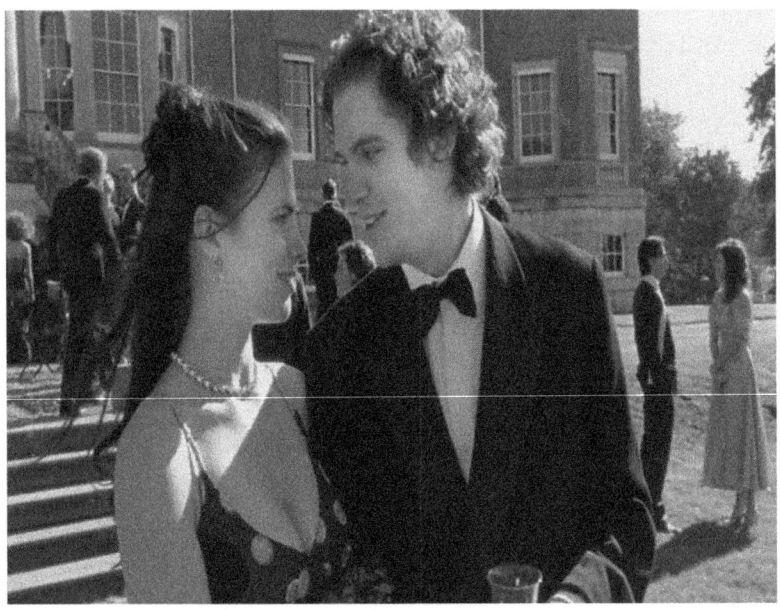

Figure 4.5 Baroque Heritage in *The Line of Beauty* (episode 1)

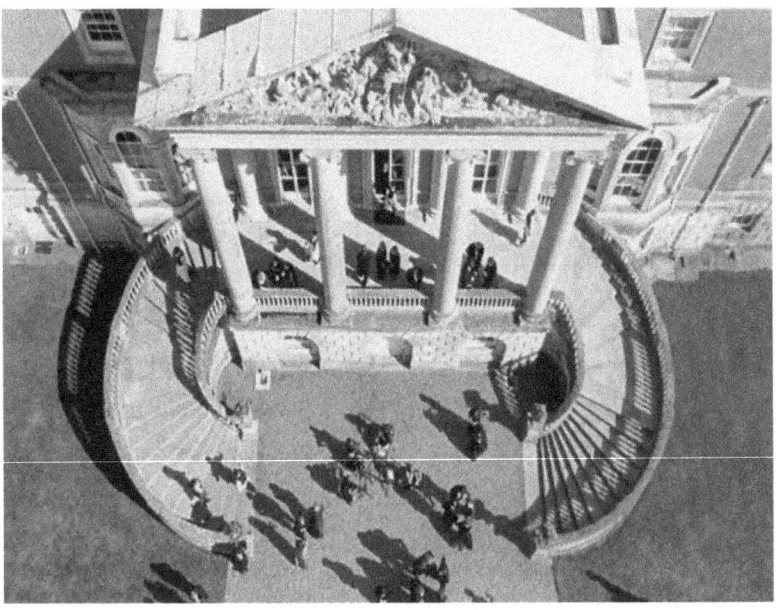

Figure 4.6 Heritage Real Estate in *The Line of Beauty* (episode 1)

AIDS Heritage in *The Line of Beauty*

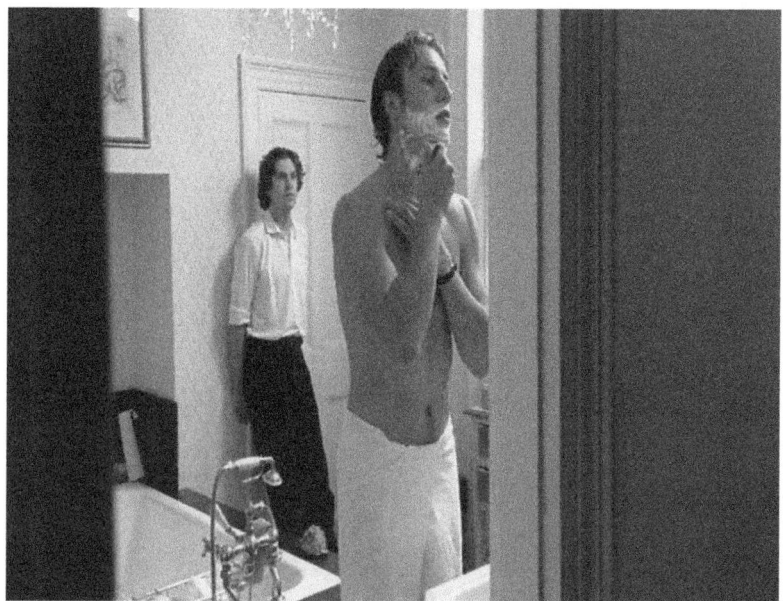

Figure 4.7 Nick steals a glance at Toby's (Oliver Coleman) buttocks in *The Line of Beauty* (episode 1)

here, [but] as to the precise arrangements, I avert my eyes.' But Nick does not avert his – indeed, all he hears and witnesses throughout his career with the Feddens become burdensome forms of knowledge that make him vulnerable and that contribute to his fall. At the party, he encounters two crass spectators that parallel his own voyeurism: Polly Tompkins (James Bradshaw), an old Oxford boy and a gratuitous perve, gossips to Nick about their mutual friends and objectifies the male waiters; Catherine's boyfriend Russel (Justin Salinger), a photographer for *The Face* magazine, exploits the Fedden connection for paparazzi shots of politicians and glamorous scenesters.

That Nick himself resembles these more grotesque, mercenary onlookers has already been suggested: earlier the camera has caught him lustfully eyeballing Toby's toweled buttocks in the bathroom (see Figure 4.7) and, in Episode Three, Nick's onlooking is intercut with, and thus likened to, the invasion of the paparazzi that envelop Gerald outside the Notting Hill house, bloodthirsty for scandal (see Figures 4.8–4.9). Later, as we shall see, the murderous gaze of the tabloid media, which has an especially disturbing valence for British audiences since the death of Diana, Princess

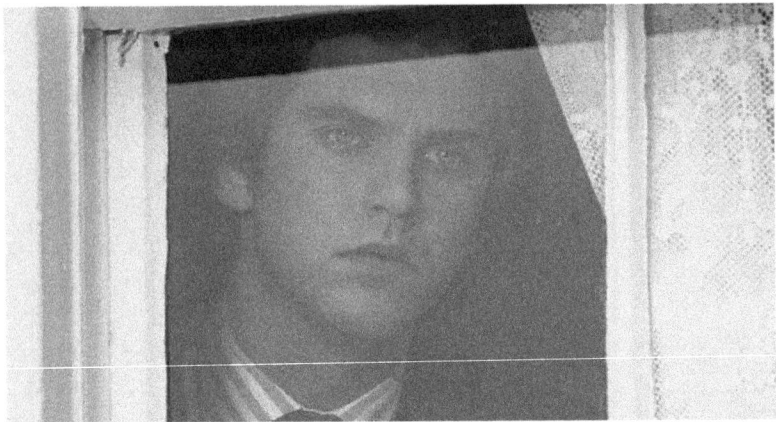

Figure 4.8 Nick watches Gerald get swamped by the media in *The Line of Beauty* (episode 3)

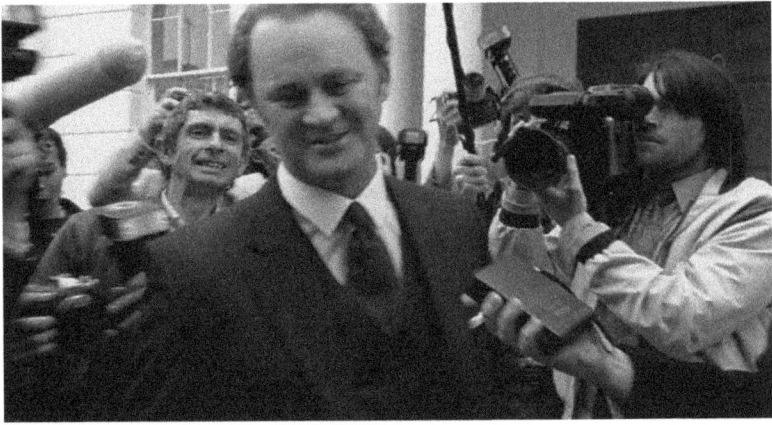

Figure 4.9 Gerald Fedden (Tim McInnerny) is enveloped by paparazzi in *The Line of Beauty* (episode 3)

of Wales in 1997, is turned back onto Nick in a powerful portrayal of the media spectacle of AIDS discussed in this book's Introduction.

In spite of these hints of danger, Nick is hypnotised by the beauty of the world inhabited by his hosts. Preferring to remain in a comfortable state of denial, he only gradually perceives its dangers. When Catherine describes her early depressive episode to Nick ('It's glittering, but it's deadly at the same time. It doesn't want you to survive it. It's totally negative'), her words hover in the air like a prolepsis of Nick's career with the Feddens, but it's a warning he doesn't heed. Like Isabel Archer in *Portrait of a Lady* (1881), Nick 'remains enamoured by the "brilliant" concealments of form upheld by the institution of the family.'[52]

But he isn't entirely or permanently dazzled. Gerald's reference to Henry James' *What Maisie Knew* (1897) in Episode One is a clue to interpreting Nick's career as an onlooker. *Masie* is a stark condemnation of parents and guardians who abandon their responsibilities towards their children – a portrait of a corrupt, decadent *fin de siècle* society told through the eyes of a child. *The Line of Beauty* is similarly concerned with themes of observation, knowledge and education. Nick's time with the Feddens rehearses the growth of Maisie's consciousness from faint glimmerings of awareness to a final, tragic comprehension of the situation, a characteristically Jamesian narrative trajectory from innocence to experience.

It is through Nick's eyes that Thatcherite excess and its ultimately murderous implications for people who contracted HIV in 1980s Britain are revealed. *The Line of Beauty* wants us to understand that passive, uncritical and consumptive forms of spectatorship may have ruinous effects. Its ambivalent identification with Nick's gaze throughout the three episodes is a central strategy for developing this awareness. In its moments of generic excess, when the spectacle of heritage circumambience may inspire the greatest viewing pleasure, the heritage gaze is always undermined, queered, repositioning the viewer to look critically.

Homeless Love

The tenuous status of the queer guest in the house of bourgeois privilege is a theme developed through the motif of admittance and tenure in the Feddens' mansion. Rather than a straightforward site of scopophilic pleasure, the heritage house is depicted as a charged symbol of inclusion and exclusion. Welcomeness is an indication of status and access, an allegory for entitlement and inclusion in the house of the nation – citizenship in the national family.

Nick's romance with Leo (Don Gilet), a black working-class civil servant, has all the excitements of first love and the frisson of racial, class and sexual transgressions practised under the Feddens' noses. Given Nick lives with the Feddens and Leo lives at home with his mother, the lovers have their first sexual encounter outdoors in the Kensington Park Road communal gardens. This scene of public sex is a very literal queering of aristocratic, heritage space. There is another scene of *al fresco* sex later on when Leo knowingly quips that they have a 'homeless love'. Shortly thereafter, Leo ends the relationship suddenly and inexplicably, leaving Nick alone, confused and devastated outside the Feddens' front door. Though it's never confirmed, early allusions suggest that Leo already has – or suspects he has – HIV, which may explain his sudden decision to leave Nick.

Jumping to 1986, episode 2 extends and further complicates the theme of the queer guest. Nick appears relaxed and comfortable in his life with the Feddens. He floats through beautiful interiors, lavish parties, cocaine and sex only faintly haunted by the spectre of AIDS. Leo seemingly forgotten, he is ensconced in a clandestine affair with glamorous Lebanese playboy and supermarket heir, Wani Ouradi (Alex Wyndham), and the two have started 'Ogee', a high-end publishing and production company named after the sinuous double curve cited by Hogarth as 'the line of beauty'. Wani is closeted, a philistine and an unapologetic snob with an insatiable appetite for cocaine, porn and sex. But despite his shortcomings, he is an object of sublime beauty and Nick remains addicted to an aesthetic fantasy of possessing him and being possessed. Ogee are planning the production of a glossy magazine and a film adaptation of Henry James' *The Spoils of Poynton* (1896/7). Originally called 'The House Beautiful', *The Spoils of Poynton* was the apotheosis of James' abiding interest in possession and possessions, in 'treating others as things even as things themselves are granted sovereign value.'[53]

On an Ogee junket to Europe, Nick and Wani join the Feddens at their *manoir* in France. This is the heritage setting par excellence, captured in luscious helicopter establishing shots and dizzying circular perspectives. However, the cracks that have already begun to appear in the surface here continue to fracture. By the huge swimming pool, Nick and Gerald exchange a loaded glance, reminding us of what Nick already knows: the MP is having a clandestine affair with his secretary, Penny Kent (Lydia Leonard). Then the Tippers arrive, rich Fedden political campaign supporters. The comedy of manners at the manoir quickly develops into a severe critique of class and homophobia. Sir Maurice Tipper (Kenneth Cranham) is a crotchety, greedy, asset-stripping 'cold blooded thug',[54] and his wife, Sally (Barbara Flynn), is smug, spoilt and ignorant. They are arch-conservative, Thatcherite powerbrokers. During dinner, news arrives that Rachel Fedden's close friend, Catherine's godfather, has died. Rachel attempts to conceal the disease that dare not speak its name:

> It was pneumonia, I'm afraid, but he hadn't been well. He picked up some extraordinary bug in the far-east last year. No one knew what it was. It was just frightfully bad luck.

In a tearful rage, Catherine protests her mother's reticence: 'Mum! For Christ sake! He had *AIDS!* He was gay! He liked anonymous sex ... Oh, it's pathetic! I mean the least we can do is tell the truth about him.'

Catherine's dissent spearheads a key discussion in the next scene during which, in one of few departures from Hollinghurst's novel, Nick comes out decisively against ignorance and homophobia. Sally Tipper casually remarks that 'with this sort of thing, I suppose everyone must have seen it coming.' Nick responds with a gentle appeal to compassion: 'I don't know, perhaps. Even if you do know it's going to happen, it doesn't make it any less awful when it does ... I think I heard you say Sir Maurice that your mother had a long final illness?' This however falls on hostile ears. Inflamed, Sir Maurice replies: 'It was utterly different, she hadn't brought it on herself!' 'No, that's true', Sally adds, 'and they're going to have to learn, aren't they? The homosexuals, I mean'. Now Nick weighs in more boldly, outing himself in a calm, assertive defense of gay men's response to AIDS: 'Actually we are learning to be safe. These days we use protection. And there are other things one can do. Oral sex for example is much less dangerous.' 'Kissing you mean?' Sally asks. But the comedy of her naivety is rapidly cut through by a vicious, visceral declaration of disgust from Maurice: 'I'm afraid what you're saying fills me with a physical revulsion. I don't see why anyone's surprised at this *AIDS business*! The whole thing's got completely out of hand! They had it coming, simple as that.'

The Tippers' reflect an ignorant, conservative view of sexuality and a vindictive, belligerent view of HIV/AIDS as a kind of punishment for sexual crimes. But this view of the plague is less religious than it is perhaps neoliberal: AIDS is a nasty 'business'; if you take a foolish risk you are likely to learn a tough lesson. This attitude conjures the transactional culture of emergent British neoliberalism, a worldview in which all human interactions – business, social, sexual – are underwritten by the logic of ownership and the market.[55]

A particularly English style of sexual reticence and bodily disgust seemed to underwrite the official response (and lack of response) to HIV/AIDS in Britain under Thatcher. In 1988, for example, the Department of Health and the Department of Education and Science censored the distribution of prevention education materials produced by its own Health Education Authority. The material was 'not sufficiently toe[ing] the "correct" moral Missionary line.'[56] The censorship of information considered erotic or pornographic or which acknowledged that homosexuality existed, along with other non-marital practices like casual sex, was part of the 'Missionary Model' of social policy on HIV/AIDS.[57] This included Section 28, which made community-based HIV/AIDS prevention and safer sex promotion very difficult. The Tippers embody precisely the type of conservatism that prevented an earlier and more concerted effort to prevent the spread of HIV.[58]

The scene is also a further intervention in heritage conventions. While classic heritage is supposedly innocent and sexually restrained, queer heritage is knowing and demonstrative. The latter is positive and unapologetic about sex, like Nick in this conversation, rather than reticent, ignorant and repulsed, like the Tippers. BBC2's amplification of the novel's critique of Thatcherite heterosexism in this scene and elsewhere in the series is a clear historical assessment of the social and legal moralism of this moment in British political culture. Under Thatcher, the mobilisation of intensified ideologies of 'the family' and 'the nation' through specific social policies were grounded in 'endless appeals to "tradition" and "heritage"'.[59] The British heritage industry – including heritage cinema – was considered to be complicit with this neoconservatism and the traditional sexual morality it encompassed. This is what makes this small augmentation of Nick's politics so significant for *The Line of Beauty* as an artifact of post-crisis culture: queer heritage is here not only implicitly *meta*-heritage (self-reflexive; staging a commentary on its own generic progenitors), it is revisionist and reparative – it speaks angrily and openly back to the violence of the not-so-distant British past. Less complicit with ruling class culture than his counterpart in the novel, BBC2's Nick refuses to remain silent. The series thus comes to resemble the 'queer heritage' described by Dyer in which coming out can be 'heroic', a 'small act of courage from the past.'[60]

Belonging

The title of episode 2, 'To Whom do you Beautifully Belong?', explicitly foregrounds the issue of belonging. It quotes the title of the second part of Hollinghurst's novel which itself quotes Henry James' 1907 play *The High Bid*. In James' play, the line is directed at a butler. In Hollinghurst's novel it draws attention to Nick's 'annihilating desire' to belong as a family member among the Feddens and his equally damaging role of 'ornamental possession' in his relationship with Wani.[61] These relationships of ownership draw attention to the dynamic in which the figure of the aesthete/artist is beholden to his patrons.[62] James was particularly interested in this theme and, interestingly, it is a theme repeated in the dynamics surrounding the domesticated, desexualised New Gay Men archetype of post-closet TV and cinema discussed in Chapter 1. This figure is frequently some kind of handy appendage to the family, a queer servant-friend or factotum who is recruited to the service of heterosexual domesticity. Nick is quite literally a 'Queer Eye' on/for the Fedden family: he monitors them, deriving his own complex pleasure from this voyeurism and from his imagined place among them, and, in exchange for room and board, his charm and aesthetic literacy are added to the family's reservoir of cultural capital. But, like Robbie in *The Next Best Thing*, his participation is restricted and when times turn sour his status becomes precarious.

In another arrangement that blurs the line between intimacy and employment, Nick's Ogee roles as editor, screenwriter, 'the 'writing man', and 'an item in a budget'[63] are remunerated, but his informal duties as Wani's lover – procuring drugs, soliciting men, keeping secrets – are an oblique form of intimate labour. Bertrand Ouradi (Andy Lucas), Wani's supermarket magnate father, refers to Nick as 'Wani's aesthete.' Nick is 'basically a servant', During observes, 'a servant to new money precisely without the English gentlemanly style, capable of unnerving coarseness and rudeness.'[64] This dynamic is never more economically conveyed than when Wani arranges lines of cocaine on the cover of a book titled *Henry James and the Question of Romance* while explaining to Nick why their relationship must remain a secret. The twin signs of Henry James and those narcotic 'lines of beauty' gesture to an economy in which intimate and material forms of possession are inextricably intertwined: sex and other intimate services are exchanged for access to drugs, money and social privilege. As Tristao, the Madeiran waiter (Bruno Lastra), who has also exchanged sex with Wani for money and drugs says, Wani 'always pay the best'.

In spite of his adoption of the role of observing outsider, Nick is frequently complicit with his social milieu. Part of what makes him so compatible with this culture's precarious arrangements of both work and intimacy is his willingness to ignore the corrupt elements of the social world he circulates in and benefits from. Nick's loyalty to Wani (which is not one of sexual fidelity) and to the Feddens is motivated by a combination of self-interest, fantasised belonging and 'an almost masochistic passivity' that During suggests is a 'characteristic quality of neoliberal subjectivity'.[65] From this perspective, Nick's complicity with these social and economic arrangements of intimacy and relationality are both a moral compromise and a survival instinct under the emergent conditions of neoconservative neoliberal culture.

'Belong' also refers to the larger issue of social belonging, a question that takes on a particular urgency when AIDS enters the narrative in Episode 3. Where does the gay man belong? Sometimes he's as an awkward interloper or a peripheral figure. At the Hawkeswood party sequence, heritage conventions telegraph his vacillation between belonging and outsiderdom. As well as showcasing a panoramic perspective on setting and sumptuous evening costumes, the circular camera rotations and panning shots show that Nick is both surrounded by people but alone in the crowd (see Figure 4.10). He floats from one space to another, sometimes included, but mostly looking on at a heterosexual world: Catherine kissing Russell, male/female dancefloor couplings, a couple copulating on the lawn outside. These exclusions dramatise the interior world of the novel's Nick, who feels

> restless and forgotten, peripheral to an event which, he remembered, had once been thought of as his party too. His loneliness bewildered him for a minute, in the bleak perspective of the bachelors' corridor: a sense close to panic that he didn't belong in this house with these people.[66]

AIDS Heritage in *The Line of Beauty*

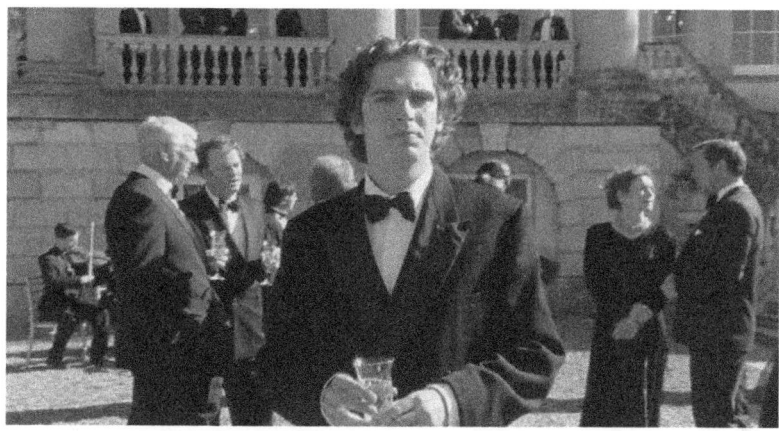

Figure 4.10 Alone in the crowd: Nick Guest (Dan Stevens) at the party in Hawkeswood in *The Line of Beauty* (episode 1)

We are reminded of Nick's guest position when Toby says: 'C'mon Guest', inviting Nick to follow him inside for the party formalities. This motif is repeated throughout the series: Nick is frequently invited to come inside the Feddens' house, reminding us of his visitor status and his incapacity to properly assimilate because of the official exclusion of homosexuality from English public life.

Rather than merely scopophilic pleasure or a guarantee of period authenticity, the high bourgeois house – the iconic visual motif of heritage cinema – is a semantically charged signifier of entitlement and inclusion in the house of the nation. Access to it demarcates those with the capacity to own literal and symbolic pieces of the national infrastructure from others who are, in effect, owned. Although Nick generally passes in the Feddens' world, there are clearer boundaries drawn around the tolerance of more visible forms of class and racial difference. When Leo visits Nick, he's not invited in warmly but greeted with a disdainful expression (see Figure 4.11). When a dinner party is interrupted by Catherine accompanied by Brentford, a black minicab driver, Gerald is shocked and yells 'What's he doing in my house?' Both of these scenes take place by the front door, the anxiously guarded line demarcating public and private, privileged and excluded. The exclusion of black working-class men warns us that the status of the gay bachelor too is likely to become precarious.

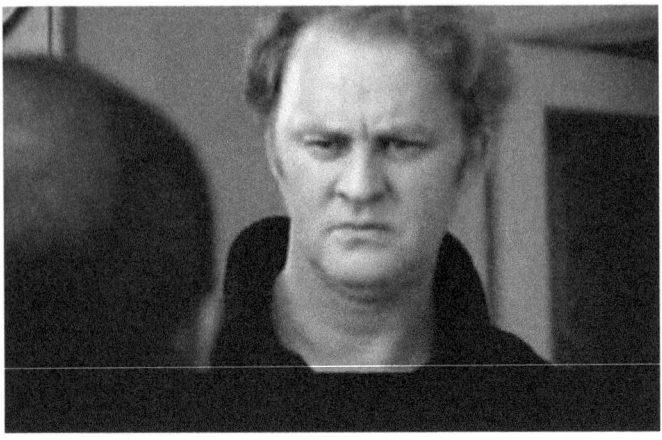

Figure 4.11 The shock of class difference: Gerard greets Leo (Don Gilet) in *The Line of Beauty* (episode 1)

Nick has neither kinship nor economic clout; he is invited to dinner, as he explains to Leo, to 'make up the numbers'.

As a guest in the house of privilege, Nick is held hostage to the mastery and monitoring of his hosts. Drawing on Jacques Derrida's work on hospitality, Daniel Hannah argues that Nick's career with the Feddens is a case study in 'the fantasy and the limitations, in language and in practice, of hospitality.'[67] He occupies a 'guest-like position' in both the private domestic and public political realms of Thatcherite Britain, realms that are 'conjoined by shared visions of a heterosexual matrix of mastery.'[68] 'So, they're easy about having a bender in their house, are they, their lordships?' Leo asks in Episode 1, and Nick never articulates his own ambiguous, semi-closeted status so well as when he replies, dryly: 'of course, they're fine about it, so long as it's never mentioned.' As the Feddens' guest – and, more figuratively, a guest in the house of the nation – Nick is compelled to selectively play down the open secret of his homosexuality as a condition of his presence. His status in the Feddens' world can be viewed as something of an allegory for the beholden position of the invited other in western culture and the limits of hospitality. As Hannah explains, for Derrida, '"hospitality"… is forever torn between "*The* law of unlimited hospitality" that demands a welcome irrespective of the guest's status and "the laws (in the plural), [that] those rights and duties that are always conditioned and conditional", seek to monitor the guest "across the family, civil society, and the State."'[69] He continues:

> In practice, hospitality – which requires the host to be "master" of a house, home, or even nation – works through a violent mastery, a taking hostage, of the guest, containing the guest's power to make the host a hostage to the law of hospitality. But if Derrida's model of torn hospitality takes the foreigner or other (*étranger*) as its ambivalent centre, *The Line of Beauty* points to the gay citizen's status within the nation-state as the ever-invited yet excluded "guest" of both the conjugal family and the family's institutional extension, the state.[70]

The Line of Beauty is a case study in 'torn hospitality'. As Hannah elaborates, 'the gay observer is retained as the perfect guest, the refined observer, in the heteronormative house of capitalist acquisition so long as evidence of his sexuality is reduced to pure aesthetic taste, so long as bodily signs of his gayness remain private, invisible'.[71]

BBC2's adaptation presents this dynamic in which the invited other always exists in a beholden and closely monitored, prohibited relationship to family and state through Nick's fraught inhabitation of heritage space. Like a butler, Nick is a custodian of the Feddens' house, monitoring its comings and goings, collecting its confidences, lingering for perhaps too long in his attic bedroom. All the while, his status in the house is tenuous and subject to unspoken constraints. When AIDS enters the narrative more forcefully in its denouement, Nick's precarious status comes into particular relief and is, finally, rendered unambiguous. The scandal of homosexuality and AIDS illustrates the limits of both tolerance and hospitality. As we shall see, this is another way that heritage *mise en scène* functions as a semiotically charged narrative space, as opposed to a merely attractive backdrop.

Eviction

Episode 3 of *The Line of Beauty* approaches the end of the 1980s. By this time two powerful, unmentionable spectres that have hitherto haunted the series have materialised in the flesh: Margaret Thatcher, invisible until she finally arrives at the Feddens' anniversary party, and AIDS. Thatcher presides over the culture with a potency that is sexual as well as political. However, like the love and the disease that, in polite company, dare not speak their name, her actual name in never mentioned. She is known as 'The Lady', 'Madam' or 'Mrs T.'

In the 1987 election Gerald narrowly retains his seat but is soon being investigated for shady finances. Nick discovers that Leo has died from AIDS, and Wani Ouradi too has AIDS. The house, in its function as the central narrative space and the embodiment of the paradoxes at the heart of Nick's story (belonging/exile; life/death), begins to crumble, and, steadily, Nick's privileges are withdrawn. Everything is unravelling as we suspected it ultimately would: Gerald's affair with his secretary is revealed and his political career is ruined; the press, now camped outside the Notting Hill mansion, discovers the connection between Nick and Wani, supermarket heir millionaire who has AIDS, and the scandals of homosexuality and epidemic disease are added to the carnage. This shocking public revelation of clandestine homosexuality in the upper echelons of the Thatcherite elite and the spectacular disease/punishment of AIDS is the straw that breaks Nick's relationship with the Feddens. The Feddens turn on Nick and blame him for both Catherine's absconding and the public revelation of Gerald's adultery. While he was cheerfully tolerated as a charming accessory in more prosperous times, now Nick is scapegoated for the family's fall from grace and expelled from the heritage house.

Nick's disgraced expulsion allegorises the panic logic of epidemic, in which gay men and others with AIDS were transformed into public enemies, social pariahs, exiles from the house of the nation. A scan of newspaper front pages in the Feddens' kitchen shows us the lurid tabloid headlines familiar from that time: 'Gay Sex Link to Minister's House', 'Peer's Playboy Son has AIDS', 'Minister's Gay Lodger: Nicholas Guest', 'Gay Sex Romps at MP's Holiday Home.' In this unostentatious way, *The Line of Beauty* reveals the extent to which the spectacle of AIDS plays a central role in the devastating end to Nick's career. The period saw a vicious backlash against gay men and lesbians in the AIDS panic that was stirred up in mainstream British media. The Feddens' handling of Nick is evocative of the way in which gay men and other AIDS 'victims' became convenient folk devils for Tory politicians 'burning off their resentments of social reforms dating back to the late 1960s.'[72] In the thick of AIDS panic, Nick's status shifts abruptly from valued insider to spurned outcast, privileged guest to contaminated pariah.

Nick's retrenchment during a period of financial and political threat (the global economic downturn and its weakening of the Tory government's political stronghold) is suggestive of the way in which the toleration of difference in the neoliberal state tends to rely upon favourable economic circumstances. Dan Stevens, who played Nick in the series, described in an interview how initially the Feddens are open to this aesthete, to this 'artistic, romantic, intellectual figure', this 'curio' with no significant purpose. However, Nick becomes a liability precisely when the economy becomes less forgiving of such extravagances: 'as the 80s progress, and the recession kicks in… they have to start chopping off all the extravagant arms of their life.'[73]

In spite of their blue-chip aristocratic and economic status, Nick's investment in the Feddens turns out to have been an insecure venture. His risky financial calculus can be read as an allegory for the paradoxes and dangers of Thatcherite neoliberalism and its somewhat conflicting strains of moralism and rampant individualism. As During argues, 'homophobia and the Thatcherite appeal to the old narrow traditions of dissenting morality is… galling because neoliberalism has another ethos too: a welcoming of risk, enterprise, independence of inherited values and hedonism, which particularly solicits a certain urban gay participation, and certainly secures Nick's participation.'[74] However, while market competitiveness, risk and entrepreneurial forms of subjectivity are idealised under neoliberal economics as the engine to advancement for all, for certain types of people labour and competition is circumscribed. *The Line of Beauty* reminds us with chilling precision that the ambitions of particular sectors of the market – openly gay men, women, black people, people with AIDS, sex workers and others – are considered illegitimate, and these illegitimacies may be strictly enforced.

The tragic finale sees Nick cast adrift. With the scandal of AIDS testing the limits of tolerance and market privilege, favour from those with congealed class privilege is rescinded. The gay bachelor is left homeless, turned out into what Agamben calls 'the state of abandonment', the non-space of bare life. This expulsion is not merely symbolic, but has material stakes that are ones of life and death. During the series denouement, we are privy to a brief, seemingly irrelevant scene of Nick having a shower. Naked, captured from behind in a middle-distance shot, he looks alone and vulnerable. This recalls a moment from episode 1 when Leo showers at the Feddens' house (see Figures 4.12–4.13). Leo is now dead, and this news has left Nick utterly devastated. We don't know whether Nick is HIV positive, but he

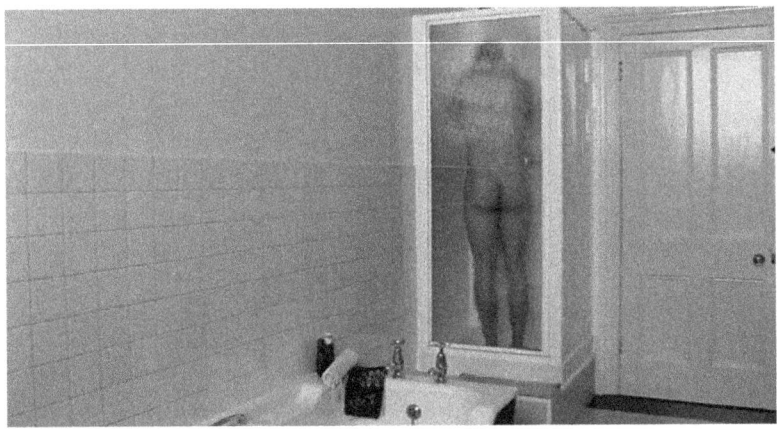

Figure 4.12 The vulnerable space of bare life in *The Line of Beauty* (episode 3)

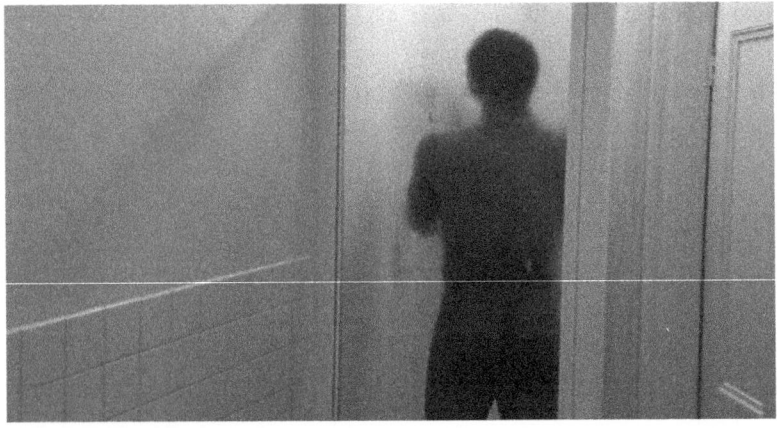

Figure 4.13 Leo showering and foreshadowing in *The Line of Beauty* (episode 1)

has lost two lovers to the disease, and shortly after the shower scene we see him getting an HIV test. The earlier shower scene foreshadows the latter. In these brief scenes, the material stakes of the spectacle of AIDS are drawn into stark relief. The vulnerable space of Nick's body becomes the space of bare life. Where will Nick go now that his 'pretend family' have ejected him and his lovers are dying or have died? Where does an aesthete belong if he's unwelcome in the house of privilege? Nick's life has been reduced to *homo sacer*, stripped of its cultural, moral and political value.

In the stylish translation of Hollinghurst's novel to the screen by BBC2, the motif of the heritage home and who is admitted into it develops a thematics of access and exclusion, extending the novel's critique of England in the era of the AIDS crisis. This knowing use of heritage conventions helps to track the status of the gay male guest in the house of bourgeois privilege, where he is ultimately confronted with the limits of tolerance. So, although *The Line of Beauty* has the stylish elegance of heritage cinema, it is far from an unmitigated indulgence in an idealised, romantic national past. It recalls the double capacity of the retrovision to capture both the attractions as well as the traumas of history. In the retrovision, as Cartmell, Hunter and Whelehan describe it, the past is reconstructed with a mixture of melancholy and fondness. This is the double capacity of nostalgic feeling: Nick's career ends in tragedy, but right up until the very end, there are heritage stylings that encourage sentimental attachments to the past. This ambivalent combination of historical feelings – of melancholy/horror combined with fondness/longing – is a paradox that, as we'll see further in the next chapter, has become a characteristic of AIDS memory. In the example of *The Line of Beauty*, the extreme proximity of murderous indifference to the sublime seductions of glamour and beauty is the climactic shock of the narrative that re-routes its comedy of manners towards Jamesian tragedy. And if, even in the final devastating scene of this drama, Nick Guest is still awed by the enigmatic façade of the high bourgeois home, this is because the past in heritage culture is still attractive, even if it was cruel. For BBC2, heritage conventions capture this ambivalent retrospective gaze: the baroque heritage retrovision, with its capacity to stir nostalgia, ambivalence and melancholy simultaneously, is a privileged genre for encapsulating these paradoxical backwards feelings. Even though style, beautiful and sublime in its forms, has become a conspicuous sign of power and heteronormative violence, we can't help but remain – like James, Hollinghurst, Nick Guest and the BBC – absolutely devoted to it.

AIDS Heritage and Post-Crisis

> It was a period of such extraordinary, violent change and of course the time in which the AIDS crisis really peaked and those are two things that have sort of weighed on my mind for a long time.... I had a sense of unfinished business, I wanted to go back and look at the period.
>
> Alan Hollinghurst[75]

In line with Dyer's formulation of a sub-genre of 'homosexual heritage', *The Line of Beauty* may be considered a form of queer heritage with a liberal, anti-homophobic political agenda. However, the symbolic work of prestige, heritage aesthetics also links BBC2's series to a popular, *national* heritage culture. If heritage, particularly in the UK, has been the stylistic idiom most closely associated with visions of the national past, then *The Line of Beauty* presents the AIDS Crisis as a national history – not only a homosexual history, but a universal history, in which all citizens are implicated. Via the pedagogical remit of the BBC and of the TV movie form, the prestige adaptation speaks directly and unapologetically to citizens of the nation as inheritors of this national legacy: AIDS and the phobic treatment of those affected by it becomes an official part of national collective memory; the national and the queer are brought together as interrelated histories.

As the next chapter will explore further, the burgeoning archive of representations of the AIDS Crisis has become its own particular current within the global 'memory boom'. More particularly, the period has become a seminal history for contemporary queer culture and politics, and particularly so for gay men. The AIDS Crisis functions as a sort of founding narrative of contemporary queer culture that is authenticating and identityc onstituting on the one hand, traumatic and lamentable on the other; it may be put to multiple political 'uses'. In describing *The Line of Beauty* as a 'memory text' I take it as axiomatic that cultural memory – a collective or localised engagement with a particular past – can function as a means of negotiating or understanding the present.

AIDS Heritage in *The Line of Beauty*

Cultural memorialisation practices and storytelling are widely understood by scholars in the field of memory studies as rituals that mediate and/or modify the past – often a troubling past – in an attempt to mollify the present or modify the future. In the next chapter, we will consider the contemporary salience of recent popular AIDS crisis memorialising further. Here, I want to conclude this chapter by returning to the idea of 'AIDS heritage', and reflecting more consciously on what this type of memory work does for political and cultural life in the present.

In this book's Introduction, we saw how a moralistic narrative fatalism frequently underwrote crisis-era representations of homosexuality and AIDS, and how this narrative was both informed by and informs a homophobic logic of diseased queer personhood. The story of 'gay AIDS' was frequently a narrative of sexual crime and punishment, a sort of 'Dorian Myth' in the likeness of Oscar Wilde's famous novel. In the previous chapter on bareback panic, we saw how new iterations of this narrative logic of crime and punishment have frequently re-emerged in the post-antiretrovirals period but in new technological and social situations – old stories resurfacing to account for new circumstances. In *The Line of Beauty*, the narrative advances through a similar, melodramatic tragic structure: a talented young man proceeds from innocence to experience in a narrative that ends with AIDS and death. Is this the same moralistic narrative logic of crisis discourse? Is Nick's story another fable of sexual crime and punishment so befitting the story of AIDS as 'gay disease', as a 'nineteenth century novelistic phenomenon,'[76] or, to quote Robert Dessaix, that 'superbly simple' Greco-Roman narrative that chronicles the career of the talented hedonist who foolishly ignores the gods, is dramatically struck down by them, suffers, cause others to suffer, and dies?[77]

Some critics have thought so. Julie Rivkin describes Hollinghurst's novel as 'a bit of a morality play,'[78] and Dascăl finds the 'extremity of its moral turn to be somewhat objectionable.'[79] Hollinghurst, she writes:

> effects a narrative unravelling so extreme that the book ends by holding to a somewhat trite and anachronistic vision of the homosexual as a figure always doomed to be unhoused and exiled from happiness, solitary and lonely, without family or friends, always nostalgic for a bosom that has always, if only secretly, rejected him.[80]

A review in *The Christian Science Monitor* provides a further example of this kind of reading:

> Rather than challenge any mainstream prejudices about homosexuals, *The Line of Beauty* confirms them. The most socially conservative reader won't be surprised to see here that gay men are emotionally oversensitive, sexually voracious, desperately lonely, and finally doomed.[81]

As these examples suggest, there's no doubt that both novel and film – and, accordingly, AIDS crisis history – may be read in this way.

I don't agree that the novel's denouement should be considered a 'moralistic turn'. *The Line of Beauty* indeed ends in tragedy, but without a precise destiny for Nick. In this, both novel and series resist the sacrificial martyrdom and the capital punishment of the PWA that brought about closure in crisis-era AIDS melodramas. *The Line of Beauty* refuses such historical fatalism. Neither does it eradicate the homosexual as a means of restoring the family. Indeed, the family is left broken, itself in profound crisis. Though one can easily imagine that the economic fortunes of the Feddens will be recouped, there is no doubt about the corruption of the institutions they represent – the white patriarchal nuclear family, the rich capitalist elite, the state.

Even more so than Hollinghurst's book, BBC2's series is unambiguous in its critique of these institutions – it wears its dim view of Thatcherite morality on its sleeve. As Swaab writes, 'the advent of AIDS, like the outbreaks of racism, cuts through the moral ambivalences of the story.'[82] If there *is* something moralistic about *The Line of Beauty*, it is that a finger is clearly being pointed at the political and economic elite. Although Nick remains somewhat complicit in the denials and disavowals that dominate that milieu, he becomes more unequivocally angry and political during key moments in the series. BBC2 gives us a (Jamesian) central consciousness with more *conscience*.

While Nick is left homeless and devastated, he is not without what might be called the agency of comprehension. Nick's story is one of a profound loss of innocence, but one with moments of frank, political resistance that are, if not defiantly activist in character, galvanising in emotional ways. As Swaab says of the final frames:

> We might feel that the ending is a blessing in disguise, traumatic but necessary if Nick is to escape into a wider and less sleazy world.... The last, visually distinctive shot is an aerial view of London's westbound roadways towards nightfall, not exactly a landscape of loss or of hope, except that it gathers Nick into a rather sombre sketch of solidarity with other lives in the metropolis.[83]

Rather than a simple moralistic trajectory of crime and punishment – that homophobic appropriation of the Wildean myth, which always leaves its queer protagonists dead as an object lesson – AIDS heritage in *The Line of Beauty* may be more profitably described as a trajectory from innocence to experience, a much more Jamesian line. If there is a 'lesson', it's not that 'they're going to have to learn', as Sally Tipper belligerently puts it. It is, rather, that there's a danger in 'making up the numbers' – that in attaching oneself to the institutions of family, money and state, the queer guest places themself in an isolated and vulnerable position. Seeking 'a place at the table', attempting to camouflage oneself within the world of privilege, may be dangerous. As we saw in Chapter 1, the New Gay Man in *The Next Best Thing* was taught a similar lesson: punished and effectively banished for his attempt to assimilate where he didn't belong. Though dissimilar stories about gay life and AIDS, *The Next Best Thing* and *The Line of Beauty* have a common obsession with the home, with the threat of being un-homed, with belonging and un-belonging, the fraught experience queer people have amidst these institutions and the way in which HIV/AIDS and its associations brings these dynamics into stark relief.

If *The Line of Beauty* is an early but exemplary case of AIDS heritage, then AIDS heritage is a category that arouses feelings that are both negative *and* reparative. AIDS memory becomes a site of mourning and painful loss, but also a site of restorative nostalgia[84] and utopian longing.[85] Arousing both nostalgic and painful feeling states, AIDS heritage is an acute example of Love's 'backwards feelings'.

But does AIDS heritage always function in this way? As the popular representation of AIDS and HIV has turned unmistakably backwards – to AIDS history, to the 'original' dramatic moment of 'The AIDS Crisis' and the response of the affected communities to that crisis – what has happened to HIV in the present? How does positioning 'crisis' as a past event function politically when we consider the present-day concerns of the post-crisis landscape of HIV? How does 'AIDS heritage' function in the realms of contemporary LGBTQI+ politics? Are AIDS retrovisions 'positive images' in the manner that this book has identified? These are large questions demanding a larger project that engages freshly with the boom in AIDS memory and AIDS history in recent years. Nonetheless, in the final chapter of this book, we shall embark on a brief consideration of these questions. What we'll find in the 'backwardsing' of AIDS and gay pasts is more complex varieties of nostalgia and more of the simultaneous orientations backwards and forwards of post-crisis culture.

5

AIDS Retrovisions

Dallas Buyers Club *and* The Normal Heart

Turning Away

After ARVs, the communities of people living with and affected by HIV were suddenly compelled to address the radically expanded temporal horizon of living with HIV from within a vastly contracted horizon of public discussion. These were the years you had to search hard for a whiff of HIV on TV screens, when HIV/AIDS plots in commercial cinemas became scarce, and when discussions of the global pandemic diminished across broadcast, print and the burgeoning digital news spaces produced in the English-speaking world. Of course there were exceptions to this overall trend, without which the preceding chapters of this book would not exist: peripheral HIV sub-plots in cinema like the one in *The Next Best Thing*, the singular and somewhat complex sero-melodrama of *Queer as Folk*, semi-regular eruptions of sex panics like the barebacking and chemsex panics discussed in Chapter 3, the strangely retrograde *Brothers & Sisters* subplot discussed in this book's Introduction and *The Line of Beauty* in both novel and screen forms, which, alongside *Angels in America,* signaled the beginning of a popular canonisation of certain – largely gay male – historical experiences of the AIDS crisis. A broad audience of media consumers may have encountered other minor dramatisations from this period that have not been mentioned in this book, like Richie (Ed Harris), the AIDS-stricken poet friend of a Clarissa Dalloway figure played by Meryl Streep in *The Hours* (2002). There was also, for example, the bohemian AIDS milieu of the screen adaptation of Broadway musical, *Rent* (2005), a glossy, faux-queer cooptation of impoverished life in East Village, New York in the late 1980s.

Small exceptions aside, after the wrap up of *Queer as Folk* in 2005 there was barely a whisper about HIV and gay male life on popular screens. Theodore Kerr calls the 12-year period stretching from the introduction of ARVs in 1996 the 'the Second Silence'. The 'first silence' was the notorious five-year period between 1981 and 1986 in which American President Ronald Regan didn't utter the word 'AIDS' in public, and against which iconic activist campaigns like Gran Fury's famous 'Silence=Death' poster reacted. During the Second Silence, Kerr writes, 'the epidemic went from explicit due to the hard work of activists and people living with HIV to make it visible, to implicit: from public to private.' HIV/AIDS cultural production in the English-speaking world went into 'undetectable crisis' mode. As I hope this book has served to demonstrate, the noiselessness of this period is not only noteworthy for its distinct contrast with what came before it. Importantly, as Kerr adds, while 'silence equals death' it 'does not equal nothingness': 'within the Second Silence, as within the First, much happened that is difficult to render for public consumption and understanding'.[2]

Many of the positive images of HIV positive and gay male life described in this book colluded with that silence in certain ways. As I argued in Chapter 1, 1990s positive imagery was motivated by the impulse to orient itself toward the future, which meant that representations of gay life worked anxiously and fastidiously to shake off its associations with death, meaninglessness, melancholy and the other negative feelings associated with the experience of AIDS. HIV and AIDS threatened to draw gay men inexorably *backwards*. Contending with the threat of this backwards drag and its seemingly unpalatable implications demanded the erection of a psychic divide between a shameful, profligate gay sexual past and a mature, future-straining present and future. If this was the 'psychology' of that moment, we also saw something of its manifestation as a narrative of history both explicitly and subtextually in the panic scripts around barebacking and chemsex. Indeed, a version of this account has existed since the first outbreaks of crisis discourse and it inheres in the homophobic fantasy that epidemic disease was a kind of divine punishment for the sexual sins of a promiscuous earlier period. An imagined divide – psychic, metaphoric, historical – between this promiscuous, hedonistic period, followed directly by AIDS (read as 'the past') and the 'mature', monogamous present has come to underwrite many representations of gay life during the post-crisis period and accounts of queer and AIDS history in neoliberal times.

Though humanities discussions of HIV/AIDS also became a much quieter field during the Second Silence, they weren't as silent as popular culture. Indeed, a number of AIDS cultural critics attempted to grapple with and interpret this silence itself. In 'Melancholia and Moralism', an essay written in 2002, Douglas Crimp diagnosed this seemingly pervasive cultural amnesia about HIV/AIDS as a form of 'melancholic disavowal'. Melancholic disavowal, he explained, was a socio-psychic response manifesting across culture but evident particularly in LGBTQI+ politics, most particularly in the rhetoric of gay neoconservatives who equated contemporary, rights-based sexual politics with maturity, while radical liberation politics were considered by them to be infantile.[3] For Crimp, the best example of this was Andrew Sullivan's controversial *New York Times* magazine article 'When Plagues End: Notes on the Twilight of an Epidemic'.[4] In this essay, the former editor of *New Republic* and neoconservative gay commentator made the argument that the experience of AIDS had brought about a shift gay politics, through which gay people began to demand recognition of their service to their country, and equal treatment under the law. According to Crimp, Sullivan couched the shift towards rights-based agendas premised on state recognition (whereas in the past there had been state *persecution* of queer people) within a 'moral narrative' in which the experience of AIDS 'made gay men grow up'. Crimp paraphrases Sullivan:

> before AIDS, gay life ... was identified with freedom from responsibility ... from the constraints of traditional norms ... in return for an acquiescence in second-class citizenship .... But with AIDS, responsibility became a central imposing feature of gay life.... People who thought they didn't care for one another found that they could. Relationships that had no social support were found to be as strong as any heterosexual marriage.[5]

Here, Crimp reads Sullivan in order to make a prescient argument about the way a historically-based 'AIDS=maturity' equation has come to underwrite the conservative turn in gay politics.[6] In the logic of this equation Crimp detects evidence of a phobic turning away from AIDS and HIV, both past and present – a 'melancholic disavowal'. The 'fearsomeness of AIDS always induced this tendency to disavowal,'[7] he observed, and yet, in the years following antiretrovirals, there was 'a drastic change, a psychic change, a change in the way we think about AIDS, or rather a change that consists in our ability to continue thinking about AIDS'.[8] Crimp argued that the traumatic experience of mass deaths, the enduring anxiety at the possibility of contracting HIV and the gnawing guilt associated with the knowledge that ongoing AIDS-related deaths were tragically occurring in so many parts of the world were all aversive feelings that together conspired to this particular way of framing history. This same collection of feelings informed the Second Silence. This turn away from AIDS has a range of motivations: 'phobic denial' ("this isn't happening"); a fantasy of prophylaxis ("this can't affect me" / "I have nothing in common with those people"); or too much pain and loss ("I can no longer bear this"). In all instances, melancholic disavowal is the coping mechanism – a way of assimilating to and remaining psychically insulated from AIDS trauma. It is 'melancholic' in the Freudian sense because it is a form of unprocessed grief: the type of psychic process that occurs when a trauma and its effects are neither resolved nor complete. 'Throughout the early 1990s', Crimp argued, 'AIDS became an increasingly unbearable and therefore more deeply repressed topic'.

Developing these ideas, Christopher Castiglia called the amnesia of post-crisis culture 'counternostalgia'. He argued that the turning away from AIDS was a kind of fantasy of prophylactic distance from the imagined excess, naivety and licence of gay liberation culture – the culture that was felt to be at fault because it helped to 'bring about' the traumatic catastrophe of the AIDS crisis. 'If the sexual revolution caused illness and one distances oneself from the sexual revolution', Castiglia explains, 'one is therefore distanced from illness.'[9] From a counternostalgic perspective, then, the late 1980s and early 1990s constituted a collective moment of 'growing up' for gay (male) culture. Later, with Christopher Reed, Castiglia came up with new names for counternostalgia, calling it both 'traumatic un-remembering' and 'degeneration', new labels that foregrounded, respectively, the centrality of trauma to this AIDS forgetfulness, and the way in which a distancing from the 'AIDS generation' came significantly from a 'post-AIDS' generation of younger gay men who came of age sexually after the crisis years.[10] Indeed, the idea that these turns – counter-nostalgic, melancholic – away from AIDS have been couched in 'generational' structures has been apparent in a number of the examples already considered in this book: *Brothers & Sisters, The Next Best Thing* and *Queer as Folk*, for example. I will return to the importance of this category of 'generation' in the Conclusion.

Both melancholic disavowal and traumatic unremembering point to the ways in which contemporary gay history has increasingly been understood in fatalistic, teleological terms whereby the AIDS crisis was imagined to be an outcome of gay liberation that has taught queer people – gay men in particular – to become grown up, responsible, 'mature' citizens of the state. In this conservative, western-centric, white gay male–centric vision of history, liberation – that carnival of erotic abandon – gave way to the AIDS crisis, a dire ecological and historical punishment for the excesses of the earlier era. Viewing things in this way may facilitate the psychic relief of distancing. Hence, the 'prophylactic' logic of counternostalgia works to support, and is in turn reinforced by, the conservative, neoliberal agenda of mainstream LGBTQI+ politics because of the latter's elevation of individualism over collectivism, and its investment in the structures of the family and the endogamous, state-recognised, married couple. Elements of queer life and queer experience that don't fit neatly into these institutions are silenced, disavowed or anxiously moralised about, alongside the embarrassment of HIV.

Turning Back

The Second Silence, however, may be over. In the current, fourth decade of the global pandemic there has been something of a re-flourishing of AIDS cultural production in the form of a return to the AIDS past. Of course, this is nothing like the attention the disease received during the plague years, but nonetheless now, overwhelmingly, the prevailing theme of positive images in Anglo-American post-crisis culture is *AIDS history*, and this theme too has become a feature of mainstream entertainment culture.

This retrospective trend was first evident in archival and conservation work, art retrospectives and scholarly histories of activism and activist media.[11] In the US this was spearheaded by some large art and archival exhibitions, including 'Why We Fight: Remembering AIDS Activism' at the New York Public Library (2014), 'NOT OVER: 25 Years of Visual AIDS' at La MaMa La Galleria, New York (2013) and 'Gran Fury: Read My Lips' at New York University's 80WSE galleries (2012). In Australia, a series of historically oriented activities accompanied the 20th International AIDS Conference in Melbourne (2014), including the National Gallery of Victoria's retrospective of the work of artist-activist David McDiarmid and 'Transmissions: Archiving HIV/AIDS', which included works re-exhibited from the influential Australian AIDS art exhibition, 'Don't Leave Me This Way' (1994). These were early indicators that the cultural interest in AIDS activist histories, AIDS art and the aesthetics of the crisis years (in fashion, design, hairstyles and so on) would be accompanied by a passionate, almost fetishistic, fascination with archival material. Archival projects, many of which have been occurring throughout the epidemic, have infused this turn to AIDS history. Indeed, in some instances they initiated it: the documentary *United in Anger* (Jim Hubbard, 2012), for example, which recounts the efforts of ACT UP activists battling corporate greed, social indifference and government neglect, is comprised largely of rare archival footage and oral histories collected by Jim Hubbard and Sarah Schulman as part of the ACT UP Oral History Project, founded in 2001.

United in Anger was one of a critical mass of documentaries released around the thirtieth anniversary of the pandemic that seemed to make official this retrospective trend. As if by some kind of design, at least four documentaries were released within months of one another: *Vito* (2011, dir. Jeffrey Schwarz), *How to Survive a Plague* (2012, dir. David France), *We Were Here* (dir. David Weissman and Bill Weber, 2011) and *United in Anger*. In *Vito*, the history of AIDS activism and the formation of ACT UP is arranged around the biography of Vito Russo, a key figure of liberation politics, AIDS activism and studies of queer film representation. *Vito* shared some of the very same archival photography footage with its contemporary, *We Were Here*, working to reinforce the iconicity of certain images and events in this burgeoning official history of the AIDS crisis. A talking-heads doco that recalls the history of San Francisco's trajectory from free love bacchanalia to epicentre of plague, *We Were Here* foregrounded the testimonies of a small handful of those who witnessed these events. *How to Survive a Plague*, which was nominated for an Academy Award for Best Documentary and thus became perhaps the most visible of these documentaries, also highlights the importance of archival material. It chronicles the actions of ACT UP and the Treatment Action Group (TAG), whose members were self-educated in biomedicine, virology and immunology, and, as the epidemic unfolded, the equally rarefied arts of publicity, lobbying and direct action. ACT UP and TAG took on bureaucrats, government leaders and drug companies in order to get AIDS into public discussion and to expedite and enhance the clinical trialing and availability of HIV drugs. Because AIDS activism paralleled the emergence of hand-held camcorders, the protagonists of this movement were able to capture big events like the civil disobedience at Wall Street and the Exchange, the shutdown of the American Food & Drug Administration, and the infamous 'die- in' protests – when thousands of protesters, including many of the sick and dying, lay down and staged mass public 'deaths' in public places like the Food and Drug Administration Headquarters in Rockville, Maryland in 1988. The footage in *How to Survive a Plague* draws from over 700 hours of found video footage, shot by 33 different people.

Although these documentaries aren't large-scale popular texts by the metric of commerce or audience numbers, the sudden documentary glut certainly made official the now ongoing trend of looking back at the plague years.[12] Since then, there has been a series of narrative films and TV series about these people and these times – not all, but mostly, focused on gay men, LGBTIQ and AIDS activists in places like London, Sydney, New York and San Francisco. Following the early pattern set by *Angels in America* and *The Line of Beauty*, some of these have been literary adaptations. The HBO adaptation of *The Normal Heart* (2014, dir. Ryan Murphy), adapted by Larry Kramer from his 1985 *roman à clef* agitprop play, and the Australian film, *Holding the Man* (2015, dir. Neil Armfield), adapted from the beloved memoir by Timothy Connigrave (1995), were both screen translations of gay male literary texts that already enjoyed some iconic status. Interestingly, the most globally popular AIDS history film of this period, the Oscar-winning and commercially successful *Dallas Buyers Club* (2013, dir. Jean Marc Vallee) was neither based on an existing text nor focused on the experience of gay men.

Although there have been a number of other films including *Test* (2014, dir. Chris Mason Johnson), set in the San Francisco dance world, the British activist film *Pride* (2014, dir. Matthew Warchus), and *When We Rise* (2017, dirs. Gus Van Sant, Dee Rees, Thomas Schlamme and Dustin Lance Black), a recent LGBTQI+ civil rights docudrama miniseries, I will focus on two examples, *Dallas Buyers Club* and *The Normal Heart,* more closely in the remainder of this chapter.

There has doubtlessly been a turn towards the past in post-crisis representations of gay men and HIV. As Avram Finkelstein writes, 'we are now witnessing the solidification of the history of AIDS'.[13] This raises questions about what gets remembered and what is unremembered. How do these AIDS retrovisions reflect and underwrite the contemporary political presence of queer people and PLHIV? As Kerr writes, 'the [AIDS crisis] Revisitation is powerful because it shares stories about the AIDS crisis that inform the world we live in now'. If we consider it axiomatic that cultural memory functions as a means of producing and negotiating a contemporary cultural presence, then what do the ways in which AIDS history is being told indicate about queer politics and culture in the present?

It will be of no surprise to readers who have made it this far that in these post-crisis (re)turns to AIDS history I find further evidence of the fraught legacies of the representational schema of AIDS crisis discourses. To draw something of a broad and schematic observation, I suggest that post-crisis culture is both romantically and nostalgically attached to the AIDS past, but simultaneously traumatised by it. If there has been a turning away and then a turning back to the history of AIDS, this is because that history is both unbearable but un-relinquishable. In post-crisis retrovisions, the AIDS past is submitted to a double vision. On the one hand, as we have seen elsewhere in post-crisis culture, AIDS is rendered as antiquated and anachronistic, abject, a spectacle, a morality tale from history, something to be kept at a safe, prophylactic distance, inconsistent with the mainstream vision of gay life formations in the present. On the other hand, there is a passionate, fascinated and 'nostalgic' investment in that past, with all of the mixed, contradictory, positive and negative valuations that category of nostalgia implies. Although this claim probably needs another entire book in order to be properly enumerated, in the brief examples that follow in this chapter and in the Conclusion, I attempt to develop this additional paradox of post-crisis – nostalgia and disavowal – as well as reflect further on the way these popular films handle the legacies of crisis culture.

Updating Sentimental Melodrama in *Dallas Buyers Club*

> The male hero is one of the most toxic myths in our lives, and the white hero is a stiff competitor.
>
> Sarah Schulman

At first glance, the various reckonings with the history of AIDS and HIV mentioned above would appear to reverse the trends of the Second Silence, the patterns of 'melancholic disavowal', 'counternostlagia' and 'traumatic unremembering'. And yet, much of what we have seen in the realms of the most popular cultural treatments of HIV/AIDS history in recent years have also worked to bolster the conservative ideological implications of these patterns.

Although not a literary adaptation or an avowed consideration of the queer experience of HIV/AIDS, the Oscar-winning and almost universally praised film *Dallas Buyers Club* was the most visible of these retrovisions and therefore it demands consideration. The film's vision of the 1980s is of a time when people living and dying with HIV/AIDS existed in a socio-political combat zone that mirrored the battles being waged in their own immune systems. Such a 'battle' may partake of some of the most clichéd of disease metaphors, as Sontag famously argued, but this is the register in which the film, as a popular Hollywood production, operates. It also reflects the narrative investments of numerous other AIDS retrovisions, which chronicle the battles of individuals and groups against both physical disease and the social dis-ease of institutionalised neglect, underpinned by structures of racism, sexism, homophobia, neo-imperialism and corporate greed. In *Buyers Club*, Oscar-winner Matthew McConaughey plays Ron Woodroof, a Texas rodeo cowboy and electrician who, on being diagnosed with full-blown AIDS and given thirty days to live, begins aggressively self-medicating with AZT, a drug still being trialed at that time. Woodroof then starts the eponymous buyers club of the film's title, through which other desperate PLWHA access black and grey market medications, mostly imported illegally from overseas, smuggled across the Mexican border, or snuck past the American Food and Drug Administration (FDA) via legal loopholes.

Dallas Buyers Club is a pacey, pleasingly filmed, satisfyingly plotted and expertly performed film. Critics fell over themselves lauding McConaughey's portrayal of the cocky, loveable rogue, Woodroof. McConaughey was explosive in the role and won the Academy Award for Best Actor. As Rayon, a sassy transgender woman enlisted by Woodroof to entice the buyers club's largely queer clientele, Jared Leto won the Academy Award for Best Supporting Actor. The film also won the award for Best Makeup and Hairstyling and gathered nominations for Best Picture, Best Original Screenplay and Best Editing. It grossed over $27 million domestically and $27.9 million internationally, the box office revenue returning over $55 million against a budget of $5 million in 182-days of a theatrical run.[14] *Dallas Buyers Club* was marketed as a 'different kind' of mainstream AIDS film: a gritty 'true' story of a working class, faggot-hating cowboy with AIDS, whose self-interested battle to rescue himself helps to pioneer alternative modes of drug distribution, and hence becomes a form of altruism or activism. There are, however, a number of problems with the retelling of AIDS history in *Dallas Buyers Club*, with implications for how the AIDS crisis is remembered.

Although the film was presented to audiences as a biographical drama, the writers and director of *Buyers Club* were reluctant to address public assertions from Woodroof's real-life friends and associates who suggested that not only was he not the homophobe the film depicts but that he may have been bisexual.[15] The film was criticised for other fabrications too, including its invention of the character of Rayon. With its straight, white male protagonist's arc from bigotry to tolerance, *Dallas Buyers Club* has the same liberal humanist formula as *Philadelphia* did in 1993. Although it could never rival the scale, commercial and cultural significance of its Hollywood precursor, *Dallas Buyers Club* managed to become a kind of new, albeit historical screen vision of that event called 'AIDS' for large global audiences as well as a contemporary neoliberal fairytale of independent triumph.

Rayon's role as Woodroof's supporting agent is objectionable. Given her chief task in the film's moral universe is to provide Woodroof with a challenge to his prejudices. Rayon becomes a dramatic instrument for the straight white male hero's evolution from aggressively heterosexual homophobe to compassionate advocate for PLWHA. This re-iterates the ideological role of gay men and other PLWHA in the sentimental pedagogy of earlier waves of AIDS popular culture, as discussed in Chapter 1: they are offered as objects of pity, fascination and kitsch sentiment to reinforce national fantasies of liberal pluralism and, in this instance, white male heroism. Rayon is portrayed as a self-destructive drug user who continues to inject drugs long after her HIV diagnosis – she suffers operatically, by her own hand, and then dies dramatically as on object lesson in self-loathing. In that sense, the character functions as an updated iteration of the sacrificial martyr figure of the coming-home-to-die dramas of the 1980s, a character whose death is a necessary narrative instrument for a certain type of closure to occur, and who needs straight people to advocate on her behalf.

The problem with this is less that Rayon becomes a throwback to the classic conventions of the Hollywood archive of 'negative images', where a more 'positive image' of a queer character with HIV should have been offered. It is, rather, that Rayon is but a more fleshed out stand-in for all of the sexual outsiders, drug users and PLWHA present only in the background of the film – the buyer's club patrons, huddled together, rendered as passive, helpless victims in need of heroic rescue. This all but ignores the history of activists who formed a significant political movement that still exists today. It ignores their very central work on redefining representation to transform the language and perception of 'AIDS victims' (passive, helpless) to 'People Living With HIV/AIDS' who have agency, capacity and political significance.

In *AIDS and its Metaphors* Sontag argued that 'the most terrifying illnesses are perceived not just as lethal, but as dehumanising.' Etymogically, the word 'patient' means 'sufferer'. As Sontag wrote, fear of disease 'is not [fear of] suffering as such'. What is feared 'most deeply' is not suffering but 'suffering that degrades', that de-humanises.[16] The recurrent images of emaciated gay men in hospital beds during the first decade of AIDS crisis did more to sustain stigmatising ideological narratives about the 'innate pathology' of homosexuality than they did to galvanise demands for a better political and medical response. Such images were the confessional centerpiece of a widely circulated, heavily moralistic, spectacular image of plague. Resistance to dehumanisation was thus central to the work of AIDS activists and this included resistance to the *representation* of such dehumanisation, alongside the dehumanising material implications of certain institutional policies and structures. For example, AIDS activist video makers and artists sought to resist the pathologising, confessional imperative of the stigmatised PWA by reframing the dynamic in which the queer/PLWHA body might speak and the listening viewer might hear, as Hallas has shown. They created representations that worked to 'reframe' the experience and presence of PLWHA and expose the ways in which their bodies were subject to the confessional pressures of dominant media that linked AIDS inexorably with racial, sexual, gendered, class, addiction and other stigma.[17] These two things – dehumanising representations and dehumanising policies – are viewed by activists as forces that work in concert, mutually reinforcing one another. To reproduce the dynamics of these images in a populist re-telling of AIDS history is to erase the efforts of these activists, and to return to an image of stigma.

Dallas Buyers Club's further failing is that its depiction of a single man in resistance to the FDA and Big Pharma also erases the agency of PLWHA and the history of pharmaceutical activism pioneered by AIDS activists that helped bring into being the drugs that keep people alive today. Vallée has said that the 2012 documentary *How to Survive a Plague* was an inspiration for scenes in which Woodroof takes on the FDA, the FBI and other government agencies,[18] but *Buyers Club* contains barely a whiff of these broader social movements. People living with and dying from HIV/AIDS are depicted as the hapless victims of unethical drug trials, desperate buyers waiting in long lines, unrepresented and uncoordinated. That these poor souls might have themselves developed a coordinated movement of political and administrative change that actually sped up the FDA's trials of HIV drugs is ignored in favour of a single man's heroic efforts and personal transformation. This makes Vallée's comment that he drew inspiration from the movements depicted in *How to Survive a Plague* that were avowedly anti-capitalist, anti-racist and critical of patriarchy (in order to flesh out the motivations of his white male heterosexual hero) seem like a disingenuous form of cooptation.

However masterful and crowd-pleasing *Dallas Buyers Club* is as an exercise in filmmaking, its elisions make it a tendentious history of American AIDS Crisis. Its narrative contrivances make the film's sentimental message of tolerance seem extremely cynical: the schematic fashion in which it valourises the buyers club and vilifies the FDA and Big Pharma suggests rigid, war-like adversaries in which Texan entrepreneurship, individualism and survival instinct join forces with the powers of moral good. It recirculates liberal mythologies in which a rabidly heterosexual buccaneer capitalist and unrepentant larrikin saves a bunch of helpless junkies and queers. It's celebration of outlaw pharmaceutical distribution and the straight, white hero who pioneered them is an ironically telling distraction from the more immediate history of western pharmaceutical companies and governments aggressively blocking access to generic AIDS drugs for the countries of Africa and the Global South in the years since 1996.[19] Access to ARVs is a huge issue in the US for people living with HIV today, but *Buyers Club* sheds little light on the contemporary scene of American HIV. It begs the question: can Hollywood make any other sort of AIDS movie?

After the Orgy: *The Normal Heart* as Teleological AIDS History

> After all our history, after all these deaths, we still don't… have a gay culture… We have our sexuality and we have made a culture out of our sexuality, and that culture has killed us. I want to say this again: We have made sex the cornerstone of gay liberation and gay culture, and it has killed us.
>
> Larry Kramer, 1997[20]

The Normal Heart received numerous Primetime Emmy award nominations: Mark Ruffalo for his mannered lead performance as the relentless Ned Weeks, Julia Roberts for her supporting actress portrayal of furiously reasonable moral compass Dr Emma Brookner, outstanding directing for Ryan Murphy of *Glee* fame, and, among others, the 'outstanding writing for a miniseries, movie or a dramatic special' nomination for Larry Kramer. Ultimately, the HBO series claimed 'Outstanding Television Movie', which it had already won at the Critics' Choice Television Awards, alongside the Best Supporting Actor in a Movie/Miniseries award for Matt Bomer. Among critics, the consensus was positive: affecting, accolade-worthy performances from a sturdy and convincing cast; a powerful, heartbreaking melodrama of anger, compassion and care; a vital contribution to the expanding film archive of the early years of the AIDS crisis in its urban

American epicenters.[21] 'The Normal Heart might be the most important movie HBO has ever made' read the title of a review on Vox.com. Willa Paskin, in Slate, wrote that 'if some of this material – scenes of lesions and deathbeds, of men being denied the right to say goodbye to their lovers – is becoming a part of the tragedy canon, so be it: it belongs.'[22] Alongside Philadelphia and Dallas Buyers Club, The Normal Heart seems destined to enter the pantheon of popular American AIDS movies.

However, Larry Kramer is a fraught figure for queer politics and culture. On the one hand, he has been a key protagonist of AIDS activism for over thirty years. He was a co-founding member of the Gay Men's Health Crisis (from which he was later expelled – the circumstances around which are dramatised in both stage and screen iterations of The Normal Heart) and after that he founded the AIDS Coalition to Unleash Power (ACT UP). That ACT UP's signature political style echoed the personal and political modus operandi of people like Kramer – unable and unwilling to temper either the message or the medium to make it palatable to the mainstream – is the stuff of numerous activist hagiographies. The man, who died in 2020, is certainly due his place in the canon of AIDS histories.

On the other hand, Kramer has long been a pugnacious ambassador for a version of gay life and gay politics that privileges monogamous love above all other forms of erotic expression. Even before HIV/AIDS, Kramer wrote furious polemics against the drugs and promiscuity of 1970s-era liberation culture. His feelings about gay men and promiscuity are well known and well matured: as recently as 2014, Kramer made characteristically scathing comments against US federal health recommendations that certain people at risk of exposure to HIV take Truvada (or PrEP), the antiretroviral drug that HIV negative people can now take as a preventative measure against seroconversion. 'Anybody who voluntarily takes an antiviral every day has got to have rocks in their heads', Kramer wrote; 'There's something to me cowardly about taking Truvada instead of using a condom. You're taking a drug that is poison to you, and it has lessened your energy to fight, to get involved, to do anything.'[23] Kramer's public position on PrEP is one of the most recent in a longand legendary political type of 'slut-shaming' of gay men, adding, in this instance, to David Duran's infamous (and since recanted) description of gay men who use PrEP as 'Truvada whores', a category that has also been reclaimed proudly by others.[24] While the argument that pharmaceutical prophylactics work to demobilise sexually active gay men as a political constituency is questionable, it's not clear how Kramer's preferred arrangement of intimacy – monogamy – lends itself to stronger political organising among gay men. Certainly decades of radical queer and feminist political thought has questioned the primacy of the couple, and recent critiques of dominant LGBTQI+ politics have argued that marriage may in fact de-politicise sexual minorities.

The liberation-to-AIDS-crisis narrative is fascinated with the brutal transformation of bodies from beautiful, proud embodiments of fleshy eroticism to frail, lesioned objects of suffering and sentiment. Such images incite complex viewing pleasures and how a screen production handles the transformation and to what end it serves is one of the questions at issue. In HBO's *The Normal Heart*, gay liberation and AIDS Crisis are connected in the historical imaginary in teleological and moralitic terms. As I outlined earlier, Crimp and others have identified negative, infantilising portrayals of gay liberation in the rhetoric used by gay neoconservatives to bolster their political claims. As Crimp argues, the 'equation of maturity with… conservative sexual politics and infantilism with… liberation politics is consistently produced through a narrative about AIDS and gay men.'[25] Such a narrative disposition towards AIDS history is evident in Murphy's adaptation of *The Normal Heart*. The film vindicates the rancorous anti-promiscuity polemics of its writer Larry Kramer, and makes the history of HIV/AIDS into a robust supporting argument for state-sanctioned monogamy, the beloved institution that has been at the centre of contemporary mainstream LGBTQI+ politics. It is, in Castiglia's terms, a counternostalgic text.

The problem of gay male promiscuity is foregrounded revealingly in the opening sequence of the film. Not yet an activist, Ned Weeks, the fictional stand-in for Kramer, disembarks from a boat at Fire Island in 1982, on the cusp of Gay Armageddon. As in so many recollections of this place at this time in queer literature, documentary and popular culture, it is depicted as a writhing cornucopia of naked bodies, early 80s styles, muscular physiques, never-ending parties and sex. The homosexual bacchanal on Fire Island has become shorthand for gay paradise on the eve of the apocalypse. Prior to this, Kramer had already published the novel *Faggots* (1978), an anti-promiscuity screed dressed up as fictional narrative. *Faggots'* protagonist, Fred Lemish, is another version of his author. He wants to find love but feels thwarted by 1970s 'fast lane' New York gay culture, and spends the novel wandering through one-night-stands, orgies and glory holes in notorious bathhouses, encountering poppers, quaaludes, PCP, LSD, pot, booze, valium, coke, and heroin en route. Because Kramer's critique of urban gay sexual and drug culture had already made him a controversial figure in the gay community, when *The Normal Heart*'s Ned Weeks arrives on the beach at Fire Island in 1982, he is lambasted by those who recognise him. Not only is he bad PR for gay liberation, he's a killjoy: 'You made us look terrible in your novel,' his friend tells him, explaining why he's become so unpopular. 'Look around you, sex is liberating!' 'All I said,' Ned responds, 'was having so much sex makes finding love impossible.' Upon this portentous utterance, Craig Donner (Jonathan Groff), a handsome and fit young man who will become the film's first AIDS casualty, drops to the sand.

This brief exchange is one of the film's small gestures to the political and identarian centrality of pleasure and desire to gay liberation politics, which of course was severely hampered by the devastating and politically hostile world that AIDS would soon bring about. As novelist and critic and author of a watershed work on these politics, *The Sexual Outlaw* (1977), John Rechy, wrote:

> Because our sex was forbidden harshly and early by admonitions of damnation, criminality, and sickness, sexual profligacy became... an essential, even central, part of our lives, our richest form of contact, at times the only one.[26]

In the literature of gay liberation, there is of course a lot more to be said about this. However HBO's *The Normal Heart* doesn't say much: although it makes it evident that these feelings were central to queer politics (and that they became a 'problem' when HIV/AIDS arrived) there is neither a substantial nor sympathetic account of why sexual freedom and experimentation had become so important for gay men at this time. Sexual community and the intimacy of strangers is not within its sights. Even well into its depiction of the AIDS crisis, *The Normal Heart* makes scant acknowledgment of the way in which informal sexual networks provided the improvised infrastructures that helped to invent and then disseminate the life-saving message and practice of safer sex with condoms, among other things.

But back to Fire Island: here, Weeks/Kramer is presented as a prescient figure, with the insight to predict what is coming and how best to respond. For him there is already something rotten about the culture gay men have made for themselves. A couple of his friends are waxing their toned torsos, upon which another of his friend's comments: 'If you can't beat them join them'. But Ned remains unconvinced. He buttons up his shirt. Later, he drifts past on orgy in the sand dunes that is the first of two dream-like, stylised sex scenes that contrast with the more conventionally realist presentation of later scenes of romantic sex between Ned and his lover Felix (Matt Bomer). The other of these is a bathhouse flashback scored and edited like a TV advertisement, situating it in the style of a commercial genre, which makes it seem depersonalised. The bathhouse flashback is glarringly out of place in an otherwise realist production. Weeks has to be reminded of the encounter because he's forgotten – repressed the memory, like *Philadelphia*'s Tom Hanks did with a similarly guilt-ridden flashback to the porn cinema where he not only cheated on his partner but also contracted HIV. The association of guilt and repression with these memories of what were 'signature' liberation-era practices has become a common trope in gay and AIDS history wring. What we will come to understand over the course of *The Normal Heart* and the thirty years of gay politics that followed its events is something that Weeks/Kramer already appears to know: there are two types of gay sex, one is 'normal' and intimate, and the other is lacking in heart. After witnessing the dreamy but somehow sinister and depersonalised orgy in the dunes, Weeks is back on the boat to New York. Over his shoulder the camera shows us that he is reading the infamous 'Rare cancer diagnosed in 41 homosexuals' article from the *New York Times* that was the very first American news report of the mysterious new disease.[27]

It has become virtually impossible to think about or celebrate gay liberation without knowing what was coming next – after the orgy. There is no seeing the beaches of Fire Island at the time without the sobering biblical story of paradise interrupted – the fall of Eden, the Genesis flood, Sodom and Gomorrah – when the inescapable penalty for mankind's crimes ensues. Worse still is to contemplate the fact that so many saw in this disaster – or were encouraged to see by the frenzy of AIDS panic – the horizon of a 'fair punishment'. The politics of *The Normal Heart* depends on and re-activates this retroactive narrative logic.

The Normal Heart was a hectoring, strident work of agitprop theatre. Ned Weeks is a mouthpiece of unapologetic rage against government inaction and the unspoken negligence of US health policy under Reagan. Weeks is also furious at the gay community for its alleged timidity and collusion with conservative organisations. Kramer's public 'outing' of closet cases in powerful places that he argued were implicated in this negligence was one of his activist strategies that was viewed as an embarrassment to the GMHC, and which led to his expulsion from the organisation.

The TV adaptation offers a break from Kramer's endless badgering in the supporting story of Dr. Emma Brooker, based on real-life Linda Laubenstein M.D. Brookner is depicted as another prophetic figure who knows from anecdotal observation that HIV/AIDS – at this early stage still 'the gay cancer' or 'GRID' – is almost certainly transmitted sexually. In spite of Weeks' warning that you simply can't instruct gay men to stop having sex ('Do you realise you are talking about millions of men who have singled out promiscuity as their main political agenda? They think sex is all they have'), Brookner is another early spokesperson against rampant sex.

In interviews, both director Ryan Murphy and lead performer Mark Ruffalo disclosed their sympathies with Kramer and the politics of *The Normal Heart*. For Ruffalo, what he admired most about Kramer was that he saw in gay men more than just sex:

> Back in '78 and '79, he was saying, "We're more than just who we're having sex with. We're an entire culture, and we will never find happiness by just putting all our eggs in the basket of, hey, look at us and look who we're fucking." He knew that in '78, and he was hated in the gay culture because of it.

For Murphy, the message was unequivocally about an emphasis on the way Kramer's thinking chimes with the (ideo)logic of the current moment in gay politics – marriage, family, recognition, rights, lifestyle comforts:

> The thing that I was very drawn to with the material was that it ends in 1984, but what it's about feels very modern to me, right now, with gay marriage in the news and people fighting to be loved and accepted for who they are… I'm married and I have

> a child. I feel like this movie really is a civil rights movie… that fight really paved the way for the life that I have today.

In their emphasis on the telos of what has become the new political mainstream in gay culture, Murphy and Ruffalo both express precisely why this text from the 1980s feels resonant to them today. HBO's film ends with Dr. Brookner conducting a marriage ceremony between Ned and his lover Felix, a deathbed wedding that presages the particular passions of gay politics today, the movement that Australians refer to as 'equal love'.

In *The Normal Heart*, early AIDS history is exploited in the service of a sexual politics that resonates with the neoconservative consensus in which marriage and the suite of privileges that come with it have become, at least until the 2015 American Supreme Court ruling that made gay marriage legal across America, the *sine qua non* of contemporary LGBTQI+ politics. That few critics even mentioned the triumph of monogamy in *The Normal Heart* is a kind of evidence of the widespread emotional reach of its historical and ideological narrative. Fire Island is in the gay past, then there was AIDS, and now 'equal love' is the new normal status quo.

Backward/Forward

The long shadows of both gay liberation and AIDS crisis continue to haunt the post-crisis present in the form of this moralistic narrative logic in which the sexual excess of liberation gave way to the punishing tragedy of AIDS. This is a difficult historical logic to wrestle free of, as we saw, for example, in Chapter 3's examination of sex panic. The 'whore culture' of liberation haunts the post-crisis present in the form of gay men who bareback and have chemsex. These men are 'throwbacks' – drawn inexorably backward into a naïve and dangerous past when they should have the maturity to know better; their behaviours indicate a pathological 'repetition', invoking feelings of 'déjà vu'.[28] This logic implies that there remains in gay male culture a perverse desire to reproduce the transgressions of the past, in spite of the irrationality and danger of these retrograde urges. The spectacle of these backward queers becomes part of the regulatory regime of neoliberal biopolitics, part of the 'logic of epidemic' that trains well-behaved subjects and punishes bad ones.

As we saw in the example of *Brothers & Sisters* that opened this book, counternostalgia has become something of an organising logic for contemporary queer culture and representation even when it is focused on the gay present. In *Brothers & Sisters*, counternostlagia is iterated through an emphasis on the differences between generations of gay men: Saul's dark, melancholic, sexually promiscuous past in opposition to Kevin and Scotty's bright, uncloseted, family-focused present and future. After antiretrovirals, we might say, popular culture has frequently struggled to contain or disavow the modes of gay life with which HIV/AIDS has become associated by rendering then as antiquated or anachronistic. Such a dynamic of disavowal can equally apply to the AIDS memory and history representations that have increasingly emerged since the late 00s.

In the Global North, the construction of HIV and the gay men associated with it as 'backwards' has doubtlessly colluded with a turning away from the pandemic in the 'rest' of the world. Even *The Line of Beauty*, in spite of its angry revisionist look back at queer history, represents AIDS as *history* – as a past event. To an extent, all these recent works of AIDS heritage and AIDS memory place the AIDS crisis in a temporal *elsewhere*. This 'pasting' of AIDS may help viewers to forget the circumstances of global poverty and privilege that informs who has access to ARVs, education and healthcare. It can foreclose the situations of global HIV/AIDS, which may otherwise seem too complex and overwhelming. If HIV/AIDS is a crisis in other, non-western parts of the world, this is because, temporally speaking, these places are 'behind' the west. If the construction of AIDS as part of an extraordinary past functions as a means of shoring up the normative gay present, it also enables both humane and liberal eyes to look forward, turning discreetly away from both past and present crises.

A turn to the past may distract the liberal gaze from looking too closely at the demands of the present. But, on the other hand, the negative feelings unavoidably present in the 'nostalgic' turn to a period of mass death among gay men (grief, loss, melancholy, shame, survivor's guilt, depression, regret, relentless yearning and desire for a lost past), may, counter-intuitively, prove to be enabling, hopeful, disruptive or sustaining of life in the mundane neoliberal present. There is, as we shall see in the Conclusion, a more reparative reading of AIDS retrovisions alongside the largely critical ones offered in this chapter. Popular AIDS histories have shown a tendency to acknowledge states and experiences that are abject, grief-ridden and wretched, sharing with other queer and feminist cultural producers a (re)turn to 'unhappy archives'[29] and 'backwards feelings' – repositories of unhappy retrospect that help to expose the injustices of the present.

A self-conscious attachment to grief, loss, melancholy and other unhappy feelings that circulate in AIDS memory practices is a potent counterpoint to the teleology of pride that has become the compulsory disposition of queer politics. The 'archive of feelings,'[30] 'counter-memories'[31] and 'retroactivisms'[32] of AIDS retrovisions may also function as incitements to hope, utopian dreaming, and a radical commitment to communitarian, coalitional, punk, anti-hegemonic ideas and practice that disrupt the status quo or help to make life bearable in the neoliberal present. If unremembering AIDS crisis makes it possible to live in a world whose political, social, media and bureaucratic structures supported and continue to support the abandonment of certain bodies, then remembering – and seeking to understand – the history of those structures may function as a powerful and galvanising form of resistance and critique. Remembering AIDS history reminds us that in the polite, democratic, liberal state, the abandonment of certain bodies is in fact knowing, compassionless and systematic; it shows us that at certain times, certain groups becomes disposable constituencies – no longer objects of official, national mourning, but homo sacer, abandoned to suffer and die. The trauma of remembering thus becomes, in fact, a terror of the present that provides a powerful disruption to the inclusion politics of mainstream LGBTQI+ culture.

Conclusion

Feeling Generational

Feelings about the notion of 'generation' in gay male culture have often been expressed in terms of unease or even outright hostility. 'Don't ask me, I flunked gay history,' Rupert Everett's character, Robbie, says dismissively to the silly old queens he works for in *The Next Best Thing*, the film discussed in Chapter 1. In this early Hollywood experiment with the representation of a queer (or, at least non-nuclear) family romance, we saw how a new homosexual archetype, the 1990s 'New Gay Man,'[1] developed in order to provide a marketable, palatable form of gay representation while disavowing the homosexual polluted with AIDS and the spectres of mortality and meaninglessness he invoked. By the start of the next decade the New Gay Man had become a recognisable type with well-established characteristics: charming, urbane, handsome, fit, Caucasian, domestically deft, disengaged from an active sex life and disconnected from the pleasure-oriented habitats of urban queer scenes. These sexual scenes were out of his orbit or, as in the case of Robbie in *The Next Best Thing*, behind him, in his past. As the quote above suggests, this figure is uneasy about – even contemptuous of – other generations of gay men. The old queens, Vernon and Ashby, are discomforting figures – amusing and benign enough to float harmlessly at the fringes of Robbie's narrative, but as homosexual relics from a no longer relevant past, they are not to be identified with.

Conclusion

Robbie's statement ('don't ask me') is a rejection of them and the culture they represent, as well as a denial that he shares any of their knowledge. The older men are throwbacks to an earlier, attenuated generation of gay men: what David Halperin calls a 'previous, abject, supposedly self-hating form of lesbian and gay male culture.'[2] Vernon and Ashby are living artifacts of a gay history from which Robbie wishes to disassociate; in this representational schema, one homosexual type is made to seem outmoded in order that the privilege of participation in normative institutions may be extended to another.

There is a further, starker example of this kind of homosexual 'foil' in the film – a contrast characterised not by age, but by HIV status and the associations lumped in with that status. Robbie's friend David, HIV positive and alone after the death of his partner, is an avatar of another type of gay life to be rejected. Facile, narcissistic, superficial, pleasure-oriented and ultimately a sad and pathetic figure because of his unwillingness to accept or adopt 'mature', 'adult' life, what David represents is also rejected by the New Gay Man so that he may proceed towards and participate in a homonormative, reproductive future (although, as we know, homophobic legal and kinship structures eventually intercept this trajectory).

Older or younger, these peripheral gay male characters are represented as figures from a sad or now largely irrelevant past – figures to renounce. *The Next Best Thing* is a good example of how normative queer participation in popular culture during the period of post-crisis has functioned through an implied or explicit renunciation of 'other' cohorts of queers, including those with HIV. Like the 'AIDS amnesia' and the unmentionable nature of HIV during the Second Silence, this trope of 'generational' difference is another example of the tendency in the popular culture of post-crisis to turn away from HIV/AIDS and its associations. In the same set of gestures and dispositions that Robbie renounces his queer forebears and his diseased queer contemporaries, he turns disgustedly away from gay history itself. In the identarian logic of Gay Redemption, *history itself* is abject. As we have also seen throughout *Positive Images,* this turn away from HIV/AIDS and its histories has often manifested in popular culture as a kind of generational struggle to contain the modes of gay life with which HIV/AIDS has become associated by rendering then as antiquated or anachronistic. The desire to render HIV a figure of the past helps to shapes the terrain of contemporary representations of gay life and its normative aspirations.

Recent work in queer studies concerned with the feelings and meanings attached to temporality and reproductive futurity can help to illuminate this desire. Heather Love's work on the 'backward feelings' surrounding queerness is one enlightening framework. In Love's observation of modern literature and culture, she points out that queers 'have been seen across the twentieth-century as a backward race'. Darwinian models that view homosexuality as a throwback to an earlier stage of human development, psychoanalytic accounts that associate homosexuality with loss, melancholia, failure and arrested development, and 'representation[s] of the AIDS crisis as a gay death wish', she points out, are all 'variations on this theme' of backwardness.[3] As something of an antidote to this, there have been queer identities that seemed to have developed almost in direct resistance to this backwardness, figures explicitly associated with modernity, cutting-edge ideas, fashions and practices – characters that strain forward. The urban aesthete dandy of the late eighteenth and early nineteenth century is one example, as are his latter-day kinfolk, the cosmopolitan global gay tourist and the in-the-know 'queer eye' lifestyle and fashion experts. These figures deploy consumption practices and forms of social and cultural capital as a way to acquire meaningfulness, modernness, citizenship and value in capitalist modernity, and perhaps also to avoid being 'left behind', to counter the backward drag. We might say that the recent turn to marriage and parenting and their attendant forms of social and economic meaningfulness and capital are a further claim on a value associated with the present and the future.

However, as Love reminds us, 'like any claim about modernity', 'the argument actually turns on backwardness – a backwardness disavowed or overcome'.[4] As emblems of the emerging economy in queer aesthetics, commodities and lifestyle markets, the gays of *Queer as Folk* – including Ben and those others living with HIV in the brave new world after antiretrovirals – became iconic figures of the new, global gay modernity.[5] But, as we have seen throughout the culture of post-crisis, when the gay male or HIV positive subject is offered as a figure of modernity, they are frequently attended by some other queer figure with a backward orientation.

Conclusion

In *Queer as Folk,* for example, the couple facing and overcoming serodiscord as an obstacle to their romatic union will ultimately abandon and forget the extremities of this unresolvable problem in order to move forward. In their wake, they leave behind dead lovers, meth users, barebackers, bug chasers and all other forms of unresolvable, disruptive difference, including the elaborately staged drama of serodifference. In the re-awakened crisis discourses of barebacking panic, or what in Chapter 3 I called 're-crisis', other backward figures (re)appear as spectacles to be avoided and renounced: the contaminated, insatiable bottom; the recalcitrant, regressive barebacker, a throwback to the chaotic hedonism of gay liberation. *Brothers & Sisters* had Saul's sad, dark, closeted, shameful past and *The Next Best Thing*'s Robbie must reject the cultures represented by David, and by Vernon and Ashby in order to make his forward claim. These figures of 'backwardness', to use Love's formulation, are unhappy anachronisms, 'representations that offer too stark an image of the losses of queer history.'[6] Robbie's whirlwind of activity is not only a flight from sex and the meaningless queer *jouissance* it represents, but a flight from the backward drag – a turning away from the messy contradictions of gay history and a concomitant disavowal of all those present-day queers who too vividly embody that history. The past, the practices associated with that past, and the abject and unhappy feelings associated with AIDS must be buried and forgotten in order to embrace the meaningfulness of reproductive futurity. As I argued in Chapter 1, the New Gay Man is *produced* through these rituals of disavowal: these denials help him to forge his identity; they are foreclosures that, in Butler's terms, are actually constitutive mechanisms of selfhood.[7] And so, the dominant positive images of post-crisis popular culture have been produced out of what we might call a 'constitutive amnesia'.

The sense that this constitutive amnesia is a problem in need of overcoming has been present in discussions of the AIDS memory 'boom' as it has developed in recent years. Moreover, this problem of forgetting has frequently been expressed in generational terms.[8] The reception of the group of AIDS documentaries in 2011–12, for example, included hints at an apparent generational schism as well as counternostalgic feelings. Sounding almost resentful, Melissa Anderson in *The Village Voice* used the frame of 'de-generation' (Casiglia and Reed's term for 'post-AIDS' gay men's turning away from their predecessors) when, in a review of *We Were Here*, she described AIDS remembering as a remedy for such generational disconnection. *We Were Here*, she writes, 'is a sober reminder of the not-too-distant past, when gays were focused not on honeymoon plans but on keeping people alive.'[9] The critic's framing of the film as a sobering, pedagogical tool for younger queers was echoed widely in reviews and other discussions – the documentaries were offered as breakers of a long silence, giving voice to 'a lost generation'.[10] *How to Survive a Plague*'s director, David France, echoed something of this sentiment when asked in an interview what he thought of 'the younger generation's views on AIDS today'. He said:

> I think the younger generation is under the impression that there's no problem… But also, they think that AIDS in history was just a terrible disease that washed in and that the government fixed it, without knowing what incredible, herculean efforts were necessary… It has fallen out of history, and I'm hoping that the movie helps put it back there, because it was transformative; it gave us the world we have today that we take for granted.[11]

In such statements there is the implication that remembering is not only a dutiful acknowledgement of the experience of generations past, but also, somehow, a means of reckoning with life in the present: if this history 'gave us the world be have today,' then reckoning with that history is part of reckoning with today. France was similarly explicit that his agenda for *How to Survive a Plague* was for it to function as something of an antidote to counternostalgia:

> I want people to know that story, and to see that story in the context of the great civil liberties movements in American history and global history… It's as revolutionary as what we saw in the civil rights movement, as what we saw in South Africa, and as what we saw recently in parts of the Arab world.[12]

Dustin Lance Black expressed similar sentiments around his recent megaseries on gay history, *When We Rise* (2017), although with a corrective, revisionist emphasis on the way in which gay liberation and AIDS activist movements were propped up by and indebted to feminist, lesbian feminist and black civil rights movements, workers' movements and the contributions of other nonwhite, non cis-gendered gay male activists whose stories have tended to be sidelined from the first wave of AIDS crisis revisitations.[13] This sentiment can be understood using Castiglia's idea of 'countermemory' – the seeking of 'competing narrative[s]' of 'resistant memory' that draw on queer history and 'knowledge of previous struggles' as a means to open up alternatives to dominant relationality in the present.[14] Examples of its kind are plentiful.

Elsewhere, activist and intellectual critiques of AIDS retrovisions have tended to frame popular AIDS histories – as I framed them in the previous chapter – as problematic history for various reasons. 'Your Nostalgia is Killing Me', for example, a poster/VIRUS project by Canadian artist Vincent Chevalier and activist–academic Ian Bradley-Perrin as part of Toronto's AIDS Action Now, provoked its audiences to reconsider the cultural responses that have been canonised as part of the AIDS historical narrative. The poster expressed indignant feelings and a resistance to the nostalgic turn in AIDS cultural production. It highlighted the marketisation and fetishisation of certain images and iconographies of the AIDS past, which, its producers felt, functioned to foreclose effective and engaged responses to the experience of HIV in the present. Making AIDS into history, as I suggested earlier, can act as a form of temporal estrangement, a kind of prophylactic distancing that disavows the present-day conditions and urgencies of HIV. As Kerr writes, the poster campaign was a protest against the negligence of nostalgia, expressing the feeling that the artist's 'current life chances as people living with HIV were being reduced by a focus on AIDS of the past. The stigma, health, and social realities that they experience were being ignored in lieu of a look back.'[15] As Pocious writes about popular film releases like *Dallas Buyers Club*, if we quarantine AIDS history from the present, we 'run the risk of contributing to a broader cultural illiteracy when it comes to the contemporary lived realities of HIV in high-income countries such as the United States or Australia.'[16]

Other critiques have been leveled at various examples of the AIDS memory boom. Some long-time activists and cultural producers have pointed out that the AIDS memory industry overlooks the already rich, extant archive of oral, literary and media texts memorialising AIDS, an epidemic that was in part defined by its having occured in an age of mass media. Such archives include game-changing forms of resistant art, performance and media, like the AIDS video work that recreated and consciously reframed the dominant discourses on AIDS.[17] As we saw in previous chapters, other critics point out that in these grand narratives the complexities of AIDS history are reduced to heroic myths of individual triumph over corporate power (*Dallas Buyers Club*), potentially moralistic fables of institutional indifference (*The Line of Beauty*), activist hagiographies that privilege the white gay male American experience (virtually all of the documentaries), or fantasies of a radical coalitional politics that may not have been as coalitional as we fondly recall (*We Were Here*, *When We Rise*). Some of these renditions have been identified as the historical rituals of a contemporary political moment in which homonormativity has co-opted equality (*The Normal Heart*).[18]

These critiques have their merits of course, but what if we were to consider the AIDS Crisis Revisitation more favourably? Problems notwithstanding, what may be the productive or enabling effects, emotionally and politically, of these retrospective trends? I suggest that certain types of sentimental and nostalgic investments in AIDS history might be viewed as creative, imaginative endeavors that reckon with the present and 'build' generational attachments in affectively queer ways.

If AIDS retrovisions have tended to demonstrate a passionate (re)turn to archives, the contexts of their reception have also shown evidence of what we might call, borrowing from the lexicon of Holocaust memory studies, a 'belated' or 'post-memorial' consciousness.[19] 'Postmemory' describes forms of individual and communal identity-formation that occurs through the 'passing down' of memories from one generation to another, but in mediated forms. In the feelings and practices that scholars of memory studies call the 'post-memorial', a historical wound is felt to be both resonant and formative in contemporary life. I propose, albeit tentatively, that a post-memorial consciousness of the history of AIDS may be considered a practice of queer kinship – a corrective to dominant homonormative politics because of its investment in a kind of sad queer retrospect and because of its emphasis on *queer lineages*. In a flourishing moment of AIDS crisis revisitation, certain examples may be deeply problematic, but others may become sites of generational feeling and ideation. Some of these generational expressions offer a celebratory *revaluation of generation* in queer culture – embracing, rather than turning away from, our history and those who came before us. With the regular repetition of the organising trope of 'generation', AIDS memory practices have the capacity to queer the concept of generation by borrowing a conventionally hetero-reproductive concept to describe an alternative model for relating with others across time. Such a speculation demands more elaborate consideration, but in the remaining pages of this book, I will offer some small examples from young gay male cultural producers in Australia that illustrate these reparative modes of generational feeling in the realms of AIDS nostalgia.

In a personal essay for Australian literary journal *The Lifted Brow*, Benjamin Riley, a journalist in his twenties, reflected on the meanings of HIV both historically and today.[20] Riley's point of departure was his own and his friend's first memories of HIV/AIDS and how these memories were weaved into later sexual and social 'coming-of-age experiences' (for want of a better description) they had as young gay men. Considering the intersections of public and private memories of the AIDS crisis and their place in the psychic universe of desire and identity for gay men today, Riley writes, 'I can't help but feel I am living somehow "after" '; 'As a gay man, my time, the moment I am helping to create, is just the echo of something bigger'. Later, Riley turns to queer politics and makes an explicit link between AIDS memory and the shift in mainstream LGBTQI+ politics from respect to respectability.

> A sense of living after… makes it tempting to view the present moment entirely through the lens of nostalgia for another time. Seeing old photos of public demonstrations and community organising in the seventies and eighties I imagine a kind of antidote to my disillusionment with contemporary gay politics. I am increasingly sentimental for a time I have not directly experienced, which in turn feeds my frustration with the present.[21]

There is much to consider here but I want to point out two key issues raised by Riley's essay. The first is that as a member of a 'post-crisis generation', Riley expresses the paradoxical feeling of being both emotionally invested in ('sentimental for'), the histories preceding and surrounding the

AIDS crisis, but simultaneously broken off from them: one cannot return, which feeds a frustration with the status quo in the present and its different organisations of community to those imagined to have existed in the past. For Riley and many others who express similar feelings, the connection to this past is stimulated by and mediated through the image. In its reflexive response to the historical archive, Riley's essay expresses an ambivalent combination of desire, loss, frustration and utopian longing, a yearning for the feeling of community and political radicalism tied to and invoked by public memories of AIDS and the queer activist histories that attended it (or, are imagined to have). This is the mode of the post-memorial nostalgic: feeling and imagination; a desire for something in the past unavailable or unmet in the present; a sense of 'coming after'.

Another example of queer generational feeling is expressed in the documentary *All the Way Through Evening* (2011), created by Rohan Spong, which pays tribute to public and private acts of mourning and remembrance. Released around the same time as the glut of documentaries discussed earlier, *All the Way Through Evening* is a story of East Village New York told through the recollections and musical rituals of eccentric pianist, Mimi Stern-Wolfe. Each year on World AIDS Day, Stern-Wolfe performs 'the Benson Concerts', a tribute to composer Eric Benson and an entire coterie of musical collaborators and friends from the East Village area that she lost to AIDS. An altogether smaller affair, produced by a young antipodean gay man, about the experiences of those from a time before him and in a place far away from where he grew up, *All the Way Through Evening* offers AIDS history from the post-memorial place of belatedness and coming-after. 'I didn't know anyone who had died and didn't know anyone who knew anyone who had died as I was growing up,' Spong said in an interview. And yet, for him, this history is powerful and important. *All the Way Through Evening* represents 'my generation trying to access that time and place, a small group of people who came and went from this one room, and now that room is empty, and the only person who's around who remembers that room is Mimi. And she's adamant that people remember'.[22] Though a post-memorial lens, Spong's work presents an archival tribute[23] in ways that strive to forge relationships across space and time. This form of post-crisis, post-memorial memory work expresses generational feelings and attachments.

Conclusion

For queer history and culture, 'generation' may be something of an awkward concept because of its pedigree in patriarchal and heterosocial structures of kinship and dynasty. Social science disciplines have also been suspicious of 'the generation' and the 'cohort' as a structure for making sense of social life. And yet it is undeniable that the idea of 'the generation' is a potent organising logic through which contemporary and historical groups and communities are arranged and imagined. Well beyond the intimate and individual spheres of family and reproductivity, generation is a metaphor though which we feel and imagine our place in culture and society; and, in a mediated culture, generational thinking is on offer in numerous places. And so, while it is sometimes a reductive or unnuanced way to comprehend social life, the mythology of generation is part of the way we conceptualise experience.

A third Australian example of generational feeling is *HEX*, an original dance performance choreographed by James Welsby that riffs explicitly on the central question of 'What does the AIDS crisis mean for people born after 1981?' (see Figure 5.1). Produced for the 2014 Next Wave Arts Festival and then re-mounted as part of the cultural program of AIDS2014 in Melbourne (before touring nationally), *HEX* pays tribute to a number of highly mediated artifacts and moments of AIDS memory. It starts with the iconic Grim Reaper TV advertisement (the moment AIDS 'broke' in the minds of many Australians) and quickly transitions into a dance montage tribute to disco and other musical genres, including iconic songs by artists that died from AIDS-related illnesses, including Peter Allen, Liberace, Klaus Nomi and Freddie Mercury. *HEX* incorporates heavily mimetic choreography and costuming, including a kind of shivering sequence that recalls the symptoms of seroconversion, pink rubber gloves that suggest sexual and medical-technological inventiveness and the intimate effects of prophylaxis (see Figure 5.2), and a violent stamping polka set to a soundtrack of shouting voices that recalls ACT UP and other AIDS protests. In heavily allegorical and affective modes, *HEX* explores and evokes the complex and contradictory feelings associated with AIDS memory: joy, sadness, terror, anger, desire, nostalgia, fatigue, intimacy, comfort and community. All of the hallmarks of the post-memorial are present in Welsby's Program Notes, including the

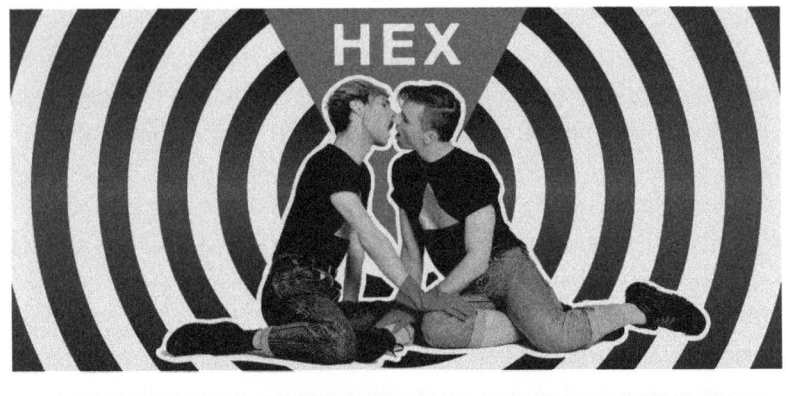

Figure 5.1 Benjamin Hancock and James Welsby in the poster for *HEX* (Next Wave Festival, Melbourne: 6–11 May 2014)

artist's mediated relationship to AIDS history, and their emotional and political attachment to that archive:

> I've known about ACT UP for a while, but the recent release of a few core-shaking documentaries made of archival footage has allowed me to take a much closer look at the movement… I'm deeply affected by the way in which such a tragedy can unite so many different people and rouse them to act together.[24]

Welsby's note self-consciously frames the work as an inter-generational dialogue, told from the perspective of a 'generation [that] has grown up in the midst of the HIV/ AIDS epidemic' but that can only understand it through 'conversations with the generations that preceded me'. Of inter-generational dialogue, he says that he 'want[s] to blur the lines between generations and question if my generation inherits queer activist history, or if we create our own. […] An important influence for me has been meeting gay men who are twenty or more years older than I am and listening to what they have to say.'[25] These ideas were extended in almost fantastical comments he offered

Conclusion

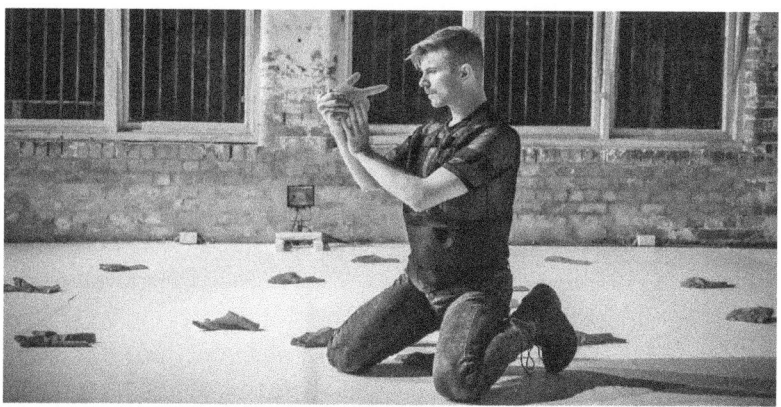

Figure 5.2 James Welsby and intimate technologies in *HEX*

about the show during an interview conducted for the AIDS2014 conference remount:

> [*HEX* is] a reflection of intergenerational relationships… I'm interested in this concept of the 'everywhen'. I've always been so fascinated with the idea of meeting my dad at twenty-six. I'm twenty-six, I wanna meet my dad at twenty-six, I wanna meet my grandfather at twenty-six, and of course that's impossible but, you know, it's not *spiritually* impossible. That's my familial lineage, but my cultural lineage is queer and so I do see people who are my biological parent's age, who are queer – I see them as my cultural parents, and we have a lineage as well: what unites us is desire and potentially social discrimination… There [are] a lot of things that unite the queer community, but it's not genetic. And so, I'm looking at the things that we have in common… and blurring the lines there. In *HEX* I wanted to make a work that was contemporary and retrospective. It's a contemporary meditation on what HIV activist history means to the generation today regardless of whether you're HIV positive or not HIV positive.[26]

I've quoted this interview in depth because, among these brief examples, it offers the clearest expression of post-memorial cultural production that reaches out to express a form of inter-generational, queer kinship. What makes this generational practice 'queer' is the way in which it participates in alternative models for transmitting culture among generations; and the way it performs these transmissions through a backward-looking, nostalgic frame of ambivalent feelings – joy, hope, desire and triumph but also fear, suffering and deep reservoirs of grief.[27]

According to Marianne Hirsch, 'postmemory' is characterised primarily by belatedness and 'coming after'. It describes 'the experience of those who grow up dominated by narratives that preceded their birth, whose own belated stories are evacuated by the stories of the previous generation, shaped by traumatic events that can be neither understood nor recreated'.[28] Hirsch's notion of postmemory was conceived in the context of the children and grandchildren of Holocaust survivors, but she suggests that it could be applicable to other contexts. Postmemory echoes some of the ambivalence in nostalgia because it entails feelings of loss and estrangement (from identity and from the past), but, on the other hand, it involves creative and imaginative forms of drawing from history. Importantly, memories are textualised – that is, experienced vicariously through the range of media that recreate historical narratives and events. As Hirsch writes, 'postmemory is a powerful and very particular form of memory precisely because its connection to its object or source is mediated not through recollection but through an imaginative investment and creation'.[29] The mediated aspect of post-crisis memory practices and their relationship to imagined forms of kinship also recalls Nancy K. Miller and Jason Tougaw's complementary idea of the 'secondary witness', a subject who reads or watches films, images and stories of historical trauma, and has an empathic response. Following from Cathy Caruth, Miller and Tougaw argue that trauma is a phenomenon of delayed response, [and] often unfolds intergenerationally; its aftermath lives on in the family – but no less pervasively in the culture at large. Storytelling can deeply affect those who have not stood directly in the path of historical trauma, who do not share bloodlines with its victims.[30] Most importantly, Miller and Tougaw argue that testimonial work reaches out to create a relational community produced through affective, testimonial speech acts.

These testimonial works, then, take us back to recent discussions in queer studies about the radical, galvanising and utopian possibilities of a posterior turn – especially toward dark, traumatic and sad pasts. For

Conclusion

Heather Love, the haste with which queer thinkers have sought to 'refunction' the unhappy and tragic experiences of the past has resulted in the failure to 'adequately reckon with their powerful legacies'.[31] Love is interested in the legacies of ugly feelings – grief, shame, melancholia – for grassroots political organising. 'I am interested,' she writes, 'in trying to imagine a future apart from the reproductive imperative, optimism, and the promise of redemption. A backward future, perhaps';[32] a future that finds its basis in a 'politics of the past'.[33] The late Jose Muñoz was perhaps the queer thinker most committed to the political promise of the nostalgic, backward gaze. In *Cruising Utopia* (2009), Muñoz champions '[a] posterior glance at different moments, objects, and spaces' that model or inspire alternative ways of being in the present.[34] Muñoz calls the energies and attitudes of the past, sentiments previously considered naïve, anachronistic, ' impractical and merely utopian' that have fallen out of favour or been usurped by other modes in the present, the 'no-longer-conscious'.[35] He suggests that drawing on the 'no-longer-conscious' may help us to imagine forms of non-normative identification in the present and produce a 'future vision' of the 'not-yet-here'.[36] In other words: drawing on the energies inspired by the past to enable radical thinking and feeling in the present. For Muñoz, the no-longer-conscious works as a kind of affective archive that ameliorates the 'disjuncture of being queer' in a present moment dominated and constrained by a 'pragmatic gay agenda'.[37]

And so, in contrast to the view of nostalgia as a dangerous feeling and a distraction from the exigencies of the present, these analyses suggest that rituals of retrovision may reach out toward the formation of new types of communities and relationships – what Bersani, following Foucault, calls 'new relational modes'.[38] One of the first to articulate this possibility in the context of archival AIDS nostalgia and link it to present-day action was Hilderbrand. This nexus of politics and nostalgia is encapsulated in his term, 'retroactivism'. Hilderbrand writes:

> As someone who was slightly too young and far too geographically isolated to participate in ACT UP's heyday, my nostalgia is tied less to the people lost than to how I imagine the queer community was united and politicised by AIDS... Nostalgia thus compensates for spatial and temporal distance, enabling a new generation to draw on activist lessons from the past.[39]

For Hilderbrand, nostalgia has the capacity inspire feelings and re-organise knowledge in a manner that might lead to action. If shared memory practices have the capacity to express and build new modes of relational feeling then those of us that are haunted by a backward gaze may find that one of the legacies of the AIDS crisis has been its potential to inspire powerful, emotional imaginings of kinship beyond normative expectations and structures. This complicates Crimp's diagnosis of melancholic disavowal and Castiglia and Reed's attribution of counternostalgia – of a culture reluctant to look back toward past or present trauma. Though the usefulness of those analyses is far from exhausted, the passionate, emotional turns to the AIDS past discussed in this chapter (and among many others both personal and public) suggest the possibilities of 're-generation' rather than 'degeneration' – the formation or strengthening of communities around feelings of loss, idealism, invention and nostalgia.

If one were to summarise the posterior gaze at AIDS history overall, a mixed set of feelings would be expressed: shame and pride; nostalgia and anxiety; lust and the terror of sex; a desire to turn toward the past and an equally potent desire to turn away. Any paradox here is no surprise, given that the historical trauma of the AIDS crisis is so recent, and given its monolithic archive of visual and material traces. As we have seen throughout *Positive Images*, the landscapes of cultural production in the years since ARVs have been nothing if not paradoxical. Some elements of the past may seem productive and enabling; others are abandoned in a steadfast avowal of the requisite for what passes as progress in the present. In AIDS retrovisions, this manifests in a range of dispositions both forward and backward: forwardnesses that can't acknowledge or sustain certain types of backwardness without the moralising force of retrospect; posterior gazes that threaten to envelope, arrest and overwhelm the subject in traumatic re-livings of the past; backward looking that enables forward momentum; backward emotions that inspire generational feeling. In all cases the past disrupts or 'haunts' the present in complex, uncanny and unresolved ways. It would seem that the only means of grappling with this 'double imperative', to borrow another of Love's phrases, is to 'face backward toward a difficult past, and simultaneously forward, towards "urgent and expanding political purposes"'.[40]

Notes

Introduction: Crisis/Post-Crisis

1. A riff on the aim of antiretroviral therapy to keep the level of virus in the blood at 'undetectable' levels, Race's phrase describes the socio-political climate in the west in which HIV/AIDS has faded from the public arena into the anonymity of private lives. See Kane Race, 'The Undetectable Crisis: Changing Technologies of Risk', *Sexualities* 4/2 (2001), pp. 167–89. I develop this term further in Chapter 2's analysis of *Queer as Folk* and the problems contemporary visual culture has with representing 'undetectable' HIV.
2. See Melanie E. S. Kohnen, 'AIDS, History, and Generation in *Brothers & Sisters*', *Flow TV* 12/8 (September 2010). https://www.flowjournal.org/2010/09/aids-history-and-generation-in-brothers-sisters/ (accessed 12 Jun 2011); David Oscar Harvey, 'Ghosts caught in our throat: of the lack of contemporary representations of gay/bisexual men and HIV', *Jump Cut: A Review of Contemporary Media* 55 (Fall 2013). https://www.ejumpcut.org/archive/jc55.2013/HarveyPoz/text.html (accessed 12 Jun 2011).
3. Harvey, 'Ghosts caught in our throat'.
4. Kohnen, 'AIDS, History and Generation'.
5. See Lisa Duggan, *The Twilight of Equality? Neoliberalism, Cultural Politics, and the Attack on Democracy* (Boston: Beacon Press, 2003).
6. 'David Marshall Grant and Ron Rifkin: HIV & Aging – Clips from Brothers & Sisters', *Youtube*, 1 November 2010. http://youtube.com/watch?v=uUCasILAcJ0 (accessed 20 June 2011).
7. Kohnen, 'AIDS, History, and Generation'.
8. Ibid.
9. Harvey, 'Ghosts caught in our throat'.
10. David Caron, *AIDS in French Culture: Social Ills, Literary Cures* (Madison, 2001), p. 103.
11. Paula Treichler, 'AIDS, Homophobia, and Biomedical Discourse: An Epidemic of Signification' in Douglas Crimp (ed.), *AIDS: Cultural Analysis, Cultural Activism* (Cambridge: MIT Press, 1988).
12. Lee Edelman, *Homographesis: Essays in Gay Literary and Cultural Studies* (New York; London: Routledge, 1994), p. 79.

13. Judith Williamson, 'Every Virus Tells a Story: The Meaning of HIV and AIDS', in Erica Carter and Simon Watney (eds), *Taking Liberties: AIDS and Cultural Politics* (London: Serpent's Tail, 1989), pp. 69–80.
14. Judith Butler, *Gender Trouble: Feminism and the Subversion of Identity* (New York: Routledge, 1990), p. 130, original emphasis.
15. Jeffrey Weeks, 'Male Homosexuality: Cultural Perspectives', in Michael W. Adler (ed.), *Diseases in the Homosexual Male* (Dordrecht: Springer, 1988), p. 1.
16. Ibid.
17. D. A. Miller, 'Sontag's Urbanity', in Henry Abelove, Michele Aina Barale and David M. Halperin (eds), *The Lesbian and Gay Studies Reader* (London; New York: Routledge, 1993), pp. 212–20.
18. 'Person Living with HIV/AIDS' (PLWHA) became the preferred term adopted by people in the positive community in the late 1980s. I use this term or 'Person Living with HIV' (PLHIV), which is more commonly used now. When I use the outmoded, stigmatising term 'Person with AIDS' (PWA) or 'AIDS victim' this is to deliberately indicate moments where the dominant gaze of early AIDS crisis discourses are in play.
19. See Gary Dowsett, 'Australian perspective on HIV/AIDS health promotion', *New South Wales Health Promotion Conference Sydney 8–10 November 1995*; David Román, 'Not-about-AIDS', *GLQ: A Journal of Lesbian and Gay Studies* 6/1 (2000), pp. 1–28.
20. Matthew Sothern, 'On Not Living with AIDS: Or, AIDS-as-Post-Crisis', *Acme: An International E-Journal for Critical Geographies* 5/2 (2006), pp. 144–62.
21. Dennis Altman, 'The Margins of Our Attention', *The Monthly* (December 2006–January 2007), p. 52.
22. Gail Bell, 'A Quiet Anniversary: AIDS 30 Years On', *The Monthly* (November 2011), pp. 44–8.
23. David Herkt, 'Degrees of Proximity in the age of HIV', *Cultural Studies Review* 21/1 (March 2015), http://epress.lib.uts.edu.au/journals/index.php/csrj/article/view/4336/4766 (accessed January 22 2016).
24. Richard Dyer, *Now You See It: Studies on Lesbian and Gay Film* (New York: Routledge, 1990), p. 275.
25. Ibid., p. 274.
26. Ellis Hanson, 'OutTakes' in Ellis Hanson (ed.), *Outtakes: Essays on Queer Theory and Film* (Durham: Duke University Press, 1999), pp. 271–87.
27. See Richard Dyer, *The Matter of Images: Essay on Representation* (London; New York: Routledge, 1993).
28. Ibid., p. 1.
29. Fran Martin, *Situating Sexualities: Queer Representation in Taiwanese Fiction, Film and Public Culture* (Hong Kong: Hong Kong University Press, 2003), p. 38. See Martin for a more detailed defence of queer textualism.

30. Robert Stam, 'The Rise of Cultural Studies', in Robert Stam and Tony Miller (eds), *Film Theory: An Introduction* (Oxford: Blackwell, 2000), p. 225.
31. Gary Dowsett and D. McInnes, 'Gay community, AIDS Agencies and the HIV Epidemic in Adelaide: Theorising "post-AIDS"', in *Out There Too: Social Research & Practice Forum* (Adelaide: HIV/AIDS Programs Unit, South Australian Health Commission, 14–15 March 1996).
32. Gary Smith and Paul Van de Ven, *Reflecting on Practice: Current Challenges in Gay and Other Homosexual Active Men's HIV Education* (Sydney: National Centre in HIV Social Research, The University of New South Wales, 2001), p. 15.
33. By 'somatechnical shifts' I mean developments and transformations in the practices and technologies of the body – 'technologies' in the sense of the machinery of scientific knowledge but also 'techniques' in the Foucauldian sense of the everyday '*dispositif*' or 'apparatuses' of the body and bodily practice that constitute the body and make it intelligible. 'Somatechnics' is a term developed by the Somatechnics Research Centre, Macquarie University in Sydney, Australia. The concept highlights the indivisible relationship of the body to the dynamics of both culture and technology, and acknowledges theoretical understandings of bodies as the materialisation of historically and culturally specific discourses and practices. See 'About Somatechnics', https://somatechnics.wordpress.com/about-somatechnics/.
34. Kane Race, *Pleasure Consuming Medicine: The Queer Politics of Drugs* (Durham: Duke University Press, 2009), p. 111.
35. Smith and Van der Ven, *Reflecting on Practice*, pp. 15–16.
36. See Michael P. Brown, *Replacing Citizenship: AIDS Activism and Radical Democracy* (New York: Guilford Press, 1997); Matthew Sothern, 'On Not Living with AIDS'.
37. See Race, 'The Undetectable Crisis'; and Race, *Pleasure Consuming Medicine*, 2009.
38. Race, *Pleasure Consuming Machine*, p. 38, original emphasis.
39. A decent list of such critiques would be long, but on pharmaceuticalisation see Race, *Pleasure Consuming Medicine*, particularly Chapter 5 for a detailed account of the subjectivisation of PLWHIV to the material culture of pharmaceuticals and the discourses of patient compliance, and, more broadly, to the 'neoliberal drug discourse [that acts] as a field of normativity that regulates and enforces so-called "healthy" consumption', or 'bionormalisation' (107). See also Marsha Rosengarten, 'Consumer activism in the pharmacology of HIV', *Body and Society* 10/1 (2004), pp. 91–107.
40. Global AIDS Update 2016, *UNAIDS*, 31 May 2016, www.unaids.org/en/resources/documents/2016/Global-AIDS-update-2016 (accessed 15 August 2016).
41. Patricia Wald, *Contagious: Cultures, Carriers, and the Outbreak Narrative* (Durham: Duke University Press: 2008), p. 238.

42. See Paul Sendziuk, *Learning to Trust: Australian Responses to AIDS* (Sydney: UNSW Press, 2003).
43. Marty Fink et al. 'Ghost Stories: an introduction', *Jump Cut: A Review of Contemporary Media* 55 (Fall 2013) http://ejumpcut.org/archive/jc55.2013/AidsHivIntroduction/index.html (accessed 25 November 2016).
44. See Christopher Castiglia and Christopher Reed, *If Memory Serves: Gay Men, AIDS, and the Promise of the Queer Past* (Minneapolis: University of Minnesota Press, 2011), pp. 10–12.
45. Harvey, 'Ghosts caught in our throat'.
46. Roger Hallas, *Reframing Bodies: AIDS, Bearing Witness, and the Queer Moving Image* (Durham: Duke University Press, 2009), p. 7.
47. Ron Becker, *Gay TV and Straight America* (New Jersey: Rutgers University Press, 2006), pp. 4–5.
48. Eve Kosofsky Sedgwick, *Between Men: English Literature and Male Homosocial Desire* (New York: Columbia University Press, 1985); *Epistemology of the Closet* (Berkeley; Los Angeles: University of California Press, 1990).
49. Becker, *Gay TV and Straight America*, p. 23.
50. Ibid.
51. Leo Bersani, *Homos* (Cambridge; London: Harvard University Press, 1995), p. 19.
52. Simon Watney, *Policing Desire: Pornography, AIDS and the Media* (London: Methuen, 1987).
53. Judith Williamson, 'Every Virus Tells a Story'.
54. Helene A Shugart, 'Reinventing Privilege: The New (Gay) Man in Contemporary Popular Media', *Critical Studies in Media Communication* 20/1 (2003), pp. 67–91.
55. Damien Riggs, '"Serosameness" or "Serodifference"? Resisting Polarised Discourses of Identity and Relationality in the Context of HIV', *Sexualities* 9/4 (2004), pp. 409–22.
56. See Race, 'The Undetectable Crisis'.
57. Michel Foucault, *The History of Sexuality, Volume I: An Introduction*. Trans. Robert Hurley (Melbourne: Penguin Books, 1976).
58. Heather Love, *Feeling Backward: Loss and the Politics of Queer History* (Cambridge; London: Harvard University Press, 2007).
59. Ann Cvetkovich, *An Archive of Feelings: Trauma, Sexuality, and Lesbian Public Cultures* (Durham: Duke University Press, 2003).
60. Julia Epstein, *Altered Conditions: Disease, Medicine, and Storytelling* (New York: Routledge, 1995), pp. 158.
61. Annabel Kanabus and Jenni Fredriksson, 'The History of AIDS up to 1986' AVERT, 12 March 2009, http://avert.org/his81_86.htm (accessed 17 August 2010).
62. Epstein, *Altered Conditions*, p. 167; Cindy Patton, *Inventing AIDS* (New York; London: Routledge, 1990), p. 112.

63. Watney, *Policing Desire*, p. 83.
64. Michel Foucault, 'On Governmentality', *Ideology and Consciousness* 6 (Autumn 1979), p. 17.
65. Watney, *Policing Desire*, p. 77.
66. See Chapter 1, note 1.
67. Watney, *Policing Desire.*, p. 78; 80.
68. Susan Sontag, *AIDS and its Metaphors* (New York: Farrar, Straus and Giroux, 1989), p. 130.
69. Quoted in ibid., p. 147.
70. Sedgwick would later trace the connection between same-sex desire and scenarios of genocide and omnicide that stretch back in western cultures to the story of Sodom and Gomorrah. See *Epistemology of the Closet*, pp. 127–30.
71. Sontag, *AIDS and its Metaphors*, p. 130.
72. Ibid., p. 110.
73. For example, see Cindy Patton, *Inventing AIDS*; Steven Epstein, *Impure Science: AIDS, Activism, and the Politics of Knowledge* (Los Angeles: University of Los Angeles Press, 1996).
74. Paula A. Treichler, *How to Have Theory in an Epidemic: Cultural Chronicles of AIDS* (Durham: Duke University Press, 1989), p. 35, original emphasis.
75. Sontag, *AIDS and its Metaphors*, p. 5.
76. Caron, *AIDS in French Culture*, p. 4.
77. Terrence Hawkes, *Metaphor* (London: Methuen, 1972), p. 60.
78. George Lakoff and Mark Johnson, *Metaphors We Live By* (Chicago: University of Chicago Press, 1980), p. 6, original emphasis.
79. Treicheler, *How to Have Theory in an Epidemic*, p. 40, original emphasis.
80. Douglas Crimp, 'AIDS: Cultural Analysis, Cultural Activism' in Douglas Crimp (ed.) *AIDS: Cultural Analysis, Cultural Activism* (Cambridge; London: MIT Press, 1988), p. 3.
81. Annamarie Jagose, *Queer Theory* (Melbourne: Melbourne University Press, 1996), p. 95.
82. See Gayle S. Rubin, 'Thinking Sex' in Henry Abelove, Michèle Aina Barale and David M. Halperin (eds), *The Lesbian and Gay Studies Reader* (New York: Routledge, 1993) [1984], pp. 3–44; Michael Warner, *The Trouble with Normal: Sex, Politics, and the Ethics of Queer Life* (Cambridge: Harvard University Press, 1999).
83. Quoted in Wald, *Contagious*, p. 240.
84. Patton, *Inventing AIDS*, pp. 116–18.
85. Duggan, *The Twilight of Equality?*, p. 177.
86. Race, 'The Undetectable Crisis', p. 38.
87. Duggan, *The Twilight of Equality?*, p. 179.
88. Watney, *Policing Desire*, p. 8.
89. Sontag, *AIDS and its Metaphors*, p. 98.

90. Jackie Stacey, *Terratologies: A Cultural Study of Cancer* (New York: Routledge, 1997), p. 44.
91. Louise Hay, *You Can Heal Your Life* (Sydney: Hay House, 1984), p. 116.
92. Stacey, *Terratologies,* p. 42.
93. Hay, *You Can Heal Your Life,* p. 139.
94. Edelman, *Homographesis,* p. 105.
95. Susan Sontag, *Illness as Metaphor* (New York, 1977), p. 56.
96. On metaphors of immunity see Patton, *Inventing AIDS,* pp. 58–64. On the 'immunophilosophy' of science and its relationship to paradigms of immunity in alternative medicine and the media see Emily Martin, *Flexible Bodies: Tracking Immunity in American Culture from the Days of Polio to The Age of AIDS* (Boston: Beacon Press, 1994). Ed Cohen has traced the conceptual history of immunity from its roots as a Roman politico-juridical concept to modern immunological understandings of immunity as a principle of organismic and human existence in *A Body Worth Defending: Immunity, Biopolitics, and the Apotheosis of the Modern Body* (Durham: Duke University Press, 2009).
97. Edelman, *Homographesis,* p. 259.
98. Ibid., pp. 9–14.
99. Ibid., p. 6.
100. Patton, *Inventing AIDS,* p. 383.
101. See Jan Zita Grover, 'Visible Lesions: Images of People With AIDS", *Afterimage* 17/1 (Summer 1989), pp. 10–16.
102. Patton, *Inventing AIDS,* p. 383.
103. Quoted in Tamsin Wilton, *Engendering AIDS: Deconstructing Sex, Text and Epidemic* (London: Sage Publications, 1996), p. 116.
104. Alan M. Brandt, 'AIDS: From Social History to Social Policy', in Elizabeth Fee and Daniel M. Fox (eds), *AIDS: The Burdens of History* (Berkeley: University of California Press, 1988), p. 152.
105. Marita Sturken, *Tangled Memories: The Vietnam War, the AIDS Epidemic, and the Politics of Remembering* (Berkeley: University of California Press, 1997), p. 150.
106. Sontag, *AIDS and its Metaphors,* p. 127; see also Caron, *AIDS in French Culture,* p. 99.
107. Sander Gilman, 'AIDS and Syphilis: The Iconography of Disease' in Douglas Crimp (ed.), *AIDS: Cultural Analysis, Cultural Activism* (Cambridge; London: MIT Press, 1988), pp. 98–9.
108. Leo Bersani, 'Is the Rectum a Grave?' in Douglas Crimp (ed.), *AIDS: Cultural Analysis, Cultural Activism* (Cambridge; London: MIT Press, 1988), p. 211.
109. Edelman, *Homographesis,* p. 105.
110. Bersani, 'Is the Rectum a Grave?', p. 212.
111. Ibid., p. 211.
112. Ibid., p. 222.

113. Brett Farmer, *Spectacular Passions: Cinema, Fantasy, Gay Male Spectatorships* (Durham: Duke University Press, 2000), p. 207.
114. Quoted in ibid., p. 206.
115. See Tim Dean, *Intimacy Unlimited: Reflections on the Subculture of Barebacking* (Chicago: University of Chicago Press, 2009).
116. Patton, *Inventing AIDS*, p. 18; p. 101.
117. Richard Meyer, 'Rock Hudson's Body' in Diana Fuss (ed.) *Inside/Out: Lesbian Theories/Gay Theories* (London: Routledge, 1991), p. 275.
118. The literature on *The Picture of Dorian Gray* makes connections between homosexuality and aristocracy, homosociality and epicene wit; rhetorical figures of periphrasis and preterition (Sedgwick, *Epistemology*, 1990), essence and identity (Ed Cohen, *Talk on the Wilde Side: Toward a Genealogy of a Discourse on Male Sexualities* (New York: Routledge, 1993)); and the psychopathologies of narcissism (Edelman, *Homographesis*, 1989) and addiction. Other scholars have noted the novel's associations of same-sex desire with: conspicuous consumption; narratives of erotic domination and apocalypse; tropes of onanism, pedagogy, corporeal textuality/legibility, Orientalism, effeminacy, the divided self; the figures of the dandy and the aesthete; references to Classicism and the pervasive theme of homosexual fatality (see in particular Jeff Nunokawa, '"All the Sad Young Men": AIDS and the Work of Mourning' in Diana Fuss (ed.), *Inside/Out: Lesbian Theories/Gay Theories* (London: Routledge, 1991), pp. 311–23; Paul Morrison, 'End Pleasure', *GLQ: A Journal of Lesbian and Gay Studies* 1/1 (November 1993), pp. 53–78).
119. Morrison, 'End Pleasure', p. 54.
120. Nunokawa, 'All the Sad Young Men', p. 311.
121. Ellis Hanson, 'Undead' in Diana Fuss (ed.), *Inside/Out: Lesbian Theories/Gay Theories* (London: Routledge, 1991), p. 324.
122. Morrison, 'End Pleasure', p. 55.
123. Oscar Wilde, *The Picture of Dorian Gray* (Melbourne: Penguin, 1985), p. 246.
124. Douglas, Crimp, 'How to Have Promiscuity in an Epidemic', in Douglas Crimp (ed.), *AIDS: Cultural Analysis, Cultural Activism* (Cambridge; London: MIT Press, 1988), p. 240.
125. Randy Shilts, *And the Band Played On: Politics, People and the AIDS Epidemic* (New York: St. Martin's Press, 1987).
126. D. M. Auerbach et. al., 'Cluster of cases of the acquired immune deficiency syndrome. Patients linked by sexual contact', *The American Journal of Medicine* 76 (1984), pp. 487–92.
127. Andrew R. Moss, 'AIDS Without End', *The New York Review of Books* (8 December 1988), http://www.nybooks.com/articles/1988/12/08/aids-without-end-2/ (accessed 3 July 2006).

128. James Miller, 'AIDS in the Novel: Getting It Straight' in James Miller (ed.), *Fluid Exchanges: Artists and Critics in the AIDS Crisis* (Toronto: University of Toronto Press, 1992), p. 257.
129. Williamson, 'Every Virus Tells a Story', p. 68.
130. Ibid., p. 70.
131. Lee Edelman, *No Future: Queer Theory and the Death Drive* (Durham: Duke University Press, 2004), p. 13.
132. Ibid., p. 14.
133. Ibid., p. 27.
134. Ibid.
135. Daniel Harris, *The Rise and Fall of Gay Culture* (New York: Hyperion, 1997), pp. 224–5. See also Sedgwick, *Epistemology of the Closet*, Chapter 3, on the cultural appropriation of male homosexuality as sentimental spectacle.
136. Benjamin Ryan, 'HIV Unplugged', in *HIVplus* (November 2004) http://hivplusmag.com/Story.asp?id=475&categoryid=1 (accessed 21 September 2009).
137. Kylo-Patrick R. Hart, *The AIDS Movie: Representing a Pandemic in Film and Television* (New York: The Haworth Press, 2000), pp. 23–32.
138. Roger Hallas, *Reframing Bodies*, p. 18.
139. See Robert J. Corber, 'Nationalising the Gay Body: AIDS and Sentimental Pedagogy in *Philadelphia*', *American Literary History* 15/1 (2003), pp. 107–33; Gabrielle Griffin, *Representations of HIV and AIDS* (Manchester: University of Manchester Press, 2001).
140. Taubin, 'The Odd Couple', p. 24.
141. Robert J. Corber, 'Nationalising the Gay Body', p. 114. For a more elaborate account of sex, citizenship and the Reagantite sentimentalisation of the public sphere, see Lauren Berlant, *The Queen of America Goes to Washington City: Essays on Sex and Citizenship* (Durham: Duke University Press, 1997).

1 Gay Redemption: Domestication and Disavowal in The Gay 90s

1. See Chapter 1, note 18.
2. Sander Gilman, 'AIDS and Syphilis: The Iconography of Disease', in Douglas Crimp (ed.), *AIDS: Cultural Analysis, Cultural Activism* (Cambridge; London: MIT Press, 1988), p. 91.
3. See Kylo-Patrick Hart, *The AIDS Movie*.
4. Daniel Harris, 'The Kitschification of AIDS', in *The Rise and Fall of Gay Culture,* p. 223.
5. Denis Allen, 'Homosexuality and Narrative', *Modern Fiction Studies* 41/3–4 (Fall-Winter 1995), p. 611.

6. Ibid., p. 610.
7. Ibid., p. 609.
8. Scott D. Paulin, 'Sex and the Singled Girl: Queer Representation and Containment in *Single White Female*', *Camera Obscura: Feminism, Culture and Media Studies* 37 (January 1996), p. 36.
9. See ibid and also Becker, *Gay TV and Straight America* among others.
10. See Shugart, 'Reinventing Privilege'.
11. Robin Wood, 'Return of the Repressed', *Film Comment* 14/4 (July–August 1978), pp. 25–32. Wood's seminal essay on horror movies and their ambivalent viewing pleasures draws on Freud's hypothesis in *Civilisation and its Discontents* (New York: Norton & Company, 1961 [1929]) to argue that 'in a society built on monogamy and the family there will be an enormous surplus of repressed sexual energy, and what is repressed must always strive to return' (80). The monster in horror, Wood argues, embodies these repressed energies. 'Otherness', he explains, 'represents that which bourgeois ideology cannot recognise or accept but must deal with… in one of two ways: either by rejecting and if possible annihilating it, or by rendering it safe and assimilating it, converting it as far as possible into a replica of itself' (73). The post-feminist theories of abjection and disavowal that I draw on in this chapter are different from the psychic model of repression that Wood draws on, however, I emulate Wood's use of these psychic processes as a heuristic for analysing popular culture.
12. See Chapter 1, note 17.
13. Edelman, *No Future*, p. 11.
14. Jess Cagle, 'The Gay 90s: America Sees Shades Of Gay; A Once-Invisible Group Finds The Spotlight', *Entertainment Weekly* (8 September 1995) http://ew.com/article/1995/09/08/special-report-gay-90s/ (accessed 7 November 2007).
15. Bruce Vilanch, 'Anything but sex', *The Advocate* 761 (9 June 1998), p. 59.
16. Paulin, 'Sex and the Singled Girl', p. 37. Queers that seemed to get the most onscreen sexual action in mainstream film culture during the 1990s were the murderous and generally psychotic lesbian/bisexual femme fatale figures of Hollywood sex thrillers. This typically insatiable, sexually polymorphous female psychopath figure developed in the 1980s and 1990s in a cycle of feminist backlash and post-feminist 'Women From Hell' films that included *Fatal Attraction* (1987), *Final Analysis* (1992), *Single White Female* and *Basic Instinct* (1992). Arguably, these films exploited the sexual anxieties that the New Gay Man was designed to assuage. See Jermyn, 'Rereading the bitches from hell: a feminist appropriation of the female psychopath', *Screen* 31/3 (Autumn 1996), pp. 251–67.
17. Becker, *Gay TV and Straight America*, p. 180.
18. Ibid.

19. Ibid., p. 172.
20. Chris Bull, 'Acting gay', *The Advocate* 671 (December 1994), p. 44.
21. Ron Becker, 'Prime-Time Television in the Gay Nineties: Network Television, Quality Audiences, and Gay Politics' in Robert Clyde Allen and Annette Hill (eds), *The Television Studies Reader* (London; New York: Routledge, 2006), p. 397.
22. Ibid., p. 391.
23. Becker, *Gay TV and Straight America*, p. 158.
24. Ibid., pp. 108–35.
25. See Amy Aronson and Michael Kimmel, 'The Saviours and the Saved: Masculine Redemption in Contemporary Films', in Peter Lehman (ed.), *Masculinity: Bodies, Movies, Culture* (New York; London: Routledge, 2001), pp. 43–50.
26. Ibid., p. 44.
27. Ibid., pp. 44–9.
28. R. Connell, *Masculinities* (Berkeley; LA: University of California Press, 2005), pp. 79–82.
29. Shugart, 'Reinventing Privilege', p. 80.
30. Ibid., p. 87.
31. Ibid., p. 83.
32. R. Connell, 'The Social Organisation of Masculinity' in Stephen M. Whitebread and Frank J. Barrett (eds), *The Masculinities Reader* (Cambridge: Polity, 2002), pp. 67–86.
33. Robert Benjamin Bateman, 'What Do Gay Men Desire? Peering Behind the Queer Eye', in James R. Keller and Leslie Stratyner (eds), *The New Queer Aesthetic on Television: Essays on Recent Programming* (North Carolina: MacFarland and Co., 2006), p. 11; see also Tania Lewis, 'He Needs to Face His Fears with These Five Queers', *Television & New Media* 8 (2007), pp. 285–311.
34. Bateman, 'What Do Gay Men Desire?', p. 10; 17.
35. Ibid., p. 13.
36. Paulin, 'Sex and the Singled Girl', p. 39.
37. Ibid., p. 39.
38. Ibid., pp. 38–9.
39. Becker, *Gay TV and Straight America*, p. 140.
40. Deborah Jermyn, 'Rereading the bitches from hell', pp. 251–67.
41. Sedgwick, *Between Men*, pp. 189–19.
42. Benjamin Kahan, '"The Viper's Traffic-Knot": Celibacy and Queerness in the 'Late' Marianne Moore', *GLQ: A Journal of Lesbian and Gay Studies* 14/4 (2008), p. 511.
43. Ibid.
44. Ibid., p. 510.

45. Ibid., p. 509.
46. Ibid., p. 511–12.
47. Mary Douglas, *Purity and Danger: An Analysis of Concepts of Pollution and Taboo*, 1966 (New York: Routledge Classics, 2002).
48. Julia Kristeva, *Powers of Horror: An Essay on Abjection*, trans. Leon S. Roudiez (New York: Colombia University Press, 1982).
49. Elizabeth Grosz, *Volatile Bodies: Towards a Corporeal Feminism* (Sydney: Allen and Unwin, 1994).
50. Judith Butler, *The Psychic Life of Power: Theories in Subjection* (Stanford: Stanford University Press, 1997).
51. Judith Butler, *Bodies That Matter: On the Discursive Limits of "Sex"* (London; New York: Routledge, 1993), p. 115.
52. Ibid., p. 116.
53. Jackie Stacey, *Terratologies*, p. 71.
54. Sigmund Freud, *Totem and Taboo* (London: Routledge, 1999) [1913].
55. Kristeva, *Powers of Horror*, pp. 12–13.
56. Ibid., p. 4.
57. Ibid., p. 3.
58. Grosz, *Volatile Bodies*, p. 71.
59. Williamson, 'Every Virus Tells a Story'.
60. Iris Marion Young, *Justice and the Politics of Difference* (New Jersey: Princeton University Press, 1990).
61. Judith Butler, *Gender Trouble*.
62. Ibid., p. 133.
63. Butler, *Bodies that Matter*, p. 243.
64. Grosz, *Volatile Bodies*, p. 76, original emphasis.
65. Young, *Justice and the Politics of Difference*, p. 156.
66. Marjorie Garber, *Vested Interests: Cross-dressing and Cultural Anxiety* (New York: Routledge, 1993), p. 16.
67. Julia Epstein, *Altered Conditions,* p. 177.
68. Ibid., p. 165.
69. Grosz, *Volatile Bodies*, p. 72.
70. Stacey, *Terratologies*, p. 79.
71. Butler, *Bodies that Matter*, pp. 113–14.
72. Ibid., p. 114.
73. Grosz, *Volatile Bodies*, p. 87.
74. Rupert Everett, *Red Carpets and Other Banana Skins* (New York: Hachette, 2006), p. 229.
75. Shugart, 'Reinventing Privilege', p. 71.
76. Susan Bordo, *The Male Body: A New Look at Men in Public and in Private* (New York: Farar, Straus and Giroux, 1999), p. 158.
77. Ibid., p. 159.

78. Shannon J. Harvey, 'The Next Best Thing', UrbanCinefile 763.
79. Dennis Lim, 'Through a Mirror Darkly', The Village Voice, 7 March 2000.
80. Rob Blackwelder, 'Homogenized by Hollywood: Madonna has Baby with Gay Friend in Disingenuous Crossover Flop The Next Best Thing', Splicedwire, 3 March 2000.
81. Roger Ebert, 'The Next Best Thing', Chicago Sun-Times, 3 March 2000.
82. Wesley Morris, 'Truly an odd couple: In appalling Next Best Thing, Madonna-Rupert pairing fascinates – like a train wreck', San Francisco Chronicle, 3 March 2000.
83. James Kendrick, 'The Next Best Thing', QNetwork Entertainment Portal, 4 November 2006.
84. Meyer, 'Rock Hudson's Body', p. 282.
85. Ibid., p. 259.
86. Ibid., pp. 262–3.
87. Ibid., p. 26, original emphasis.
88. Ibid., p. 275.
89. Ibid., pp. 264–5.
90. Ibid., p. 265.
91. Mary Douglas, Purity and Danger, p. 2.
92. See Vito Russo, The Celluloid Closet: Homosexuality in the Movies (New York: Harper & Row, 1981); Richard Dyer, The Matter of Images, p. 19.
93. Edelman, No Future, p. 143.
94. Ibid., p. 75.
95. Williamson, 'Every Virus Tells a Story'.
96. Edelman, No Future, p. 27.
97. Nick Davis, 'The Next Best Thing', Nicks Flick Picks, 4 November 2006.
98. Christopher Null, 'The Next Best Thing', ACM Filmcritic, 29 February 2000.
99. Patton, Inventing AIDS, p. 118.
100. Bersani, Homos, p. 212.
101. Love, Feeling Backward, p. 131.

2 Positive Men Are from Mars, Negative Men Are from Venus: Sero-Melodrama in *Queer As Folk*

1. Walter Chaw, '*Queer as Folk*', Film Freak Central DVD Review, http://filmfreakcentral.net/dvdreviews/queersasfolk.htm (accessed 16 January 2009).
2. Glynn Davis, Queer as Folk (London: BFI Publishing, 2007), p. 121.
3. Kathleen P. Farrell, 'HIV on TV: Conversations with Young Gay Men', Sexualities 9/2 (2006) pp. 193–213. Farrell collected and analysed the responses of gay male American undergraduates to the dramatisation of

serodiscord in Series 2 of *Queer as Folk* in order to better understanding how young gay men might interpret these stories and incorporate them into their own lives. Her findings suggest TV drama is a potentially productive space for communicating the complicated messages of HIV prevention, stigma reduction and living with and understanding HIV. Farrell's focus on audiences makes a productive counterpart to this chapter's mostly textual and contextual analysis of the series.

4. Ibid. p. 197.
5. Ryan, 'HIV Unplugged'.
6. Ibid.
7. Wilton, *Engendering AIDS*, p. 42.
8. Riggs, '"Serosameness" or "Serodifference"?'
9. José Esteban Muñoz, 'Queer Minsrels for the Straight Eye: Race as Surplus in Gay TV', *GLQ: A Journal of Lesbian and Gay Studies* 11/1 (2005), p. 102.
10. Bobby Noble, 'Queer as Box: Boi Spectators and Boy Culture on Showtime's *Queer as Folk*' in Merri Lisa Johnson (ed.), *Third Wave Feminism and Television: Jane Puts it in a Box* (London: I.B.Tauris 2007), p. 147.
11. Warner, *The Trouble with Normal*, p. 34.
12. Peter Brooks, *The Melodramatic Imagination: Balzac, Henry James, Melodrama, and the Mode of Excess* (New Haven: Yale University Press, 1995 [1976]), p. 2.
13. Robin Nelson, *State of Play: Contemporary "High-End" TV Drama* (Manchester: Manchester University Press, 2007), pp. 7–8.
14. John Caldwell, *Production Culture: Industrial Reflexivity and Critical Practice in Film/Television* (Durham: Duke University Press, 2008), p. 54.
15. Trisha Dunleavy, 'Strategies of Innovation in "High-End" TV Drama: The Contribution of Cable', *Flow*, 6 March 2009, http://flowtv.org/?p=257418 (accessed 6 August 2009).
16. Nelson, *State of Play*, p. 22.
17. Sally R Munt, 'Shame/pride dichotomies in *Queer as Folk*', *Textual Practice* 14/3 (2000), p. 531.
18. Dennis Hensley, 'Inside *Queer as Folk*', *The Advocate* (21 Nov 2000), p. 50.
19. This includes: Chaw, '*Queer as Folk*'; Davis, *Queer as Folk*, p. 1; Noble, 'Queer as Box', p. 147; Holleran, 'Brief History of a Media Taboo', *Gay and Lesbian Review Worldwide* 8/2 (2001), p. 14; Hensley, 'Inside *Queer as Folk*', p. 47 among various others.
20. Quoted in Davis, *Queer as Folk*, p. 120.
21. Andrew Holleran, 'Brief History of a Media Taboo', p. 14.
22. Quoted in Rebecca Beirne, 'Embattled Sex: Rise of the Right and Victory of the Queer in *Queer as Folk*' in James R. Keller and Leslie Stratyner (eds), *The New Queer Aesthetic on Television: Essays on Recent Programming* (North Carolina: McFarling and Co., 2006), p. 43.

23. See Susan Fraser, 'Poetic World-Making: *Queer as Folk*, Counterpublic Speech and the "Reader"', *Sexualities* 9/2 (2006), p. 152–70; Mary Lou Rasmussen and Jane Kenway, 'Queering the Youthful *Cyberflâneur*', *Journal of Gay and Lesbian Issues in Education* 2/1 (2004), pp. 47–63; Esther Peeren, 'Queering the Straight World: The Politics of Resignification in *Queer as Folk*' in James R. Keller and Leslie Stratyner (eds), *The New Queer Aesthetic on Television: Essays on Recent Programming* (North Carolina: McFarling and Co., 2006), p. 63. According to Warner's 2002 formulation, a 'counterpublic' is a 'scene where a dominated group aspires to re-create itself as a public and in doing so finds itself not only in conflict with the dominant social group but with norms that constitute the dominant culture as public.' Warner, *Publics and Counterpublics* (New York: Zone Books, 2002), p. 112.
24. Jaap Kooijman, 'They're Here, They're Queer, and Straight American Loves it', *GLQ: A Journal of Lesbian and Gay Studies* 11/1 (2005), p. 107.
25. See Mary Rasmussen and Kenway, 'Queering the Youthful *Cyberflâneur*', pp. 47–63.
26. Beirne, 'Embattled Sex', pp. 43–4.
27. Fraser, 'Poetic World-Making', pp. 152–70.
28. Noble, 'Queer as Box', p. 164. As Noble summarises, Bérubé's five white-washing strategies are: 'the deployment of race analogies; the mirroring of white normativity as a tactic of winning credibility; excluding people of colour from controlling images or representations; the marketing of gay as white and middle class within commodity capitalism; and the assumption of the white shield that camouflages unearned and unmarked privilege' (164).
29. Noble, 'Queer as Box', p. 151; see also Beirne, 'Embattled Sex', pp. 99–107.
30. See for example Noble, 'Queer as Box' for a re-appraisal of anal receptivity in *Queer as Folk*.
31. Davis, *Queer as Folk*, p. 119.
32. David Alderson, 'Queer Cosmopolitanism: Place, Politics, Citizenship and *Queer as Folk*', *New Formations* 55/1 (Spring 2005), p. 75.
33. Rushbrook quoted in ibid., p. 77.
34. Bobby Benedicto, 'The Haunting of Gay Manila: Global Space-Time and the Specter of Kabaklaan', *GLQ: A Journal of Lesbian and Gay Studies* 14/2–3 (2008), p. 319.
35. Eric O. Clarke, *Virtuous Vice: Homoeroticism and the Public Sphere* (Durham: Duke University Press, 2000).
36. Noble, 'Queer as Box', p. 147. For a more equivocal view of the series' relationship to a commodified global gay modernity see Beirne, 'Embattled Sex'.
37. Benedicto, 'The Haunting of Gay Manila', p. 319. See also Heidi Nast, 'Queer Patriarchies, Queer Racisms, International' *Antipode* 34/5 (2002), pp. 874–909.
38. Noble, 'Queer as Box', p. 164.

39. Esther Peeren, 'Queering the Straight World', pp. 59–60.
40. Davis, *Queer as Folk*, p. 124.
41. See for example, Brooks, *The Melodramatic Imagination*, 1995 [1976]), p. 2; Christine Gledhill, 'The Melodramatic Field: An Investigation' in Christine Gledhill (ed.), *Home is Where the Heart Is* (London: BFI Publishing, 1987), pp. 5–39.
42. See Mark Davis, 'HIV Prevention Rationalities and Serostatus in the Risk Narratives of Gay Men', *Sexualities* 5/3 (2002), pp. 282–3; Barry Adam, 'Constructing the Neoliberal Sexual Actor: Responsibility and care of the self in the discourse of barebackers', *Culture, Heath and Sexuality* 7/4 (2005), pp. 333–46.
43. Quoted in Davis, 'HIV Prevention Rationalities and Serostatus', p. 285.
44. Ibid., p. 283.
45. Race, 'The Undetectable Crisis', p. 179.
46. Ibid., p. 174; p. 171.
47. Race, *Pleasure Consuming Medicine*, p. 24.
48. Ibid., p. 24.
49. Bardella Claudio, 'Pilgrimages of the Plagued: AIDS, Body and Society', *Body & Society* 8 (2002), p. 97.
50. Race, *Pleasure Consuming Medicine*, p. 24.
51. Race, 'The Undetectable Crisis', p. 76.
52. Ibid., pp. 178–80
53. Ibid., p. 178.
54. Asha Persson, 'Incorporating Pharmakon: HIV, Medicine, and Body Shape Change', *Body & Society* 10/4 (2004), p. 47.
55. Certain types of ARVs have had side effects for some people that include visually apparent symptoms including lipoatrophy (an accumulation of fat in certain body parts) and lipodystrophy (fat loss). These can produce body shape changes including distended belly, enlarged breasts in women, a mound of fat lodged at the back of the neck, flat buttocks, stick-like arms and legs, loss of subcutaneous fat on the legs which produces bulging veins, and sunken cheeks (Persson 52). These particular drugs are now less frequently prescribed.
56. Matthew Sothern, 'On Not Living with AIDS', p. 146.
57. Ibid., pp. 145–6.
58. Ibid., p. 157.
59. Ibid., p. 146.
60. Quoted in Bardella, 'Pilgrimages of the Plagued', p. 88.
61. Ibid., p. 88.
62. Andrew Sullivan, 'When Plagues End: Notes on the Twilight of an Epidemic', *New York Times Magazine* (10 November 1996), http://www.nytimes.com/1996/11/10/magazine/when-plagues-end.html (accessed 4 July 2009).
63. There are now a number of recognised approaches to conception when one or more partners are HIV-positive, including artificial insemination, timed

unprotected intercourse, the process known as sperm washing and the reduction of viral load to undetectable levels. These significantly reduce the chances of transmitting HIV to an embryo.
64. Marcia Ian, 'When is a Body Not a Body? When It's a Building' in Joel Sanders (ed.), *Stud: Architectures of Masculinity* (Princeton: Princeton University Press, 1996), p. 191.
65. Ibid., p. 189.
66. Ibid., p. 192–3.
67. See Race, *Pleasure Consuming Medicine* for a more fulsome discussion of which drugs are deemed licit and illicit in public culture and their relationships with male homosexuality, queer culture and HIV.
68. Riggs, '"Serosameness" or "Serodifference"?', p. 417.
69. Ibid., p. 418.
70. Ibid., p. 415.
71. *Men are from Mars, Women are from Venus* (New York: HarperCollins, 1992) was the first of an enormously popular self-help book franchise by American writer and relationship counsellor John Gray, who advises on improving heterosexual relationships through an understanding of gendered emotional and communication styles. As the title implies, men and women are viewed as beings from different planets with alien communication styles and ineluctable differences.
72. Riggs, '"Serosameness" or "Serodifference"?', p. 412.
73. Michael Kackman, 'Quality Television Melodrama and Cultural Complexity', *Flow* 7 April 2009. http://flowtv.org/2010/03/flow-favorites-quality-television-melodrama-and-cultural-complexity-michael-kackman-university-of-texas-austin/ (accessed 12 April 2009).
74. Geoffrey Nowell-Smith, 'Minelli and Melodrama' in Bill Nichols (ed.), *Movies and Method Vol 2* (Berkeley, 1985), p. 193.
75. Persson, 'Incorporating Pharmakon', p. 62.
76. Warner, *The Trouble with Normal*, p. 60.
77. Nelson, *State of Play*, p. 20.
78. Kackman, 'Quality Television Melodrama'.
79. Ibid.
80. Ibid., emphasis added.
81. Ibid., emphasis added
82. See Brooks, *The Melodramatic Imagination*.

3 Crisis Re-Runs: Barebacking, *Chemsex* and Post-Crisis Sex Panic

1. Tim Robey, '*Chemsex* review: 'Seriously Sobering', *The Telegraph*, 3 December 2015, http://www.telegraph.co.uk/film/Chemsex/review/ (accessed 8 April 2016).

2. Emma Reynolds, '*Chemsex*: Inside the alarming trend for risky, drug-fuelled group sex', *News.com*, available at http://www.news.com.au/lifestyle/real-life/chemsex-inside-the-alarming-trend-for-risky-drugfuelled-group-sex/news-story/88bdb86dd790dfe3abe7e411e86f6429 (accessed 8 April 2016).
3. Stanley Cohen, *Folk Devils and Moral Panics* (Great Britain, 1972), p. 10.
4. Stephen A Russell, 'Dangerous Liaisons: inside the world of *Chemsex*" *SBS* 15 April 2015, http://www.sbs.com.au/topics/sexuality/article/2016/03/31/dangerous-liaisons-inside-world-chemsex (accessed 21 June 2017).
5. On the pleasures and cultures of care around illicit drug use and the virtual impossibility of speaking about these in any forum that considers itself 'public' or 'healthy' see Race, *Pleasure Consuming Medicine*. As Race argues, to speak of pleasure or of the techniques people invent to protect themselves and others would involve 'an account of pleasures that exceed normative forms' (p. 138–9).
6. For a more elaborate discussion of the lingua of sex panic in *Chemsex* see Kagan, 'How to take Drugs in a Chemsex Epidemic', *The Lifted Brow* 30, 2016. See also Race, '*Chemsex* review: gay sex and drug use demand more careful forms of attention', *The Conversation*, http://theconversation.com/chemsex-review-gay-sex-and-drug-use-demand-more-careful-forms-of-attention-51586 (accessed 8 December 2015).
7. By all accounts the first discussion of barebacking in a mainstream Australian publication was an article by gay journalist Steve Dow in the *Sydney Morning Herald* in 2003. Dow characterised barebacking as a mode of sexual outlawry imported from America via the internet and used it to flagellate local AIDS educators and organisations. See Dow, 'Denial becomes the new language of casual sex', *Sydney Morning Herald*, 3 July 2003.
8. For example, see Laura Kipnis, *How to Become a Scandal: Adventures in Bad Behavior* (Metropolitan Books: New York, 2010).
9. Janice M. Irvine, 'Transient Feelings: Sex Panics and the Politics of Emotions', *GLQ: A Journal of Lesbian and Gay Studies* 14/1 (2008), pp. 16–20.
10. Linda Singer, *Erotic Welfare: Sexual Theory and Politics in The Age of Epidemic* (London: Routledge, 1993).
11. Kane Race, 'Engaging in a culture of barebacking: Gay men and the risk of HIV prevention', in K. Hannah-Moffat and P. O'Malley (eds), *Gendered Risk* (London: Glasshouse Press, 2007), p. 11.
12. 'Viral sex' refers to 'risky sex between men' wherein 'safe sex practices' (like condom use) are ignored. What constitutes 'safe' or 'safer' has always been contested and has changed as new technologies and practices have emerged and new understandings of these have developed. Tomso argues that 'viral sex' may be understood as an act of biopolitical resistance to state power. See 'Viral Sex and the Politics of Life', *South Atlantic Quarterly* 107/2 (Spring 2008), pp. 265–85.

13. J. P. Cheuvront, 'High-Risk Sexual Behaviour in the Treatment of HIV-Negative Patients', in *Journal of Gay & Lesbian Psychotherapy* 6/3 (2002), p. 8.
14. Dean, *Intimacy Unlimited*.
15. Paul Morris, 'No Limits: Necessary Danger in Male Porn', Lecture, World Pornography Conference, University City, California, 6–9 August 1998. https://queerrhetoric.wordpress.com/2010/06/22/no-limits-necessary-danger-in-male-porn/ (accessed 10 January 2017).
16. Michael Graydon, 'Don't bother to wrap it: Online Giftgiver and Bugchaser newsgroups, the social impact of gift exchanges and the "carnivalesque"', *Culture, Health and Sexuality* 9/3 (May–June 2007), p. 280.
17. See special issue "Bareback sex and queer theory across three national contexts (France, UK, USA)", *Sexualities* 18/1–2 (2015).
18. Mark J. Blechner, 'Intimacy, Pleasure, Risk, and Safety: Discussion of Cheuvront's "High-Risk Sexual Behaviour in the Treatment of HIV-Negative Patients"', *Journal of Gay and LesbianPsychotherapy* 6/3 (2002), p. 31.
19. Benjamin Junge, 'Bareback Sex, Risk, and Eroticism: Anthropological Themes (Re-) Surfacing in the Post-AIDS Era' in Ellen Lewin and Willian L. Leap (eds), *Out in Theory: The Emergence of Lesbian and Gay Anthropology* (Urbana and Chicago, 2002), pp. 189–90.
20. On this fraught distinction and its articulation by men who enjoy watching barebacking pornography see Florian Vörös, 'Raw fantasies: An interpretative sociology of what bareback porn does and means to French gay male audiences', in R. Borba, B. Falabella Fabrício, D. Pinto and E.S. Lewis (eds), *Queering Paradigms IV* (Bern, 2014), pp. 321–43.
21. Donna M. Orange, 'High-Risk Behaviour or High-Risk Systems? Discussion of Cheuvront's "High-Risk Sexual Behaviour in the Treatment of HIV-Negative Patients", *Journal of Gay and Lesbian Psychotherapy* 6/3 (2002), p. 48.
22. Race, 'Engaging in a culture of barebacking', p. 106.
23. Ibid., p. 111.
24. See Rubin, 'Thinking Sex'.
25. See Gregory Tomso, 'Bug Chasing, Barebacking, and the Risks of Care', *Literature and Medicine* 23/1 (Spring 2004), p. 89.
26. Foucault, *The History of Sexuality*.
27. Quoted in Dennis Altman, 'Political Sexualities: Meanings and Identities in the Time of AIDS' in Richard G. Parker and John Gagnon (eds), *Conceiving Sexualities: Approaches to Sex Research in a Postmodern World* (New York: Routledge, 1996), p. 105.
28. Tomso, 'Bug Chasing, Barebacking, and the Risks of Care,' p. 90.
29. Dean, *Intimacy Unlimited*, p. 4.
30. A. A. Moskowitz and Me. E. Roloff, 'The Ultimate High: Sexual addiction and the bug chasing phenomenon', *Sexual Addition and Compulsivity* 14/1 (2007), p. 22.
31. Ibid., p. 26.

32. R. Tewksbury '"Click here for HIV": An analysis of internet-based bug chasers and bug givers', *Deviant Behaviour* 27/4) (2006), p. 390.
33. See Nicolas Sheon and Aaron Plant, 'Protease Dis-Inhibitors? The Gay Bareback Phenomenon', *HIV InSight*, 11 Nov 1997; Susan Kippax and Kane Race, 'Sustaining Safe Practice: Twenty Years On', *Social Science and Medicine* 57/1 (2003), pp. 1–12; Michael Shernoff, 'Condomless Sex: Gay Men, Barebacking, and Harm Reduction', *Social Work* 51/2 (April 2006), pp. 106–13.
34. Race, 'Revaluation of risk among gay men', *Social Research Issues Paper* 1 (Aug 2003), National Centre in HIV Social Research, available here http://sprc.unsw.edu.au/media/File/SRIP01.pdf (accessed 12 June 2005), p. 1, emphasis added.
35. Sharif Mowlabocus, *Gaydar Culture: Gay Men, Technology and Embodiment in the Digital Age* (Abingdon: Ashgate, 2010), p. 158.
36. Walt Odets, *In the Shadow of the Epidemic: Being Negative in the Age of AIDS* (Durham: Duke University Press, 1995).
37. Eric Rofes, *Dry Bones Breathe: Gay Men Creating Post-AIDS Identities and Cultures* (New York: Harrington Park, 1998).
38. Oliver Davis, 'Introduction to "Bareback sex and queer theory across three national contexts"', *Sexualities* 18/1–2 (2015), p. 121.
39. Pierre Bourdieu, *The Logic of Practice* (Trans. by Richard Nice) (Stanford University Press, Stanford, 1990 [1980]).
40. Michele L. Crossley, 'The Perils of Health Promotion and the "Barebacking" Backlash', *Health: An Interdisciplinary Journal for the Social Study of Health, Illness and Medicine* 6/1 (2002), p. 49.
41. Ibid.
42. Ibid., p. 57.
43. Michele L. Crossley, 'Making sense of "barebacking": Gay men's narratives, unsafe sex and the "resistance habitus"', *The British Journal of Social Psychology* 43/2 (2004), p. 236.
44. Sheon and Plant, 'Protease Dis-Inhibitors?'.
45. Crossley, 'Making sense of "barebacking"', p. 236.
46. Cited in ibid., p. 236.
47. Ibid., p. 239.
48. Shernoff, 'Condomless Sex', p. 108.
49. See Sedgwick *Epistemology of the Closet*, Chapter 1 for an explanation of the distinction between 'minoritising' and 'universalising' analyses.
50. Barry Adam, 'Constructing the neoliberal sexual actor', p. 334.
51. A. Carballo-Diéguez, 'HIV, barebacking and gay men's sexuality', *Journal of Sex Education and Therapy* 26/3 (2001), p. 229.
52. Michael Graydon, 'Don't bother to wrap it', p. 282.
53. Damien Ridge, '"It was an incredible thrill": The social meanings and dynamics of younger men's experience of barebacking in Melbourne', *Sexualities* 7/3 (2001), p. 265.

54. G. Dowsett, H. Williams, A. Ventuneac and A. Carballo-Diéguez, '"Taking it like a man": Masculinity and barebacking online', *Sexualities* 11/1–2 (2008), p. 131.
55. Ibid., pp. 130–5.
56. Byron Lee, 'It's a question of breeding: Visualising queer masculinity in bareback pornography', *Sexualities* 17/1–2 (2014), pp. 100–20.
57. Dean, *Unlimited Intimacy*.
58. David M. Halperin, *What Do Gay Men Want? An Essay on Sex, Risk, and Subjectivity* (Michigan: University of Michigan Press, 2007).
59. Dowsett et al., '"Taking it like a man"'.
60. Tomso, 'Viral Sex and the Politics of Life'.
61. Adam, 'Constructing the neoliberal sexual actor', p. 334.
62. J. Medew, 'Officials failed to alert police about HIV man', *The Age*, 21 March 2007, p. 3
63. Ibid.
64. I. Gould, 'HIV accused "slept with 200"', *Sydney Star Observer*, 12 October 2007.
65. Medew, 'Officials failed'.
66. Julia Medew, 'Monash team starts mapping HIV rise', *The Age*, 14 May 2007, p. 1; Julia Medew, 'Officials failed'; Julia Medew and Karen Kissane. 'Gays in HIV "bug chase"' *The Age* 23 April 2007, p. 1; Karen Kissane and Julia Medew, 'Dance with Death', *The Age*, 21 April 2007, p. 5; Bredan Roberts, 'Deadly party game: Gays deliberately infected with HIV, court told', *Herald Sun*, 21 March 2007, p. 3.
67. For example Medew, 'Officials'; Medew and Kissane, 'Gays in HIV "bug chase"'; Medew and Kissane 'Dance with Death'; Roberts, 'Deadly Party Game'. The reports discussed in this chapter were mostly sourced from *The Age*, *The Herald Sun* and *The Australian* newspapers. Owned and published by Fairfax Media, *The Age* is a broadsheet newspaper targeted at an 'influential and discerning audience' that at that time had a reach of approximately 668,000 readers per week (*'The Age*: Audience'). Its competitor, *The Herald Sun*, a morning tabloid published by The Herald and Weekly Times (a subsidiary of News Limited, itself a subsidiary of News Corp.), was then and remains the highest circulating daily newspaper in Australia. *The Australian* is also owned by News Corp. and is the biggest selling national newspaper in Australia, although with figures substantially below top-selling local (that is, state-based) newspapers.
68. 'Man Held HIV Parties – court told', *Herald Sun*, 20 Mar 2007, available at http://heraldsun.com.au/news/victoria/man-held-hiv-parties-court-told/story-e6frf7kx-1111113189029 (accessed 16 July 2008).
69. Roberts, 'Deadly Party Game'.
70. Natasha Robinson, 'Five years to tell police of HIV case', the *Australian*, 23 March 2007, p. 4.
71. Natasha Robinson, 'Accused HIV man most evil in years, says doctor', *The Age*, 23 March 2007.

72. Ibid.
73. Natasha Robinson, 'Chain of Indifference', the *Australian*, 2 April 2007, Features Section, p. 10.
74. Natasha Robinson, "HIV Man 'tricked sex slave'", the *Australian*, 29 March 2007, p. 7.
75. Robinson, 'Accused HIV Man'.
76. Robinson, 'Chain of Indifference'.
77. Ibid.
78. Robinson, 'Accused HIV Man'.
79. Ibid.
80. See Wald, *Contagious*.
81. Thomas Shevory, *Notorious H.I.V: The Media Spectacle of Nushawn Williams* (Minneapolis: University of Minnesota Press, 2004), p. ix.
82. Hanson, 'Undead', p. 325.
83. Hallas, *Reframing Bodies*, p. 6.
84. Crimp, 'How to Have Promiscuity in an Epidemic', p. 241.
85. Brendan Roberts, 'Seedy world unravels', *Herald Sun*, 31 March 2007, p. 25.
86. Simon Watney, 'Hollywood's Homosexual World', *Screen* 23/3–4 (1982), p. 109.
87. Edelman, *Homographesis*, p. 114.
88. Laura Mulvey, 'Visual Pleasure and Narrative Cinema', *Screen* 16/3 (1975), pp. 6–18.
89. Quoted in Irvine, 'Transient Feelings', p. 20.
90. Guy Davidson, '"Contagious Relations": Simulation, Paranoia, and the Portmodern Condition in William Freidkin's *Cruising* and Felice Picano's *The Lure*', *GLQ: A Journal of Lesbian and Gay Studies* 11/1 (2005), p. 58.
91. Ibid.
92. Ibid., p. 26.
93. Irvine., p. 28.
94. Ibid., p. 19.
95. Foucault, *The History of Sexuality*, p. 57.
96. Irvine, 'Transient Feelings', p. 10.
97. Kissane and Medew, 'Dance with Death'.
98. Conceived by advertiser Simon Reynolds, the controversial Grim Reaper TV campaign aired in Australia in 1987. The advertisement depicted the Grim Reaper knocking down men, women and children positioned as 'pins' in a bowling alley. The campaign was considered highly successful at raising community awareness around HIV/AIDS, but was also heavily criticised for its alleged potential to demonise gay men and PLWHA.
99. Sendziuk, *Learning to Trust*.
100. John Heard, 'Gays are too proud to confront AIDS, still the real killer', the *Australian*, 1 December 2006, p. 12.
101. Davidson, '"Contagious Relations"', p. 33.

102. Irvine, 'Transient Feelings', p. 24.
103. Ibid., p. 1.
104. Ibid., p. 2.
105. Ibid., p. 11.
106. See Lauren Berlant, *The Queen of America Goes to Washington City*; Michael Warner, *Publics and Counterpublics*.
107. Singer, *Erotic Welfare*, p. 27.
108. Ibid.
109. Ibid.
110. Annabel Stafford, 'HIV-positive visitors may be tracked or banned', *The Age*, 11 May 2007, p. 2.
111. Suellen Hinde, 'Refugees "must face HIV tests": Sex charges prompt call by minister', *Sunday Herald Sun*, 1 July 2007, p. 21.
112. See Daniel Reeders, 'The Impact of Criminalisation on Community-Based HIV Prevention', in Sally Cameron and John Rule (eds), *The Criminalisation of HIV Transmission in Australia: Legality, Morality and Reality* (NAPWA Monograph, 2009), pp. 134–45.
113. Julia Medew and C. Nader, '"Risky" HIV carriers to be reported: Doctor-patient privacy under threat', *The Age*, 25 July 2007, p. 5.
114. Julia Medew, 'Monash team starts mapping HIV rise.'
115. The use of the criminal justice system as a means of governing HIV is a relatively recent phenomenon in the Global North. In American states that currently have HIV transmission laws, the vast majority stipulate that it is a crime for HIV positive people to have sex without first disclosing their HIV status, regardless of condom use or whether there is risk of the transmission of HIV. The movement against criminalisation argues, among other things, that this stipulation is counter to the objectives of public health because it enhances stigma and hence the likelihood of HIV testing and treatment. See Matthew Weait, *Intimacy and Responsibility: The Criminalisation of HIV Transmission* (New York: Routledge, 2007).
116. John Russell, 'Bio-Power and Biohazards: A projective system reading of gay men's community-based HIV prevention', *Culture, Health & Sexuality* 7/2 (March 2005), p. 145.
117. Dean, *Unlimited Intimacy*, p. 47.
118. Tomso, 'Bug Chasing, Barebacking, and the Risks of Care', p. 89.
119. William Haver, *The Body of this Death: Historicity and Sociality in the Time of AIDS* (Stanford: Stanford University Press, 1996), p. 3.
120. See Nguyen Tan Hoang, *A View from the Bottom: Asian American Masculinity and Sexual Representation* (Durham: Duke University Press, 2014).
121. Dean, *Unlimited Intimacy*, p. 50.
122. Ibid., p. 56.

123. Ibid., p. 51.
124. See Mowlabocus et al. on the historical and industrial travails of the condom code in gay male porn in 'Porn Laid Bare: Gay men, pornography and bareback sex', *Sexualities* 16/5–6 (2013), pp. 523–47.
125. See Stuart Scott, 'The Condomlessness of Bareback Sex: Responses to the unrepresentability of HIV in Treasure Island Media's *Plantin' Seed* and *Slammed*', *Sexualities* 18/1–2 'Bareback sex and queer theory across three national contexts (France, UK, USA)' 2015, pp. 210–23.
126. Mowlabocus et al.
127. Heard, 'Gays are too proud to confront AIDS'.

4 AIDS Heritage in *The Line of Beauty*

1. Reghina Dascăl, 'The Long Shadow of the Lady', *Gender Studies* 5 (2006), p. 240.
2. Simon During, 'Queering Thatcher: Whatever happened to politics and culture in the 1980s?', *JOMEC Journal* 3 (June 2013), p. 6.
3. Jackie Stacey, 'Promoting Normality: Section 28 and the Regulation of Sexuality', in S. Franklin, C. Lury and J. Stacey (eds), *Off-Centre: Feminism and Cultural Studies* (London: HarperCollins, 1991), p. 286.
4. Eckart Voigts-Virchow, 'Introduction' in Eckart Voigts-Virchow (ed.), *Janespotting and Beyond: British Heritage Retrovisions Since the Mid-1990s* (Tübingen: Gunter Narr Verlag Tübingen, 2004), p. 14.
5. See Andrew Higson, 'Re-Presenting the National Past: Nostalgia and Pastiche in the Heritage Film', in Lester Friedman (ed.), *Fires Were Started: British Cinema and Thatcherism* (Minneapolis: University of Minnesota Press, 1993), pp. 109–29.
6. Deborah Cartmell, I. Q. Hunter and Imelda Whelehan, *Retrovisions: Reinventing the Past in Film and Fiction* (London: Pluto Press, 2001), p. 2.
7. Lucas Hilderbrand, 'Retroactivism', *GLQ: A Journal of Lesbian and Gay Studies* 12/2 (2006), p. 308.
8. Love, *Feeling Backward*, p. 18.
9. Ibid., p. 8.
10. Ibid., p. 19.
11. From *An Early Frost* (1985) onwards, the movie of the week was something of a privileged form for the mainstream depiction of AIDS. See Elaine Rapping's *Movie of the Week* (London, 1992) for an account of the TV movie as a national ideological apparatus that functions pedagogically and helps to determine what and how nations construct and conceptualise matters of collective importance.

12. Timothy Corrigan, 'Which Shakespeare to Love? Film, Fidelity, and the Performance of Literature', in Jim Collins (ed.), *High-pop: Making Culture into Popular Entertainment* (Oxford: Blackwell Publishers, 2002), p. 157.
13. Jim Collins, 'High-Pop: An Introduction' in Jim Collins (ed.), *High-Pop*, p. 6.
14. BBC, 'Building Public Value', *BBC.co.uk*, 1994, http://bbc.co.uk/info/policies/text/bpv.html (accessed 15 July 2008).
15. Colm Tóibín, 'The Comedy of Being English', *The New York Review of Books* 52/1 (13 January 2005), http://www.nybooks.com/articles/2005/01/13/the-comedy-of-being-english/ (accessed 19 November 2009).
16. 'Alan Hollinghurst', *GLBTQ: Encyclopedia of Gay, Lesbian, Bisexual, Transgender and Queer Culture*, 2006, http://glbtq.com/literature/hollinghurst_a.html (accessed 2 July 2008).
17. See Held pp. 119–22.
18. Thomas Schatz, *Hollywood Genres: Formulas, Filmmaking and the Studio System* (New York: Random House, 1981), pp. 36–41.
19. Sarah Street, *British National Cinema* (London; New York: Routledge, 1997), p. 102.
20. Richard Dyer, 'Homosexual Heritage' in *The Culture of Queers* (London; New York: Routledge, 2002), p. 204.
21. The classic Leftist critique of heritage cinema is best encapsulated in Andrew Higson's since-revised 'Re-Presenting the National Past'. Claire Monk was another key protagonist in early debates. See also Higson, *English Heritage, English Cinema: Costume Drama since 1980* (Oxford; New York: Oxford University Press, 2003); Ginette Vincendeau, *Film/Literature/Heritage: A Sight and Sound Reader* (London, 2001), Voigts-Virshow, 2004 and Belén Vidal, *Heritage Film: Nation, Genre and Representation* (New York: Columbia University Press, 2012).
22. Higson, 'Re-Presenting the National Past', p. 115.
23. Ibid., p. 117.
24. Ibid., pp. 117–18.
25. Ibid., p. 117.
26. Barbara Schaff, 'Still Lives – Tableaux Vivants: Art in British Heritage Films', in Eckart Voigts-Virchow (ed.), *Janespotting and Beyond*, p. 128.
27. Martin A. Hipsky, 'Anglophil(M)ia: Why Does America Watch Merchant-Ivory Movies?', *Journal of Popular Film and Television* 22 (1994), p. 102.
28. Ibid., p. 103.
29. Pam Cook, *Fashioning the Nation: Costume and Identity in British Cinema* (London: BFI Publishing, 1994); Hipsky, p. 115.
30. Dyer, 'Homosexual Heritage', p. 206.
31. Claire Monk, 'Sexuality and the Heritage', *Sight and Sound* 5/10 (Oct 1995), p. 3.

32. Carolin Held, 'From "Heritage Space" to "Narrative Space": Anti-Heritage Aesthetics in the Classic TV Serials *Our Mutual Friend* and *Vanity Fair*', in Eckart Voigts-Virchow, *Janespotting and Beyond*, p. 114.
33. Claire Monk, quoted in ibid., p. 113.
34. Ben Gook, 'Really-existing Nostalgia? Remembering East Germany in Film', *Traffic* 10 (January 2008), p. 125.
35. Frederic Jameson, 'Postmodernism, or The Cultural Logic of Late Capitalism', *New Left Review* 146 (July–August 1984), pp. 72–91.
36. See for example Svetlana Boym, *The Future of Nostalgia* (New York: Basic Books, 2001); and Susannah Radstone, *The Sexual Politics of Time: Confession, Nostalgia, Memory* (London; New York: Routledge, 2007).
37. Pam Cook, *Fashioning the Nation*, p. 4.
38. Jason Goldman, '"The Golden Age of Gay Porn": Nostalgia and the Photography of Wilhelm von Gloeden', *GLQ: A Journal of Lesbian and Gay Studies* 12/2 (2006), p. 250.
39. Boym, *The Future of Nostalgia*, p. 49.
40. Monk, 'Sexuality and the Heritage'.
41. Vidal, *Heritage Film*, p. 4.
42. Giorgio Agamben, *Homo Sacer: Sovereign Power and Bare Life*, Trans. Daniel Heller-Roazen (Stanford: Stanford University Press, 1998).
43. Love, *Feeling Backwards*, p. 27.
44. Quoted in ibid., p. 27.
45. Quoted in ibid, p. 14.
46. Ibid., p. 4.
47. Ibid., p. 27.
48. Dascăl, 'The Long Shadow of the Lady', p. 242.
49. Alan Hollinghurst, *The Line of Beauty* (London, Picador 2004), p. 48.
50. Ibid.
51. Held, 'From "Heritage Space" to "Narrative Space"', p. 118.
52. Daniel Hannah, 'The Private Life, the Public Stage: Henry James in Recent Fiction', *Journal of Modern Literature* 30/3 (Spring 2007), p. 88.
53. Lee Clark Mitchell, ' "To suff er like chopped limbs": The Dispossessions of *The Spoils of Poynton*', *The Henry James Review* 26 (2005), p. 21. In BBC2's adaptation, *The Spoils of Poynton* reference acts as a self-reflexive joke about the 1980s penchant for adapting British literary classics in heritage-style films. As I argue elsewhere, *The Spoils* is the key intertextual reference for understanding the character of Hollinghurst's critique of Thatcherite culture and neoliberalism. See Dion Kagan, 'Possessions and dispossession: homo economicus and neoliberal sociality in *The Line of Beauty*', *Continuum: Journal of Media & Cultural Studies* 28/ 6 (2014), pp. 797– 807.
54. Hollinghurst, *The Line of Beauty*, p. 447.
55. Kagan, 'Possessions and dispossession'; and During, 'Queering Thatcher'.

56. Simon Watney, 'Taking Liberties: An Introduction' in Erica Carter and Simon Watney (eds), *Taking Liberties: AIDS and Cultural Politics* (London: Serpent's Tail 1989), p. 22.
57. Ibid., p. 21.
58. Ibid., pp. 24–6.
59. Ibid., p. 23.
60. Dyer, 'Homosexual Heritage', p. 209.
61. Hannah, 'The Private Life, the Public Stage', p. 89.
62. Julie Rivkin, 'Writing the Gay 80s with Henry James: David Leavitt's *A Place I've Never Been* and Alan Hollinghurst's *The Line of Beauty*', *The Henry James Review* 26/3 (Fall 2005), p. 8.
63. Hollinghurst, *The Line of Beauty*, p. 223.
64. During, 'Queering Thatcher', p. 9.
65. Ibid., p. 9.
66. Hollinghurst, *The Line of Beauty*, p. 75.
67. Hannah, 'The Private Life, the Public Stage', p. 85.
68. Ibid., p. 86.
69. Ibid., p. 77.
70. Ibid., p. 85.
71. Ibid.
72. Gregory Woods, '"It's My Nature": AIDS Narratives and the Moral Re-Branding of Queerness in the mid-1990s' in Robin Griffiths (ed.), *British Queer Cinema* (London; New York: Routledge, 2006), p. 172.
73. Locksley Hall, 'Dan Stevens on *The Line of Beauty*', *After Elton*, 13 October 2006, http://afterelton.com/archive/elton/people/2006/10/danstevens.html (accessed 23 July 2008)
74. During, 'Queering Thatcher', p. 10.
75. Quoted in Dascăl, 'The Long Shadow of the Lady', p. 241.
76. Morrison, 'End Pleasure', p. 55.
77. Robert Dessaix, 'Death to Art: Reflections on AIDS, Art and Susan Sontag' *(and so forth)* (Sydney: PanMacmillan 1998), pp. 274–5.
78. Rivkin, 'Writing the Gay 80s', p. 7.
79. Dascăl, 'The Long Shadow of the Lady', p. 252.
80. Ibid.
81. Ron Charles, 'Lines of Beauty and Depravity', *The Christian Science Monitor*, 26 October 2004, http://csmonitor.com/2004/1026/p14s01-bognhtml (accessed 23 July 2008).
82. Peter Swaab, '*The Line of Beauty*' *Film Quarterly* 60/3 (2007), p. 14.
83. Ibid., p. 11.
84. Boym, *The Future of Nostalgia*.
85. José Esteban Muñoz, *Cruising Utopia: The Then and There of Queer Futurity* (New York: NYU Press, 2009).

5 AIDS Retrovisions: *Dallas Buyers Club* and *The Normal Heart*

1. Theodore Kerr, 'AIDS 1969: HIV, History, and Race', *Drain* special edition on 'AIDS and Memory' (2017), http://drainmag.com/aids-1969-hiv-history-and-race (accessed 21 April 2017).
2. Ibid.
3. Douglas Crimp, *Melancholia and Moralism* (Cambridge: MIT Press, 2002), p. 4.
4. Andrew Sullivan, 'When Plagues End' pp. 52–62, 76–7, 84.
5. Crimp, *Melancholia and Moralism*, p. 5.
6. See also Richard Goldstein, *Homocons: The Rise of the Gay Right* (London; New York: Verso, 2003); Warner, *The Trouble with Normal*.
7. Crimp, *Melancholia and Moralism*, p. 9.
8. Ibid., p. 16.
9. Christopher Castiglia, 'Sex Panics, Sex Publics, Sex Memories', *Boundary* 27/2 (2000), pp. 161–2.
10. Christopher Castiglia and Christopher Reed, *If Memory Serves*.
11. For example, see Ann Cvetkovich, *An Archive of Feelings: Trauma, Sexuality, and Lesbian Public Cultures* (Durham: Duke University Press, 2003); Deborah Gould, *Moving Politics: Emotion and ACT Ups Fight Against AIDS* (Chicago: University of Chicago Press, 2009); Roger Hallas, *Reframing Bodies*.
12. Dion Kagan, 'How to Have Memories in an Epidemic: Recent Documentaries about HIV/AIDS', *Kill Your Darlings* April 2013, pp. 141–56.
13. Avram Finkelstein, 'AIDS 2.0', *POZ*, 10 January 2013, https://www.poz.com/article/avram-finkelstein-23355-3691 (accessed 7 May 2016).
14. '*Dallas Buyers Club* Box Office', *The Numbers*, http://www.the-numbers.com/movie/Dallas-Buyers-Club#tab=box-office (accessed 7 August 2015).
15. Forrest Wickman, 'Was *Dallas Buyers Club*'s Ron Woodroof gay or bisexual?' *Slate*, 17 January 2014, http://www.slate.com/blogs/browbeat/2014/01/17/was_dallas_buyers_club_s_ron_woodroof_gay_or_bisexual_friends_and_doctor.html (accessed 2 March 2014).
16. Sontag, *AIDS and its Metaphors*, p. 123.
17. Hallas, *Reframing Bodies*, p. 12.
18. David Edelstein, 'Outlaw Pharmacology', *New York Magazine*, 27 October 2013, http://nymag.com/movies/reviews/dallas-buyers-club-about-time-2013-11/ (accessed 2 March 2014).
19. Emily Bass, 'How to Survive a Footnote: AIDS activism in the "after" years', *n+1* 23 (Fall 2015), https://nplusonemag.com/issue-23/annals-of-activism/how-to-survive-a-footnote/ (accessed 4 April 2016).
20. Larry Kramer, 'Sex and Sensibility', *The Advocate*, 27 May 1997, p. 65.

21. Critical review aggregator Rotten Tomatoes records a score of 94 per cent fresh out of a total of 48 counted reviews and offers a consensus summary: 'Thanks to Emmy-worthy performances from a reputable cast, *The Normal Heart* is not only a powerful, heartbreaking drama, but also a vital document of events leading up to and through the early AIDS crisis'. 'The Normal Heart', *Rotten Tomatoes*, https://www.rottentomatoes.com/m/the_normal_heart/ (accessed 13 June 2017).
22. Willa Paskin, '"By 1984 You Could Be Dead": HBO and Ryan Murphy's tremendously moving *The Normal Heart*', *Slate*, 22 May 2014, available at http://www.slate.com/articles/arts/television/2014/05/ryan_murphy_s_hbo_version_of_the_normal_heart_reviewed.html (accessed 12 June 2015).
23. Patrick Healy, 'A Lion Still Roars, With Gratitude: Larry Kramer Lives to See His "Normal Heart" Filmed for TV', *The New York Times*, 21 May 2014, https://www.nytimes.com/2014/05/25/arts/television/larry-kramer-lives-to-see-his-normal-heart-filmed-for-tv.html?_r=0 (accessed 13 June 2017).
24. Adam Zeboski, '#TruvadaWhore goes viral', *HIV Equal*, 24 June 2014, http://www.hivequal.org/hiv-equal-online/truvadawhore-goes-viral (accessed 3 June 2017).
25. Crimp, *Mourning and Melancholia*, p. 3.
26. Cited in Jim Downs, 'How "the 70s" became a morality play', *Gay & Lesbian Review Worldwide* 13/2 (2006), p. 8.
27. Lawrence K. Altman, 'Rare cancer diagnosed in 41 homosexuals', *The New York Times*, 3 July 1981, http://www.nytimes.com/1981/07/03/us/rare-cancer-seen-in-41-homosexuals.html (accessed 13 June 2017).
28. Crossley, 'Making sense of "barebacking"', p. 236.
29. 'Unhappy archives' is Sara Ahmed's term. See *The Promise of Happiness* (Durham, Duke University Press, 2010), pp. 17–19.
30. This phrase comes from the title of Ann Cvetkovich's book, *An Archive of Feelings*.
31. 'Countermemory' is Castiglia's term for a queer political consciousness in which history and memory are deliberately drawn on to expose the inadequacies of contemporary LGBTQI+ narratives of progress and to provide a locus of identification for queer radicals in the present.
32. Hilderbrand, 'Retroactivism'.

Conclusion: Feeling Generational

1. Shugart, 'Reinventing Privilege'.
2. David Halperin, *How to Be Gay* (Boston: Harvard University Press, 2012), p. 49.
3. Love, *Feeling Backward*, p. 6.
4. Ibid., p. 7.

5. Benedicto, 'The Haunting of Gay Manila', p. 319.
6. Love, *Feeling Backward*, p. 17.
7. Butler, *Bodies That Matter*, p. 115.
8. I have been placing 'generation' in scare quotes in order to draw attention to the way that, as a concept, it calls upon heterosexual structures of biological reproduction, kinship, genealogy and consanguinity. I suggest that part of the effect of AIDS memorial practices may be to place some deconstructive pressure on those meanings of the concept and to recreate it in queerer terms.
9. Melissa Anderson, '*We Were Here*: Five San Franciscans Remember the AIDS Crisis', *The Village Voice*, 7 September 2011, https://www.villagevoice.com/2011/09/07/we-were-here-five-san-franciscans-remember-the-aids-crisis/ (accessed 13 June 2017).
10. Jake Weinraub, '*We Were Here* Captures the Voices of a Generation Lost to HIV/AIDS', *The Wrap*, 15 July 2011 http://www.thewrap.com/review-we-were-here-captures-voices-generation-lost-hivaids-29145/ (accessed 2 December 2014).
11. Anderson, V. '*How to Survive a Plague*: Undeniable Witness – interview with David France', *A&U Magazine: America's AIDS Magazine*, 8 October 2012, http://aumag.org/2012/10/08/how-to-survive-a-plague/ (accessed 12 June 2013).
12. Kagan, 'How to Have Memories in an Epidemic', pp. 146–7.
13. 'Dustin Lance Black: ABC's *When We Rise*', *The Treatment*, http://www.stitcher.com/podcast/college-radio-workshop/kcrws-the-treatment/e/dustin-lance-black-abcs-when-we-rise-49366290 (accessed 12 March 2017).
14. Castiglia and Reed, *If Memory* Serves, p. 55.
15. Theodore Kerr, 'On Organising, and "Your Nostalgia Is Killing Me"', *The Visual AIDS blog*, 1 March 2014, https://www.visualaids.org/blog/detail/on-organizing-and-your-nostalgia-is-killing-me (accessed 21 April 2017).
16. Joshua Pocius, 'HIV/AIDS on screen: by focusing on history, we ignore the present', *The Conversation*, 21 July 2014, http://theconversation.com/hiv-aids-on-screen-by-focusing-on-history-we-ignore-the-present-28972 (accessed 2 February 2015).
17. See Hallas, *Reframing Bodies*, 2009.
18. Dion Kagan, 'After the Orgy: The (New) *Normal Heart*', *The Lifted Brow* 24 (2014), pp. 44–5.
19. Marriane Hirsch, 'The Generation of Postmemory' in Karen Beckman and Lilianne Weissberg (eds), *On Writing with Photography* (Minnesota: University of Minnesota Press, 2013), pp. 202–30.
20. Benjamin Riley, 'Objects in History: AIDS as Cultural Singularity', *The Lifted Brow* 25 (2015), pp. 49–53.
21. Ibid., p. 51.

22. '*All the Way Through Evening*: Rohan Spong Interview', *Time Out* http://www.au.timeout.com/melbourne/gay-lesbian/features/2043/all-the-way-through-evening-rohan-spong-interview (link no longer working).
23. Stern-Wolfe has an apartment-sized archive of musical concert and other footage captured on VHS and thus *All the Way Through Evening* is another work that foregrounds the chronicling and archiving of AIDS history in this now superseded visual technology.
24. James Welsby, 'Between Suffering and Celebration', *Next Wave Festival 2014 Magazine*, p. 11, available at https://issuu.com/nextwave2014festival/docs/nw_publication-v2 (accessed 21 June 2017).
25. Ibid.
26. 'James Welsby HEX', *YouTube*, posted by Act Up Queensland, 29 July 2014, https://www.youtube.com/watch?v=4FAh79gfZdw (accessed 21 June 2017).
27. Parallel arguments about the transmissibility of queer kinship and knowledge exist in Tim Dean's anthropological and ethnographic notion of 'viral consanguinity' applied to practices and cultures of barebacking in *Unlimited Intimacy*, and Alyson Campbell and Dirk Gindt's notion of 'viral dramaturgies' in Alyson Campbell and Dirk Gindt (eds) *HIV and AIDS in Twenty-First Century Performance: An International Collection* (Palgrave, UK, 2018). Welsby's work would most certainly constitute an example of 'viral dramaturgy' in the sense offered by Campbell and Gindt.
28. Marianne Hirsch, *Family Frames: Photographs, Narratives and Post-Memory* (London: Harvard University Press, 1997), p. 22.
29. Ibid., p. 22.
30. Nancy K. Miller and Jason Tougaw, 'Introduction: Extremeties', *Extremities: Trauma, Testimony, and Community* (Champaign: University of Illinois Press, 2002), p. 9.
31. Love, *Feeling Backward*, p. 19.
32. Ibid., p. 147.
33. Ibid., p. 21.
34. José Esteban Muñoz, *Cruising Utopia*, p. 22.
35. Ibid., p. 20 and p. 4.
36. Ibid., p. 12.
37. Ibid., p. 10.
38. See Leo Bersani, 'Sociality and Sexuality', *Critical Inquiry* 26: 4 (Summer, 2000), pp. 641–56.
39. Hilderbrand, p. 311.
40. Love, *Feeling Backward*, p. 19.

Bibliography

'About Somatechnics', Somatechnics Blog, https://somatechnics.wordpress.com/about-somatechnics/Somatechnics Research Centre (accessed July 2015).

Act Up Queensland, 'James Welsby HEX', *YouTube*, 29 July 2014, https://www.youtube.com/watch?v=4FAh79gfZdw (accessed 21 June 2017).

Adam, Barry D., Winston Husbands, James Murray and John Maxwell, 'AIDS Optimism, Condom Fatigue, or Self- Esteem? Explaining Unsafe Sex Among Gay and Bisexual Men', *The Journal of Sex Research* 42/3 (August 2005), pp. 238–248.

——, 'Constructing the Neoliberal Sexual Actor: Responsibility and care of the self in the discourse of barebackers', *Culture, Heath and Sexuality* 7/4 (2005), pp. 333–46.

Agamben, Giorgio, *Homo Sacer: Sovereign Power and Bare Life*, Trans. Daniel Heller-Roazen (Stanford: Stanford University Press, 1998).

'*The Age*: Audience' *Fairfax Media* 2008, http://adcentre.com.au/theage.aspx?show=audience (link no longer working).

Ahmed, Sara, *The Cultural Politics of Emotion* (New York: Routledge, 2004).

——, *The Promise of Happiness* (Durham: Duke University Press, 2010).

'Alan Hollinghurst', *GLBTQ: Encyclopedia of Gay, Lesbian, Bisexual, Transgender and Queer Culture*, http://glbtq.com/literature/hollinghurst_a.html (link no longer working).

'Alarming jump in HIV infections', *The Age*, 7 October 2006, p. 7.

Alderson, David, 'Queer Cosmopolitanism: Place, Politics, Citizenship and *Queer as Folk*', *New Formations* 55/1 (Spring 2005), pp. 73–88.

Allen, Dennis, 'Homosexuality and Narrative', *Modern Fiction Studies* 41/3-4 (Fall–Winter 1995), pp. 609–34.

Altman, Dennis, 'The Margins of Our Attention', *The Monthly* (December 2006–January 2007), pp. 52–8.

——, 'Political Sexualities: Meanings and Identities in the Time of AIDS' in Richard G. Parker and John Gagnon (eds), *Conceiving Sexualities: Approaches to Sex Research in a Postmodern World* (New York: Routledge, 1996), pp. 96–106.

Altman, Lawrence K., 'Rare cancer diagnosed in 41 homosexuals', *New York Times*, 3 July 1981, http://www.nytimes.com/1981/07/03/us/rare-cancer-seen-in-41-homosexuals.html (accessed 13 June 2017).

Bibliography

Anderson, Melissa, '*We Were Here*: Five San Franciscans Remember the AIDS Crisis', *The Village Voice*, 7 September 2011, https://www.villagevoice.com/2011/09/07/we-were-here-five-san-franciscans-remember-the-aids-crisis/ (accessed 13 June 2017).

Anderson, V., '*How to Survive a Plague*: Undeniable Witness – interview with David France', *A&U Magazine: America's AIDS magazine*, 8 October 2012, http://aumag.org/2012/10/08/how-to-survive-a-plague/ (accessed 12 June 2013).

Aronson, Amy and Michael Kimmel, 'The Saviours and the Saved: Masculine Redemption in Contemporary Films' in Peter Lehman (ed.), *Masculinity: Bodies, Movies, Culture* (New York and London: Routledge, 2001), pp. 43–50.

Auerbach, D. M., Jaffe Darrow and J. Curran, 'Cluster of cases of the acquired immune deficiency syndrome: Patients linked by sexual contact', *The American Journal of Medicine* 76 (1984), pp. 487–92.

Bardella, Claudio, 'Pilgrimages of the Plagued: AIDS, Body and Society', *Body & Society* 8 (2002), pp. 79–105.

Bateman, Robert Benjamin, 'What Do Gay Men Desire? Peering Behind the *Queer Eye*' in James R. Keller and Leslie Stratyner (eds), *The New Queer Aesthetic on Television: Essays on Recent Programming* (North Carolina: McFarland & Co., 2006), pp. 9–19.

BBC, 'Building Public Value', *BBC.co.uk*, http://bbc.co.uk/info/policies/text/bpv.html.

Becker, Ron, *Gay TV and Straight America* (New Jersey: Rutgers University Press, 2006)

——, 'Prime-Time Television in the Gay Nineties: Network Television, Quality Audiences, and Gay Politics' in Robert Clyde Allen and Annette Hill (eds), *The Television Studies Reader* (London: Routledge, 2006), pp. 389–403.

——, 'Prime-Time Television in the Gay Nineties: Network Television, Quality Audiences, and Gay Politics', *The Velvet Light Trap* 42 (1998), pp. 36–47.

Beirne, Rebecca Clare, 'Embattled Sex: Rise of the Right and Victory of the Queer in *Queer as Folk*' in James R. Keller and Leslie Stratyner (eds), *The New Queer Aesthetic on Television: Essays on Recent Programming* (North Carolina: McFarland & Co., 2006), pp. 43–58.

Bell, Gail, 'A Quiet Anniversary: AIDS 30 Years On', *The Monthly* (November 2011), pp. 44–8.

Benedicto, Bobby, 'The Haunting of Gay Manila: Global Space-Time and the Specter of Kabaklaan', *GLQ: A Journal of Lesbian and Gay Studies* 14/2–3 (2008), pp. 317–38.

Berlant, Lauren, *The Queen of America Goes to Washington City: Essays on Sex and Citizenship* (Durham: Duke University Press, 1997).

Bersani, Leo, *Homos* (Cambridge: Harvard University Press, 1995).

Bibliography

——, 'Is the Rectum a Grave?' in Douglas Crimp (ed.), *AIDS: Cultural Analysis, Cultural Activism* (Cambridge: MIT Press, 1988), pp. 197–222.

——, 'Sociality and Sexuality', *Critical Inquiry* 26/4 (Summer, 2000), pp. 641–56.

Blackwelder, Rob, 'Homogenized By Hollywood: Madonna has Baby with Gay friend in Disingenuous Crossover Flop *The Next Best Thing*', splicedwire 3 Mar 2000 http://splicedwire.com/00reviews/nextbest.html (accessed 4 November 2006).

Blechner, Mark J. 'Intimacy, Pleasure, Risk, and Safety: Discussion of Cheuvront's "High-Risk Sexual Behaviour in the Treatment of HIV-Negative Patients", *Journal of Gay and Lesbian Psychotherapy* 6/3 (2002), pp. 27–33.

Bordo, Susan, *The Male Body: A New Look at Men in Public and in Private* (New York: Farar, Straus and Giroux, 1999).

Bourdieu, Pierre, *Distinction: A Social Critique of Judgement and Taste* (London: Routledge, 1984).

——, *The Logic of Practice*, Trans. Richard Nice (Stanford: Stanford University Press, 1990 [1980]).

Boym, Svetlana, *The Future of Nostalgia* (Basic Books: New York, 2001).

Brandt, Alan M., 'AIDS: From Social History to Social Policy' in Elizabeth Fee and Daniel M. Fox (eds), *AIDS: The Burdens of History* (Berkeley: University of California Press, 1988), pp. 147–71.

Brown, Michael P., *Replacing Citizenship: AIDS Activism and Radical Democracy* (New York: Guilford Press, 1997).

Brooks, Peter, *The Melodramatic Imagination: Balzac, Henry James, Melodrama, and the Mode of Excess* (New Haven: Yale University Press, 1995 [1976]).

Bull, Chris, 'Acting gay', *The Advocate* 671 (27 December 1994), p. 44.

Butler, Judith, *Bodies That Matter: On the Discursive Limits of "Sex"* (London: Routledge, 1993).

——, *Gender Trouble: Feminism and the Subversion of Identity* (London: Routledge, 1990).

——, *The Psychic Life of Power: Theories in Subjection* (Stanford: Stanford University Press, 1997).

Cagle, Jess, 'The Gay 90's: America Sees Shades of Gay; A Once-Invisible Group Finds The Spotlight', *Entertainment Weekly* (8 September 1995), http://ew.com/article/1995/09/08/special-report-gay-90s/ (accessed 7 November 2007).

Caldwell, John. *Production Culture: Industrial Reflexivity and Critical Practice in Film/Television* (Durham: Duke University Press, 2008).

Campbell, Alyson and Dirk Gindt (eds), *HIV and AIDS in Twenty-First Century Performance: An International Collection* (Palgrave: London, 2018).

Carballo-Diéguez, Alex, 'HIV, barebacking and gay men's sexuality', *Journal of Sex Education and Therapy* 26/3 (2001), pp. 225–33.

Caron, David, *AIDS in French Culture: Social Ills, Literary Cures* (Madison: University of Wisconsin Press, 2001).

Bibliography

——, *The Nearness of Others: Searching for Tact and Contact in The Age of HIV* (Minneapolis: University of Minnesota Press, 2014).

Cartmell, Deborah, I. Q. Hunter and Imelda Whelehan, *Retrovisions: Reinventing the Past in Film and Fiction* (London and Sterling: Pluto Press, 2001)

Castiglia, Christopher, 'Sex Panics, Sex Publics, Sex Memories', *Boundary* 27/2 (2000), pp. 149–75.

Castiglia, Christopher and Christopher Reed. *If Memory Serves: Gay Men, AIDS, and the Promise of the Queer Past* (Minneapolis: University of Minnesota Press, 2011).

Charles, Ron, 'Lines of Beauty and Depravity', *The Christian Science Monitor*, 26 October 2004, http://csmonitor.com/2004/1026/p14s01-bognhtml (accessed 23 July 2008).

Chaw, Walter, 'Queer as Folk', *Film Freak Central DVD Review* http://filmfreakcentral.net/dvdreviews/queerasfolk.htm (accessed 16 January 2009).

Cheuvront, J.P., 'High-Risk Sexual Behaviour in the Treatment of HIV-Negative Patients', *Journal of Gay & Lesbian Psychotherapy* 6/3 (2002): pp. 7–25.

Clarke, Eric O., *Virtuous Vice: Homoeroticism and the Public Sphere* (Durham: Duke University Press, 2000).

Cohen, Ed., *A Body Worth Defending: Immunity, Biopolitics, and the Apotheosis of the Modern Body* (Durham: Duke University Press, 2009).

——, *Talk on the Wilde Side: Toward a Genealogy of a Discourse on Male Sexualities* (New York: Routledge, 1993).

Collins, Jim, 'High-Pop: An Introduction' in Jim Collins (ed.), *High-Pop: Making Culture into Popular Culture* (Oxford: Blackwell Publishers, 2002).

Connell, R., 'The Social Organisation of Masculinity' in Stephen M. Whitebread and Frank J. Barrett (eds), *The Masculinities Reader* (Cambridge: Polity, 2002), pp. 67–86.

——, *Masculinities* (Berkeley and LA: University of California Press, 2005).

Cook, Pam, *Fashioning the Nation: Costume and Identity in British Cinema* (London: BFI Publishing, 1994).

Corber, Robert J., 'Nationalising the Gay Body: AIDS and Sentimental Pedagogy in *Philadelphia*', *American Literary History* 15/1 (2003), pp. 107–33.

Corrigan, Timothy, 'Which Shakespeare to Love? Film, Fidelity, and the Performance of Literature', in Jim Collins (ed.), *High-pop: Making Culture into Popular Entertainment* (Oxford: Blackwell, 2002), pp. 155–81.

Crimp, Douglas, 'AIDS: Cultural Analysis, Cultural Activism' in Douglas Crimp (ed.), *AIDS: Cultural Analysis, Cultural Activism* (Cambridge: MIT Press, 1988), pp. 3–16.

——, 'How to Have Promiscuity in an Epidemic' in Douglas Crimp (ed.), *AIDS: Cultural Analysis, Cultural Activism* (Cambridge: MIT Press, 1988), pp. 237–71.

——, *Melancholia and Moralism: Essays on AIDS and Queer Politics* (Cambridge: MIT Press, 2002)

Bibliography

Crossley, Michele L., 'The Perils of Health Promotion and the 'Barebacking' Backlash', *Health: An Interdisciplinary Journal for the Social Study of Health, Illness and Medicine* 6/1 (2002), pp. 47–68.

———, 'Making sense of "barebacking": Gay men's narratives, unsafe sex and the "resistance habitus"', *The British Journal of Social Psychology* 43/2 (2004), pp. 225–44.

Cvetkovich, Ann, *An Archive of Feelings: Trauma, Sexuality, and Lesbian Public Cultures* (Durham: Duke University Press, 2003).

'Dallas Buyers Club Box Office', *The Numbers*, http://www.the-numbers.com/movie/Dallas-Buyers-Club#tab=box-office (accessed 7 August 2015).

Dascăl, Reghina, 'The Long Shadow of the Lady', *Gender Studies* 5 (2006), pp. 240–53.

'David Marshall Grant and Ron Rifkin: HIV & Aging – Clips from *Brothers & Sisters*', *Youtube*, 1 November 2010 http://youtube.com/watch?v=uUCasILAcJ0 (accessed 20 June 2011).

Davidson, Guy, ' "Contagious Relations": Simulation, Paranoia, and the Portmodern Condition in William Freidkin's *Cruising* and Felice Picano's *The Lure*', *GLQ: A Journal of Lesbian and Gay Studies* 11/1 (2005), pp. 23–64.

Davis, Glynn, *Queer as Folk* (London: BFI publishing, 2007).

Davis, Mark, 'HIV Prevention Rationalities and Serostatus in the Risk Narratives of Gay Men', *Sexualities* 5/3 (2002), pp. 281–99.

Davis, Nick, 'The Next Best Thing', *Nicks Flick Picks,* http://nicksflickpicks.com/nextbest.html (accessed 4 November 2006).

Davis, Oliver, Introduction to 'Bareback sex and queer theory across three national contexts (France, UK, USA)', special issue of *Sexualities* 18/1-2 (2015), pp. 12–126.

Dean, Tim, *Intimacy Unlimited: Reflections on the Subculture of Barebacking* (Chicago: University of Chicago Press, 2009).

Dessaix, Robert, 'Death to Art: Reflections on AIDS, Art and Susan Sontag' *(and so forth)* (Sydney: Pan MacMillan, 1998), pp. 272–93.

Douglas, Mary, *Purity and Danger: An Analysis of Concepts of Pollution and Taboo* (New York: Routledge Classics, 2002 [1966]).

Dow, Steve, 'Denial becomes the new language of casual sex', *Sydney Morning Herald*, 3 July 2003, http://smh.com.au/articles/2003/07/02/1056825457732.html (10 July 2011).

Dowling, Linda, 'Esthetes and Effeminati, *Raritan: A Quarterly Review* 12 (1993), pp. 52–68.

Downs, Jim, 'How "the 70s" became a morality play', *Gay & Lesbian Review Worldwide* 13/2 (2006), p. 8.

Dowsett, Gary and D. McInnes, 'Gay community, AIDS Agencies and the HIV Epidemic in Adelaide: Theorising "post-AIDS"', *Out There Too: Social Research*

Bibliography

& *Practice Forum Adelaide March 14–15 1996* (Adelaide: HIV/AIDS Programs Unit, South Australian Health Commission, 1996).

———, Herukhuti Williams, Ana Ventuneac and Alex Carballo-Diéguez, '"Taking it Like a Man": Masculinity and Barebacking Online', *Sexualities* 11/1–2 (February 2008), pp. 121–41.

Duggan, Lisa, *The Twilight of Equality? Neoliberalism, Cultural Politics, and the Attack on Democracy* (Boston: Beacon Press, 2003).

Dunleavy, Trisha, 'Strategies of Innovation in 'High-End' TV Drama: The Contribution of Cable', *Flow* 6, March 2009, http://flowtv.org/?p=2574 (accessed 18 August 2009).

During, Simon, 'Queering Thatcher: Whatever happened to politics and culture in the 1980s?', *JOMEC Journal* 3 (June 2013) https://publications.cardiffuniversitypress.org/index.php/JOMEC/article/view/318 (accessed 17 March 2015).

'Dustin Lance Black: ABC's *When We Rise*', *The Treatment*, http://www.stitcher.com/podcast/college-radio-workshop/kcrws-the-treatment/e/dustin-lance-black-abcs-when-we-rise-49366290 (accessed 12 March 2017).

Dyer, Richard, *Now You See it: Studies on Lesbian and Gay Film* (New York: Routledge, 1990)

———, 'Homosexual Heritage' in *The Culture of Queers* (London: Routledge, 2002).

———, *The Matter of Images: Essay on Representation* (London: Routledge, 1993).

Ebert, Roger, '*The Next Best Thing*', *Chicago Sun-Times* (3 March 2000), http://rogerebert.suntimes.com/apps/pbcs.dll/article?AID=/20000303/REVIEWS/3030307/1023 (accessed 4 November 2006).

Edelman, Lee, *Homographesis: Essays in Gay Literary and Cultural Studies* (New York: Routlege, 1994).

———, *No Future: Queer Theory and the Death Drive* (Durham: Duke University Press, 2004).

Edelstein, David, 'Outlaw Pharmacology', *New York Magazine*, 27 October 2013, http://nymag.com/movies/reviews/dallas-buyers-club-about-time-2013-11/ (accessed 12 May 2017).

Epstein, Julia, *Altered Conditions; Disease, Medicine, and Storytelling* (New York: Routledge, 1995).

Epstein, Steven, *Impure Science: AIDS, Activism, and the Politics of Knowledge* (Berkeley: University of Los Angeles Press, 1996).

Everett, Rupert, *Red Carpets and Other Banana Skins* (New York: Hachette, 2006).

Farmer, Brett, *Spectacular Passions: Cinema, Fantasy, Gay Male Spectatorships* (Durham: Duke University Press, 2000).

Farrell, Kathleen P., 'HIV on TV: Conversations with Young Gay Men', *Sexualities* 9/2 (2006), pp. 193–213.

Fink, Marty, Alexandra Juhasz, David Oscar Harvey with Bishnupriya Ghosh, 'Ghost stories: an introduction', *Jump Cut: A Review of Contemporary Media*, No. 55

Bibliography

(Fall 2013), http://ejumpcut.org/archive/jc55.2013/AidsHivIntroduction/index.html (accessed 25 November 2016).

Finkelstein, Avram, 'AIDS 2.0', *POZ*, 10 January 2013, https://www.poz.com/article/avram-finkelstein-23355-3691 (accessed 25 Nov 2014).

Foucault, Michel, 'On Governmentality', *Ideology and Consciousness* 6 (Autumn 1979), pp. 5–22.

——, *The History of Sexuality, Volume I: An Introduction*, trans. Robert Hurley (Melbourne: Penguin Books, 1976).

Fraser, Suzanne, 'Poetic World-Making: *Queer as Folk*, Counterpublic Speech and the "Reader"', *Sexualities* 9/2 (2006), pp. 152–70.

Freud, Sigmund, *Civilization and its Discontents* (New York: Norton & Company, 1961 [1929]).

——, *Totem and Taboo* (London: Routledge, 1999 [1913]).

Garber, Marjorie, *Vested Interests: Cross-dressing and Cultural Anxiety* (New York: Routledge, 1993).

Gilman, Sander, 'AIDS and Syphilis: The Iconography of Disease' in Douglas Crimp (ed.), *AIDS: Cultural Analysis, Cultural Activism* (Cambridge: MIT Press, 1988), pp. 87–108.

Gledhill, Christine, 'The Melodramatic Field: An Investigation' in Christine Gledhill (ed.), *Home is where the Heart is: Studies in Melodrama and the Woman's Film* (London: British Film Institute, 1987), pp. 5–39.

Global AIDS Update 2016, *UNAIDS*, 31 May 2016, www.unaids.org/en/resources/documents/2016/Global-AIDS-update-2016 (accessed 15 August 2016).

Goldman, Jason, '"The Golden Age of Gay Porn": Nostalgia and the Photography of Wilhelm von Gloeden', *GLQ: A Journal of Lesbian and Gay Studies* 12/2 (2006), pp. 237–58.

Goldstein, Richard, *Homocons: The Rise of the Gay Right,* (London and New York: Verso, 2003).

Gook, Ben, 'Really-existing Nostalgia? Remembering East Germany in Film', *Traffic* 10 (January 2008), pp. 123–42.

Gould, Deborah, *Moving Politics: Emotion and ACT Ups Fight Against AIDS* (Chicago: University of Chicago Press, 2009).

Gould, Ian, 'HIV accused "slept with 200"', *Sydney Star Observer* 12 October 2006, p. 7

Gray, John, *Men Are from Mars, Women Are from Venus: A Practical Guide for Improving Communication and Getting What You Want in Your Relationships* (New York: HarperCollins, 1992).

Graydon, Michael, 'Don't bother to wrap it: Online Giftgiver and Bugchaser newsgroups, the social impact of gift exchanges and the "carnivalesque"', *Culture, Health and Sexuality* 9/3 (May–June 2007), pp. 277–92.

Bibliography

Griffin, Gabrielle, *Representations of HIV and AIDS: Visibility Blues* (Manchester: Manchester University Press, 2001).

Grosz, Elizabeth, *Volatile Bodies. Towards a Corporeal Feminism* (Sydney: Allen and Unwin, 1994).

Grover, Jan Zita, 'Visible Lesions: Images of People With AIDS', *Afterimage* 17/1 (Summer 1989), pp. 10–16.

Hall, Locksley, 'Dan Stevens on *The Line of Beauty*', *After Elton*, 13 October 2006, http://afterelton.com/archive/elton/people/2006/10/danstevens.html (accessed 23 July 2008).

Hallas, Roger, *Reframing Bodies: AIDS, Bearing Witness, and the Queer Moving Image* (Durham: Duke University Press, 2009).

Halperin, David M., *How to be Gay* (Boston: Harvard University Press, 2012).

——, *What Do Gay Men Want? An Essay on Sex, Risk, and Subjectivity* (Michigan: University of Michigan Press, 2007).

Hannah, Daniel, 'The Private Life, the Public Stage: Henry James in Recent Fiction', *Journal of Modern Literature* 30/3 (Spring 2007), pp. 70–94.

Hanson, Ellis, 'OutTakes' in Ellis Hanson (ed.), *Outtakes: Essays on Queer Theory and Film* (Durham: Duke University Press, 1999), pp. 271–87.

——, 'Undead' in Diana Fuss (ed.), *Inside/Out: Lesbian Theories/Gay Theories* (London: Routledge, 1991), pp. 324–40.

Harris, Daniel, *The Rise and Fall of Gay Culture* (New York: Hyperion, 1997).

Hart, Kylo-Patrick R., *The AIDS Movie: Representing a Pandemic in Film and Television* (The Haworth Press: New York, 2000).

Harvey, David Oscar, 'Ghosts caught in our throat: on the lack of contemporary representations of gay/bisexual men and HIV', *Jump Cut: A Review of Contemporary Media* 55 (Fall 2013).

Harvey, Shannon J., '*The Next Best Thing*', *UrbanCinefile* 763, 4 November 2006 http://urbancinefile.com.au/home/view.asp?a=3622&s=Reviews (accessed 4 November 2006).

Haver, William, *The Body of this Death: Historicity and Sociality in the Time of AIDS* (Stanford: Stanford University Press, 1996).

Hawkes, Terrence, *Metaphor* (London: Methuen, 1972).

Hay, Louise, *You Can Heal Your Life* (Hay House: Sydney, 1984).

Heard, John, 'Gays are too proud to confront AIDS, still the real killer', *The Australian*, 1 December 2006, p. 12.

Held, Carolin, 'From "Heritage Space" to "Narrative Space": Anti-Heritage Aesthetics in the Classic TV Serials *Our Mutual Friend* and *Vanity Fair*' in Eckart Voigts-Virchow (ed.), *Janespotting and Beyond: British Heritage Retrovisions Since the Mid-1990s* (Tübingen: Gunter Narr Verlag Tübingen, 2004), pp. 113–23.

Hensley, Dennis, 'Inside *Queer as Folk*', *The Advocate* 21, November 2000, pp. 46–52.

Bibliography

Herkt, David, 'Degrees of Proximity in *The* Age of HIV', *Cultural Studies Review* 21/1 (March 2015).

Higson, Andrew, 'Re-Presenting the National Past: Nostalgia and Pastiche in the Heritage Film' in Lester Friedman (ed.), *Fires Were Started: British Cinema and Thatcherism* (Minneapolis: University of Minnesota Press, 1993), pp. 109–29.

——, *English Heritage, English Cinema: Costume Drama since 1980* (Oxford: Oxford University Press, 2003).

Hilderbrand, Lucas, 'Retroactivism', *GLQ: A Journal of Lesbian and Gay Studies* 12/2 (2006), pp. 303–17.

Hinde, Suellen, 'Refugees "must face HIV tests": Sex charges prompt call by minister', *Sunday Herald Sun*, 1 July 2007, p. 21.

Hipsky, Martin A., 'Anglophil(M)ia: Why Does America Watch Merchant-Ivory Movies?', *Journal of Popular Film and Television* 22 (1994), pp. 98–108.

Hirsch, Marriane, 'The Generation of Postmemory' in Karen Beckman and Lilianne Weissberg (eds), *On Writing with Photography* (Minnesota: University of Minnesota Press, 2013), pp. 202–30.

——, *Family Frames: Photographs, Narratives and Post-Memory* (London: Harvard University Press, 1997).

Holleran, Andrew, 'Brief History of a Media Taboo', *Gay and Lesbian Review Worldwide* 8/2 (2001), pp. 12–14.

Hollinghurst, Alan, *The Line of Beauty*. London: Picador, 1994.

Ian, Marcia, 'When is a Body Not a Body? When It's a Building' in Joel Sanders (ed.) *Stud: Architectures of Masculinity* (Princeton: Princeton University Press, 1996), pp. 189–205.

Irvine, Janice M., 'Transient Feelings: Sex Panics and the Politics of Emotions', *GLQ: A Journal of Lesbian and Gay Studies* 14/1 (2008), pp. 1–40.

Jagose, Annamarie, *Queer Theory* (Melbourne: Melbourne University Press, 1996).

Jameson, Frederic, 'Postmodernism, or The Cultural Logic of Late Capitalism', *New Left Review* 146 (July–August 1984), pp. 72–91.

Jermyn, Deborah, 'Rereading the Bitches From Hell: a feminist appropriation of the female psychopath', *Screen* 31/3 (Autumn 1996), pp. 251–67.

Junge, Benjamin, 'Bareback Sex, Risk, and Eroticism: Anthropological Themes (Re)Surfacing in the Post-AIDS Era' in Ellen Lewin and Willian L. Leap (eds), *Out in Theory: The Emergence of Lesbian and Gay Anthropology* (Urbana and Chicago: University of Illinois Press, 2002), pp. 186–221.

Kackman, Michael, 'Quality Television Melodrama and Cultural Complexity', *Flow* 7 (April 2009) http://flowtv.org/2010/03/flow-favorites-quality-television-melodrama-and-cultural-complexity-michael-kackman-university-of-texas-austin/ (accessed 12 April 2009).

Kagan, Dion, 'After the Orgy: *The* (New) *Normal Heart*', *The Lifted Brow* 24 (2014), pp. 44–5.

Bibliography

———, 'Homeless Love: Heritage and Aids in BBC2's *The Line of Beauty*.' *Literature/Film Quarterly*, 39/4, 2011, pp. 276–96

———, 'How to Have Memories in an Epidemic: Recent Documentaries about HIV/AIDS', *Kill YourDarlings* 13, April 2013, pp. 141–52.

———, 'How to take Drugs in a Chemsex Epidemic', *The Lifted Brow* 30, 2016.

———, 'Possessions and dispossession: homo economicus and neoliberal sociality in *The Line of Beauty*', *Continuum: Journal of Media & Cultural Studies* 28/6 (2014): 797–807.

———, 'Re-crisis': Barebacking, sex panic and the logic of epidemic", *Sexualities* 18:7 (2015), pp. 817–37

Kahan, Benjamin, "'The Viper's Traffic-Knot':" Celibacy and Queerness in the "Late" Marianne Moore', *GLQ: A Journal of Lesbian and Gay Studies* 14/4 (2008), pp. 509–35.

Kanabus, Annabel and Jenni Fredriksson, 'The History of AIDS up to 1986', *AVERT* 12 (March 2009) http://avert.org/his81_86.htm (accessed 17 August 2010).

Kendrick, James, 'The Next Best Thing', *QNetwork Entertainment Portal* http://qnetwork.com/index.php?page=revFiew&id=577.

Kerr, Theodore, 'On Organizing, and "Your Nostalgia Is Killing Me"', *The Visual AIDS blog*, 1 March 2014 https://www.visualaids.org/blog/detail/on-organizing-and-your-nostalgia-is-killing-me (accessed 12 August 2015).

Kipnis, Laura, *How to Become a Scandal: Adventures in Bad Behavior* (Metropolitan Books, New York, 2010).

Kippax, Susan and Kane Race, 'Sustaining Safe Practice: Twenty Years On', *Social Science and Medicine* 57/1 (2003), pp. 1–12.

Kissane, Karen and Julia Medew, 'Dance with Death', *The Age*, 21 April 2007, Sec. Insight, p. 5.

Kohnen, Melanie E. S., 'AIDS, History, and Generation in *Brothers & Sisters*', *Flow TV* 12, 8 September 2010, http://flowtv.org/2010/09/aids-history-and-generation-in-brothers-sisters/ (accessed 12 June 2011)

Kooijman, Jaap, 'They're Here, They're Queer, and Straight American Loves it', *GLQ: A Journal of Lesbian and Gay Studies* 11/1 (2005), pp. 106–9.

Kramer, Larry, *Faggots* (New York: Grove Press, 1978).

———, 'Sex and Sensibility', *The Advocate*, 27 May 1997, pp. 59–70.

Kristeva, Julia, *Powers of Horror: An Essay on Abjection*. Trans. Leon S. Roudiez (New York: Columbia University Press, 1982).

Lakoff, George and Mark Johnson, *Metaphors We Live By* (Chicago: University of Chicago Press, 1980).

Lee, Byron, ' "It's a question of breeding": Visualising queer masculinity in bareback pornography', *Sexualities* 17/1–2 (2014), pp. 100–20.

Lewis, Lynette and Michael Ross, *A Select Body: The Gay Dance Party Subculture and the HIV/AIDS Pandemic* (New York: Castell, 1995).

Bibliography

Lewis, Tania, 'He Needs to Face His Fears with These Five Queers', *Television & New Media* 8 (2007), pp. 285–311.

Lim, Dennis, 'Through a Mirror Darkly', *The Village Voice*, 7 March 2000, http://villagevoice.com/2000-03-07/film/through-a-mirror-darkly/1 (accessed 23 July 2006).

Love, Heather, *Feeling Backward: Loss and the Politics of Queer History* (Cambridge: Harvard University Press, 2007).

'Man Held HIV Parties – court told', *Herald Sun*, 20 March 2007, http://heraldsun.com.au/news/victoria/man-held-hiv-parties-court-told/story-e6frf7kx-1111113189029 (accessed 13 October 2007).

Martin, Emily, *Flexible Bodies: Tracking Immunity in American Culture from the Days of Polio to The Age of AIDS*. Boston: Beacon Press, 1994.

Martin, Fran, *Situating Sexualities: Queer Representation in Taiwanese Fiction, Film and Public Culture* (Hong Kong: Hong Kong University Press, 2003).

Medew, Julia, '"Lock him up" warning on HIV man: Court hears of psychiatrist's plea', *The Age*, 23 March 2007, p. 3.

———, 'Monash team starts mapping HIV rise', *The Age*, 14 May 2007, p. 1.

———, 'Officials failed to alert police about HIV man', *The Age*, 21 March 2007, p. 3.

Medew, Julia, and Karen Kissane, 'Gays in HIV "bug chase"', *The Age*, 23 April 2007, p. 1.

Medew, Julia, and Carol Nader, '"Risky" HIV carriers to be reported: Doctor-patient privacy under threat', *The Age*, 25 July 2007, p. 5.

Meyer, Richard, 'Rock Hudson's Body' in Diana Fuss (ed.), *Inside/Out: Lesbian Theories/Gay Theories* (London: Routledge, 1991), pp. 258–88.

Miller, D. A., 'Sontag's Urbanity', in Henry Abelove, Michele Aina Barale and David M. Halperin (eds), *The Lesbian and Gay Studies Reader* (London: Routledge, 1993), pp. 212–20.

Miller, James. "AIDS in the Novel: Getting It Straight," in James Miller (ed.) *Fluid Exchanges: Artists and Critics in the AIDS Crisis,* (Toronto: University of Toronto Press, 1992), pp. 258–71.

Miller, Nancy K. and Jason Tougaw, *Extremities: Trauma, Testimony, and Community* (Champaign: University of Illinois Press, 2002).

Mitchell, Lee Clark, '"To suffer like chopped limbs": The Dispossessions of *The Spoils of Poynton*', *The Henry James Review* 26 (2005), pp. 20–38.

Monk, Claire, 'Sexuality and the Heritage', *Sight and Sound* 5/10 (October 1995), pp. 33–4.

Morris, Paul, 'No Limits: Necessary Danger in Male Porn', Lecture, World Pornography Conference, University City, California, 6–9 August 1998. https://queerrhetoric.wordpress.com/2010/06/22/no-limits-necessary-danger-in-male-porn/ (accessed 10 January 2017).

Morris, Wesley, 'Truly an odd couple: In appalling *Next Best Thing*, Madonna-Rupert pairing fascinates – like a train wreck', *San Francisco Chronicle* 3 March

2000 http://sfgate.com/cgibin/article.cgi?f=/e/a/2000/03/03/WEEKEND6536. dtl#ixzz1ZJ9KdsBx (link no longer working).

Morrison, Paul, 'End Pleasure', *GLQ: A Journal of Lesbian and Gay Studies* 1/1 (November 1993), pp. 53–78.

Moskowitz, David A. and Michael E. Roloff, 'The Ultimate High: Sexual Addiction and the Bug Chasing Phenomenon', *Sexual Addition and Compulsivity* 14 (2007), pp. 21–40.

Moss, Andrew R., 'AIDS Without End', *The New York Review of Books*, 8 December 1988, http://nybooks.com/articles/archives/1988/dec/08/aids-without-end-2/ (accessed 3 July 2006).

Mowlabocus, Sharif, *Gaydar Culture: Gay Men, Technology and Embodiment in the Digital Age* (Abingdon: Ashgate, 2010).

——, Justin Harbottle and Charlie Witzelon, 'Porn Laid Bare: Gay men, pornography and bareback sex', *Sexualities* 16/5–6 (2013), pp. 523–47.

Mulvey, Laura, 'Visual Pleasure and Narrative Cinema', *Screen* 16/3 (1975), pp. 6–18.

Muñoz, José Esteban, *Cruising Utopia: The Then and There of Queer Futurity* (New York: NYU Press, 2009).

——, 'Queer Minsrels for the Straight Eye: Race as Surplus in Gay TV', *GLQ: A Journal of Lesbian and Gay Studies* 11/1 (2005), pp. 101–2.

Munt, Sally R., 'Shame/pride dichotomies in *Queer As Folk*', *Textual Practice* 14/3 (2000), pp. 531–46.

Nast, Heidi, 'Queer Patriarchies, Queer Racisms, International', *Antipode* 34/5 (2002), pp. 874–909.

Nelson, Robin, *State of Play: Contemporary "High-End" TV Drama* (Manchester: Manchester University Press, 2007).

Noble, Bobby, 'Queer as Box: Boi Spectators and Boy Culture on Showtime's *Queer as Folk*', in Merri Lisa Johnson (ed.) *Third Wave Feminism and Television: Jane Puts it in a Box* (London: I.B.Tauris, 2007), pp. 147–65.

Nowell-Smith, Geoffrey, 'Minelli and Melodrama' in Bill Nichols (ed.) *Movies and Method Vol 2* (Berkeley: University of California Press, 1985), pp. 190–4.

Null, Christopher, 'The Next Best Thing', *ACM Filmcritic*, 29 February 2000 http://filmcritic.com/reviews/2000/the-next-best-thing/ (link no longer working).

Nunokawa, Jeff, '"All the Sad Young Men": AIDS and the Work of Mourning', in Diana Fuss (ed.), *Inside/Out: Lesbian Theories/Gay Theories* (London: Routledge, 1991), pp. 311–23.

Odets, Walt, *In the Shadow of the Epidemic: Being Negative in The Age of AIDS* (Durham: Duke University Press, 1995).

Orange, Donna M., 'High-Risk Behaviour or High-Risk Systems? Discussion of Cheuvront's "High-Risk Sexual Behaviour in the Treatment of HIV-Negative Patients"' *Journal of Gay and Lesbian Psychotherapy* 6/3 (2002), pp. 45–50.

Patton, Cindy, *Globalising AIDS* (Minneapolis: University of Minnesota Press, 2002).

Bibliography

———, *Inventing AIDS* (New York: Routledge, 1990).

———, 'Visualizing Safe Sex: When Pedagogy and Pornography Collide' in Diana Fuss (ed.), *Inside/Out: Lesbian Theories/Gay Theories* (London: Routledge, 1991), pp. 373–86.

Paulin, Scott D., 'Sex and the Singled Girl: Queer Representation and Containment in *Single White Female*', *Camera Obscura: Feminism, Culture and Media Studies* 37 (January 1996), pp. 32–69.

Peeren, Esther, 'Queering the Straight World: The Politics of Resignification in *Queer as Folk*' in James R. Keller and Leslie Stratyner (eds), *The New Queer Aesthetic on Television: Essays on Recent Programming* (North Carolina: McFarland & Co., 2006), pp. 59–74.

Persson, Asha, 'Incorporating Pharmakon: HIV, Medicine, and Body Shape Change', *Body & Society* 10/4 (2004), pp. 45–67.

Pocius, Joshua, 'HIV/AIDS on screen: by focusing on history, we ignore the present', *The Conversation*, 21 July 2014, http://theconversation.com/hiv-aids-on-screen-by-focusing-on-history-we-ignore-the-present-28972 (accessed 2 February 2015).

Race, Kane, 'Engaging in a culture of barebacking: Gay men and the risk of HIV prevention', in K. Hannah-Moffat and P. O'Malley (eds), *Gendered Risk* (London: Glasshouse Press, 2007), pp. 99–126.

———, '*Chemsex* review: gay sex and drug use demand more careful forms of attention', *The Conversation*, 8 December 2015, http://theconversation.com/chemsex-review-gay-sex-and-drug-use-demand-more-careful-forms-of-attention-51586 (accessed 8 December 2015).

———, *Pleasure Consuming Medicine: The Queer Politics of Drugs* (Durham: Duke University Press, 2009).

———, 'Revaluation of risk among gay men', *Social Research Issues Paper* 1 (August 2003), National Centre in HIV Social Research, http://sprc.unsw.edu.au/media/File/SRIP01.pdf (accessed 12 June 2005).

———, 'The Undetectable Crisis: Changing Technologies of Risk', *Sexualities* 4/2 (2001), pp. 167–89.

Radstone, Susannah, *The Sexual Politics of Time: Confession, Nostalgia, Memory* (London: Routledge, 2007).

Rapping, Elayne, *The Movie of the Week: Private Stories, Public Events* (London: University of Minnesota Press, 1992).

Rasmussen, Mary Lou and Jane Kenway, 'Queering the Youthful Cyberfâneur', *Journal of Gay and Lesbian Issues in Education* 2/1 (2004), pp. 47–63.

Reeders, Daniel, 'The Impact of Criminalisation on Community-Based HIV Prevention' in Sally Cameron and John Rule (eds), *The Criminalisation of HIV Transmission in Australia: Legality, Morality and Reality*, NAPWA Monograph 2009, pp. 134–45.

Bibliography

Ridge, Damien, '"It was an Incredible Thrill": The Social Meanings and Dynamics of Younger Men's Experience of Barebacking in Melbourne', *Sexualities* 7 (2004), pp. 259–79.

Riggs, Damien, '"Serosameness" or "Serodifference"? Resisting Polarised Discourses of Identity and Relationality in the Context of HIV', *Sexualities* 9/4 (2004), pp. 409–22.

Riley, Benjamin, 'Objects in History: AIDS as Cultural Singularity', *The Lifted Brow* 25 (2015), pp. 49–53.

Rivkin, Julie, 'Writing the Gay 80s with Henry James: David Leavitt's *A Place I've Never Been* and Alan Hollinghurst's *The Line of Beauty*', *The Henry James Review* 26/3 (Fall 2005), pp. 282–92.

Roberts, Brendan, 'Deadly Party Game: Gays deliberately infected with HIV, court told', *Herald Sun*, 21 March 2007, p. 3.

———, 'HIV Infection fantasies', *Herald Sun*, 22 March 2007, p. 9.

———, 'Seedy world unravels', *Herald Sun*, 22 March 2007, p. 25.

Robey, Tim, '*Chemsex* review: 'Seriously Sobering', *The Telegraph*, 3 December 2015, http://www.telegraph.co.uk/film/Chemsex/review/ (accessed 8 April 2016).

Robinson, Natasha, 'Accused HIV man most evil in years, says doctor', *The Australian*, 23 March 2007.

———, 'Accused "set out to spread his HIV"', *The Australian*, 21 March 2007.

———, 'Chain of Indifference', *The Australian* 2 April 2007. Sec. Features, p. 10.

———, 'Five years to tell police of HIV case', *The Australian*, 23 March 2007, p. 4.

———, 'HIV Man "tricked sex slave"', *The Australian*, 29 March 2007, p. 7.

Rofes, Eris, *Dry Bones Breathe: Gay Men Creating Post-AIDS Identities and Cultures*. New York: Harrington Park, 1998.

Rosengarten, Marsha, 'Consumer activism in the pharmacology of HIV', *Body and Society* 10/1 (2004), pp. 91–107.

Rowe, Michael, 'The Queer Report', *The Advocate*, 15 April 2003, pp. 40–7.

Rubin, Gayle S., 'Thinking Sex' in Henry Abelove, Michele Aina Barale and David M. Halperin (eds), *The Lesbian and Gay Studies Reader* (London: Routledge, 1993 [1984]), pp. 3–44.

Russell, John, 'Bio-Power and biohazards: A projective system reading of gay men's communith-based HIV prevention', *Culture, Health & Sexuality* 7/2 (March 2005), pp. 145–58.

Russell, Stephen A., 'Dangerous liaisons: inside the world of *Chemsex*", *SBS*, 15 April 2015, http://www.sbs.com.au/topics/sexuality/article/2016/03/31/dangerous-liaisons-inside-world-chemsex (accessed 21 June 2017).

Russo, Vito, *The Celluloid Closet: Homosexuality in the Movies* (New York: Harper & Row, 1981).

Ryan, Benjamin, 'HIV Unplugged, *HIV plus* 1 October 2004, https://www.hivplus-mag.com/issue-features/2004/10/01/hiv-unplugged (accessed 21 September 2009).

Bibliography

Schaff, Barbara, 'Still Lives – Tableaux Vivants: Art in British Heritage Films' in Eckart Voigts-Virchow (ed.), *Janespotting and Beyond: British Heritage Retrovisions Since the Mid-1990s* (Germany: Gunter Narr Verlag Tübingen, 2004), pp. 125–34.

Schatz, Thomas, *Hollywood Genres: Formulas, Filmmaking and the Studio System* (New York: Random House, 1981).

Sedgwick, Eve Kosofsky, *Between Men: English Literature and Male Homosocial Desire* (New York: Columbia University Press, 1985).

———, *Epistemology of the Closet* (Berkeley: University of California Press, 1990).

Scott, Stuart, 'The Condomlessness of Bareback Sex: Responses to the unrepresentability of HIV in Treasure Island Media's *Plantin' Seed* and *Slammed*', Sexualities, special issue: 'Bareback sex and queer theory across three national contexts (France, UK, USA)' 18/122 (2015), pp. 210–33.

Sendziuk, Paul, *Learning to Trust: Australian Responses to AIDS* (Sydney: UNSW Press, 2003).

Sheon, Nicolas and Aaron Plant, 'Protease Dis-Inhibitors? The Gay Bareback Phenomenon', 11 November 1997, http://managingdesire.org/sexpanic/ProteaseDisinhibitors.html (link no longer working).

Shernoff, Michael, 'Condomless Sex: Gay Men, Barebacking, and Harm Reduction', *Social Work* 51/2 (April 2006), pp. 106–13.

Shevory, Thomas H., *Notorious H.I.V: The Media Spectacle of Nushawn Williams* (Minneapolis: University of Minnesota Press, 2004).

Shilts, Randy, *And the Band Played On: Politics, People and the AIDS Epidemic* (New York: St. Martin's, 1987).

Shugart, Helene A., 'Reinventing Privilege: The New (Gay) Man in Contemporary Popular Media', *Critical Studies in Media Communication* 20/1 (2003), pp. 67–91.

Singer, Linda, *Erotic Welfare: Sexual Theory and Politics in The Age of Epidemic* (London: Routledge, 1993).

Sitze, Adam, 'Denialism', *The South Atlantic Quarterly* 103/4 (Fall 2004), pp. 769–811.

Smith, Gary and Paul Van de Ven, *Reflecting on Practice: Current Challenges in Gay and Other Homosexually Active Men's HIV Education* (Sydney: National Centre in HIV Social Research, The University of New South Wales, 2001).

Sontag, Susan, *AIDS and its Metaphors* (New York: Farrar, Straus and Giroux, 1989).

———, *Illness as Metaphor* (New York: Farrar, Straus and Giroux, 1977).

Sothern, Matthew. 'On Not Living with AIDS: Or, AIDS-as-Post-Crisis', *Acme: An International E-Journal for Critical Geographies* 5/2 (2006), pp. 144–62.

Spong, Rohan, *All the Way Through Evening*: Rohan Spong Interview, *Time Out*, http://www.au.timeout.com/melbourne/gay-lesbian/features/2043/all-the-way-through-evening-rohan-spong-interview (link no longer working).

Stacey, Jackie, 'Promoting Normality: Section 28 and the Regulation of Sexuality' in S. Franklin, C. Lury and J. Stacey (eds), *Off-Centre: Feminism and Cultural Studies* (London: HarperCollins, 1991), pp. 284–304.

Bibliography

——, *Terratologies: A Cultural Study of Cancer* (New York: Routledge, 1997).
Stafford, Annabel, 'HIV-positive visitors may be tracked or banned', *The Age*, 11 May 2007, p. 2.
Stam, Robert, 'The Rise of Cultural Studies' in Robert Stam and Tony Miller (eds), *Film Theory: An Introduction* (Oxford: Blackwell, 2000), pp. 223–9.
Street, Sarah, *British National Cinema* (London: Routledge, 1997).
Sturken, Marita, *Tangled Memories: The Vietnam War, the AIDS Epidemic, and the Politics of Remembering* (Berkeley: University of California Press, 1997).
Sullivan, Andrew, 'When Plagues End: Notes on the Twilight of an Epidemic', *New York Times Magazine* November 10 1996, http://www.nytimes.com/1996/11/10/magazine/when-plagues-end.html (accessed 4 July 2009).
Swaab, Peter, 'The Line of Beauty', *Film Quarterly* 60/3 (2007), pp. 10–15.
Tewksbury, Richard, ' "Click here for HIV": An Analysis of Internet-based Bug Chasers and Bug Givers', *Deviant Behaviour* 27 (2006), pp. 379–95.
Tóibín, Colm, 'The Comedy of Being English', *The New York Review of Books* 52/1 (13 January 2005), http://www.nybooks.com/articles/2005/01/13/the-comedy-of-being-english/ (accessed 19 November 2009).
Tomso, Gregory, 'Bug Chasing, Barebacking, and the Risks of Care', *Literature and Medicine* 23/1 (Spring 2004), pp. 88–111.
——, 'Viral Sex and the Politics of Life', *South Atlantic Quarterly* 107/2 (Spring 2008), pp. 265–85.
Treichler, Paula A., *How to Have Theory in an Epidemic: Cultural Chronicles of AIDS* (Durham: Duke University Press, 1989).
——, 'AIDS, Homophobia, and Biomedical Discourse: An Epidemic of Signification' in Douglas Crimp (ed.), *AIDS: Cultural Analysis, Cultural Activism* (Cambridge: MIT Press, 1988), pp. 31–70.
Vidal, Belén, *Heritage Film: Nation, Genre and Representation* (Columbia University Press, New York: 2012).
Vilanch, Bruce, 'Anything but sex', *The Advocate* 761 (9 June 1998), p. 59.
Vincendeau, Ginette, *Film/Literature/Heritage: A Sight and Sound Reader* (London: BFI Publishing, 2001).
Vörös, Florian, 'Raw Fantasies: An Interpretative Sociology of what Bareback Porn does and means to French Gay Male Audiences', in R. Borba, B. Falabella Fabrício, D. Pinto et E.S. Lewis (eds), *Queering Paradigms IV* (Bern, Peter Lang, 2014), pp. 321–43.
Wald, Patricia, *Contagious: Cultures, Carriers, and the Outbreak Narrative* (Durham: Duke University Press, 2008).
Warner, Michael, *Publics and Counterpublics* (Zone Books, New York: 2002).
——, *The Trouble with Normal: Sex, Politics, and the Ethics of Queer Life* (Cambridge: Harvard University Press, 1999).
Watney, Simon, 'Hollywood's Homosexual World', *Screen* 23/3-4 (1982), pp. 107–21.
——, *Policing Desire: Pornography, AIDS and the Media* (London: Methuen, 1987).

Bibliography

——, 'The Spectacle of AIDS' in Douglas Crimp (ed.), *AIDS: Cultural Analysis, Cultural Activism* (Cambridge: MIT Press, 1988), pp. 71–86.

——, 'Taking Liberties: An Introduction' in Erica Carter and Simon Watney (eds), *Taking Liberties: AIDS and Cultural Politics* (London: Serpent's Tail, 1989), pp. 11–57.

Weait, Matthew, *Intimacy and Responsibility: The Criminalisation of HIV Transmission* (New York: Routledge, 2007).

Weeks, Jeffrey, 'Male Homosexuality: Cultural Perspectives' in Michael W. Adler (ed.), *Diseases in the Homosexual Male* (Dordrecht: Springer, 1988).

Weinraub, Jake, '*We Were Here* Captures the Voices of a Generation Lost to HIV/AIDS', *The Wrap*, 15 July 2011, http://www.thewrap.com/review-we-were-here-captures-voices-generation-lost-hivaids-29145/ (accessed 2 December 2014).

Welsby, James, 'Between Suffering and Celebration', *Next Wave Festival 2014 Magazine*, p. 11, https://issuu.com/nextwave2014festival/docs/nw_publication-v2 (accessed 21 June 2017).

Wickman, Forrest, 'Was *Dallas Buyers Club*'s Ron Woodroof gay or bisexual? Friends and doctor say maybe, so why did the movie make him straight?', *Slate*, 17 January 2014, http://www.slate.com/blogs/browbeat/2014/01/17/was_dallas_buyers_club_s_ron_woodroof_gay_or_bisexual_friends_and_doctor.html (accessed 2 March 2014).

Williamson, Judith, 'Every Virus Tells a Story: The Meaning of HIV and AIDS', in Erica Carter and Simon Watney (eds), *Taking Liberties: AIDS and Cultural Politics* (London: Serpent's Tail, 1989).

Wilde, Oscar, *The Picture of Dorian Gray* (Penguin: Melbourne, 1985).

Wilton, Tamsin, *Engendering AIDS: Deconstructing Sex, Text and Epidemic* (London: Sage Publications, 1996).

Wood, Robin, 'Return of the Repressed', *Film Comment* 14/4 (July–August 1978), pp. 25–32.

Woods, Gregory, '"It's My Nature": AIDS Narratives and the Moral Re-Branding of Queerness in the mid-1990s' in Robin Griffiths (ed.), *British Queer Cinema* (London; New York: Routledge, 2006), pp. 171–82.

Young, Iris Marion, *Justice and the Politics of Difference* (New Jersey: Princeton University Press, 1990).

Zeboski, Adam, '#TruvadaWhore goes viral', *HIV Equal*, 24 June 2014, http://www.hivequal.org/hiv-equal-online/truvadawhore-goes-viral (accessed 3 May 2017).

Film and Television References

Ally McBeal, Fox Network, 1997–2002
All the Way Through Evening, Dir. Rohan Spong, 2011.
Angels in America, Dir. Mike Nichols, HBO, 2003.
The Birdcage, Dir. Mike Nichols. MGM Home Entertainment, 1996.
'Brat-Sitting,' *Queer as Folk: The Complete 1–5 Season*, Writ. Ron Cowen, Daniel Lipman and Del Shores, Dir. Kari Skogland, Showtime, 2000–5.
Breaking Bad, Sony Pictures Home Entertainment, 2008–13.
Brideshead Revisited, Dirs. Charles Sturridge and Michael Lindsay-Hogg, AcornMedia, 1981.
Brideshead Revisited, Dir. Julian Jarrold, Miramax, 2008.
Carol, Dir. Todd Haynes, StudioCanal, 2015.
Chicago Hope, Columbia Broadcasting System, 1994–2000.
Cruising, Dir. William Friedkin, Warner Home Video, 1980.
Dallas Buyers Club, Dir. Jean-Marc Vallée, Focus Features, 2013.
Darling, Dir. John Schlesinger, Warner Home Video.
An Early Frost, Dir. John Erman, National Broadcasting Company, 1985.
Ellen, American Broadcasting Company, 1994–8.
'The End of the Street', Writ. Andrew Davies, *The Line of Beauty,* Dir. Saul Dibb. BBC, 2006.
ER, NBC, Warner Bros. Television 1994–2009.
Far From Heaven, Dir. Todd Haynes, Focus Features, 2002.
Four Weddings and Funeral, Dir. Mike Newell, Polygram Video, 1993.
Girls, HBO, 2012–17.
Glee, Fox Network, 2009–15.
Holding the Man, Dir. Neil Armfield, Transmission Films, 2015.
How to Survive a Plague, Dor. David France, Sundance Selects, 2012.
In and Out, Dir. Frank Oz, Paramount Home Entertainment, 1997.
Irreversible, Dir. Gaspar Noé, Accent Film Entertainment, 2002.
It's My Party, Dir. Randal Kleiser, Chapel Distribution, 1996.
The Last of England, Dir. Derek Jarman, 1987.
'The Leper (Hath the Babe Not Eyes?),' Writ. Ron Cowen, Daniel Lipman and Blair Fell, Dir. Michael DeCarlo, *Queer as Folk: The Complete 1–5 Season*, Showtime, 2000–5.
Life Goes On, American Broadcasting Company, 1989–93.

Film and Television References

'The Love Chord,' Writ. Andrew Davies, *The Line of Beauty*, Dir. Saul Dibb. BBC, 2006.

'Love for Sale,' Writ. Ron Cowen, Daniel Lipman and Michael MacLennan, Dir. Alex Chapple, *Queer as Folk: The Complete 1–5 Season,* Showtime, 2000–5.

Mad About You, Sony Pictures Home Entertainment, 1992–9.

Melrose Place, Paramount Home Entertainment, 1992–9.

A Midsummer Night's Dream, Dir. Michael Hoffman, Twentieth Century Fox, 1999.

'Mixed Blessings,' Writ. Ron Cowen, Daniel Lipman, Matt Pyken and Michael Berns, Dir. Bruce McDonald, *Queer as Folk: The Complete 1–5 Season*, Showtime, 2000–5.

My Best Friend's Wedding, Dir. P. J. Hogan, TriStar Pictures, 1997.

The Next Best Thing, Dir. John Schlesinger, Paramount Pictures, 2000, DVD.

The Normal Heart, Dir. Ryan Murphy, HBO, 2014.

NYPD Blue, Fox Television Network, 1993–2005.

The Object of my Affection, Dir. Nicholas Hytner, 20th Century Fox, 1998.

'On the Road Again,' Writ. Jon Robin Baitz, David Marshall Grant and Geoffrey Nauffts, Dir. Ken Olin. ABC, 2010.

'One Ring to Rule Them All,' Writ. Ron Cowen, Daniel Lipman and Brad Fraser, Dir. Bruce McDonald. *Queer as Folk: The Complete 1–5 Season*, Showtime, 2000–5.

One Night Stand, Dir. Mike Figgis, New Line Cinema, 1997.

Orlando, Dir. Sally Potter, Umbrella Entertainment, 1992.

Our Sons, John Erman, American Broadcasting Company, 1991. Television.

A Passage to India, Dir. David Lean, Columbia Tristar, 1984.

Philadelphia, Dir. Jonathan Demme, Columbia TriStar, 1993.

A Place for Annie, Dir. John Gray, American Broadcasting Company, 1994.

The Portrait of a Lady, Dir. Jane Campion, Polygram, 1996.

Pride and Prejudice, Dir. Simon Langton, BBC Video, 1995.

Queer as Folk (UK series), Dir. Sarah Harding and Charles McDougall, Acorn Media Group, 1999.

Queer Eye for the Straight Guy, Bravo, 2003–7.

Reality Bites, Dir. Ben Stiller, Universal Home Video, 1994.

A Room with a View, Dir. James Ivory, Umbrella Entertainment, 1985.

Roseanne, Paramount Television, 1988–97.

The Ryan White Story, Dir. John Herzfed, American Broadcasting Company, 1989.

'Sick, Sick, Sick,' Writ. Ron Cowen, Daniel Lipman, Matt Pyken and Michael Berns, Dir. Alex Chapple, *Queer as Folk: The Complete 1–5 Season*. Showtime, 2000–5.

Single White Female, Dir. Barbet Schroeder, Columbia TriStar, 1992.

Six Feet Under, Home Box Office Home Video, 2001–5.

Something to Live For, Dir. Tom McLoughlin, American Broadcasting Company, 1992. DVD.

The Sopranos, Home Box Office Home Video, 1999–2007. DVD.

Film and Television References

Spin City, American Broadcasting Company, 1996–2002. Television.
'Stop Hurting Us,' Writ. Ron Cowen, Daniel Lipman and Michael MacLennan. Dir. Bruce McDonald. *Queer as Folk: The Complete 1–5 Season* Showtime, 2000–5.
Stella Dallas, Dir. Douglas Sirk, Home Box Office, 1937.
Test, Dir. Chris Mason Johnson, Variance Films, 2014.
Thirtsomething, Shout Factory, 1987–91.
'To Whom Do You Beautifully Belong,' Writ. Andrew Davies, *The Line of Beauty*, Dir. Saul Dibb. BBC, 2006.
United in Anger, Dir. Jim Hubbard, 2012.
Vito, Dir. Jeffrey Schwarz, HBO, 2011.
We Were Here, Dirs. David Weissman and Bill Weber, 2011.
Weeds, Showtime, 2005–12.
When We Rise, Dirs. Gus Van Sant Dee Rees Thomas Schlamme and Dustin Lance Black American Broadcasting Company, 2017.
Will and Grace, Universal Pictures, 1998–2006.

Index

abjection 52, 60, 61–3, 70–4, 80, 83–7
Academy Award 45, 207, 210
ACT UP 206–7, 214, 231–2, 235
adaptation 168–70
Adam, Barry 138, 143
addiction 42, 120, 129
aesthete 41, 187, 193, 195, 224
Agamben, Giorgio 173, 194
Age newspaper 53, 154–7, 256n.67
Ahmed, Sara 157
AIDS
  activism 16, 32
  as anachronism 19, 75–7, 222–3
  body 52, 71, 77, 85, 195, 215
  conflation with gay liberation 27, 43
  conflation with homosexuality 8–9, 17, 27–8
  end of 17
  spectacle of 20–2, 27–9, 57, 183, 192
  visual iconography of 40
AIDS activist history 206–7, 211–13, 214–19
AIDS and its Metaphors (1989) 29, 211–12
AIDS crisis 21, 26–47, 174
  afterlives of 19, 160–2, 219–21
  Australian response to 18
  historical significance of 196
  revisitation of 2, 208, 213, 228
AIDS cultural criticism 14, 16, 29–33
AIDS history 15, 20, 24, 206–21
  moral narrative of 203–5
  narratives structures of 25, 162, 197, 215–19
  teleology of 6, 202–3, 219
AIDS memory 167–8, 195, 196–200, 225
AIDS monster 23, 147–52, 158
AIDS panic 21, 28, 127, 157–9, 193
AIDS service organisations (ASOs) 16, 109–10
AIDS victim 27, 28, 37, 150, 211
Alderson, David 97
All the Way Through Evening (2011), 230
Allen, Dennis 50
Altman, Dennis 10
American Food and Drug Administration (FDA), 210, 212
amnesia 19, 204, 223–5
anality 38–9, 68, 85, 135, 141, 152
And the Band Played On (1988), 42–3, 148
Anderson, Melissa, 225–6
Angels in America (2003) 2, 24, 201, 207
antiretrovirals (ARVs)
  changes instigated by 9, 14–17, 90, 138–9, 201
  global availability of 17
  introduction of 1, 9, 46
  patient compliance with 16–17, 32
  representation of 83

Index

archives 206, 228
Aronson, Amy 55, 64
artificiality, trope of 68–70
As Good as It Gets (1997) 53
Australian newspaper 156
AZT 210

backwards or feeling backwards
   7, 77, 167, 195, 200, 202,
   219–21, 222–36
backwards turn 25, 222–36
Bardella, Claudio 106
bare life 193–5
barebacking
   definition of 135–42
   media representation of 130–3, 145
   panic surrounding 33, 132–3
   porn 40, 134
   research into 137–44
   sexology of 137–44
   subcultures of 134–5, 150, 152
Bateman, Robert 56–7
BBC/BBC2 24, 169
Becker, Ron 20, 54, 56, 58, 66
Beirne, Rebecca 96
belonging 173, 183–91
Benedicto, Bobby 98
Benetton 44
Bersani, Leo 21, 31, 37–9, 235
Bérubé, Allan 97
biomedicine 15–17, 29–30
biopolitics 27–9, 32–3, 103, 132, 144, 157–9, 219
Black, Dustin Lance 208, 226–7
Blechner, Mark J., 136
blood 36, 61–2, 86–7, 108, 114, 120
bodily fluids 36, 61–3, 73, 141

Bordo, Susan 64
Bordowitz, Gregg 31
Bourdieu, Pierre 140
Boym, Svetlana 173
Bradley-Perrin, Ian 227
breeding 145, 150
Brideshead Revisited (1945) 177
British cinema 170
Britishness 168–9
Brooks, Peter 100
Brothers & Sisters (2006–11) 3, 19, 201, 205, 225
Buchanan, Pat 29
buddy comedy 21, 55, 67, 71
bug chasing 23, 121, 130–3, 145, 151
Butler, Judith 8, 60, 62, 63, 172, 225
buyers club 209–13
Byron, Lee 144

camp 67, 75, 77
Campion, Jane 173
cancer 29, 34
Carballo-Diéguez, A. 143
Carol (2015) 173
Caron, David 8, 30
Cartmell, Deborah 166–7, 195
Caruth, Cathy 234
Castiglia, Christopher 204–5, 215
celebrity 40
celibacy 52, 53–60, 66
Celluloid Closet, The (1981) 12
cesspool 37
Chao, Walter 96
Chemsex (2015) 23, 125–30, 149, 153
Cheuvront, J. P. 134
Chevalier, Vincent 227
cholera 36–7

Index

citizenship 97–8
class 190
closet, the 40, 49
Cohen, Stanley 128
Collins, Jim 168
coming out 3, 49–52, 187
condoms 117, 133–45
confessional mode 47–51,
  126–9, 211–12
Cook, Pam 172
Corber, Robert 45
counternostalgia 204–5, 220, 226
counterpublic 96–7, 250n.23
Crimp, Douglas 30–1, 174, 203–5,
  215, 236
crisis discourse 18–21, 26–46
Crossley, Michele, L. 140–3, 162
Cruising (1980) 57, 153
Cruising Utopia (2009) 235
cultural capital 56, 171, 178–9, 187, 224
Cvetkovich, Ann 25, 157

Dallas Buyers Club (2013) 24, 45, 165,
  207–13, 214, 227
Dascăl, Reghina 165, 197
Davidson, Guy 153
Davies, Andrew 169
Davis, Glynn 97
Davis, Oliver 139
Dean, Tim 138, 160–1, 266n.27
death
  drive 44, 81
  representation of 77–80
  wish 42–3, 60
decadence 41–3
decadent literature 27, 149
Derrida, Jacques 190–1
Dessaix, Robert 197

developing world 17, 220
disavowal 19, 21–2, 53, 60, 63, 68,
  75–87, 110–11, 225
disco 104–7, 231
disease
  characterological model of 27,
    33–6
  representation of 14, 36–8
documentary 24, 125–30, 206–7, 225
domesticity 6, 21, 28, 46, 47, 52, 55–60,
  65, 71–3, 222
Douglas, Mary 60, 74
Dowsett, Gary 14–15, 143
drugs
  intravenous 26, 118–20, 125–30
  methamphetamine 125–30
  recreational use of 106, 216
  steroids 112–14
Dugas, Gaëtan 42–3
Duggan, Lisa 32, 157
Dunleavy, Trisha 94
Duran, David 214
During, Simon 165, 193
Dyer, Richard 12, 14, 172, 187, 196

Early Frost, An (1985) 45, 90
Edelman, Lee 8, 35–6, 43, 52, 81–2
effeminacy 56, 71, 77
Ellen (1994–8), 53
Ellis, Havelock 35
epidemic,
  representation of 2, 7–8, 14–17,
    26–7, 36–8, 108–10, 127–32,
    148–9, 153, 156, 157–9, 192, 202–3
epidemiology 16
Epstein, Julia 62
Everett, Rupert 54, 53–4, 66, 69–70, 75,
  79, 84–5, 222

Index

Faggots (1978) 215–16
Fairman, William 125, 129
Falwell, Jerry, 29
Farmer, Brett 39
Farrell, Kathleen 90
fatality, 42–3
Finkelstein, Avram 208
Fire Island 215–17
folk devil 33, 128, 150, 153, 193
Foucault, Michel 23, 27, 59, 153, 235
   History of Sexuality, The 23, 137
Four Weddings and a Funeral
   (1993), 55
France, David 206, 226
Fraser, Suzanne 96
Freudian 48, 52, 61, 142, 204
funeral 78
futurity 7, 44, 52, 58, 68, 80, 85,
   202, 223

Gaines, Jane 172
gardening 69–71
Gay 90s 5, 11, 21–2, 46, 52–4,
   55–60, 85
gay liberation 27, 141–3,
   215–19, 219–21
Gay Men's Health Crisis (GMHC)
   214, 218
gay neoconservatism 203–5, 219
gay pride 3, 11–12, 77, 221
gay redemption 21–2, 51–2, 66–68,
   70–4, 85
generation
   degeneration 205, 225–6
   feeling of 149, 222–36
   generational difference 4–8, 93, 220
Gilman, Sander 37
GLAAD 12, 55

global gay 97–8, 224
Gogarty, Max 125, 129
Goldman, Jason 173
Gook, Ben 172
Gothic 41, 149, 169, 179
Gran Fury 202, 206
Grant, Cary 64
Grant, David Marshall 6
Graydon, Michael 143
Great Gatsby, The (1925) 177
GRID 8, 26, 218
Grim Reaper 154, 231
Grindr 125–6
Grosz, Elizabeth 60
guest, theme of 177–82, 184, 189–91

Hallas, Roger 19, 151, 212
Halperin, David 223
Hannah, Daniel 190–1
Hanson, Ellis 13, 149
Harris, Daniel 45, 49
Hart, Kylo-Patrick 45
Harvey, David Oscar 4–5
Haver, William 160
Hawkes, Terrence 30
Hay, Louise 34–5
haunting 7, 18–19, 87, 235
hedonism 57, 60, 75, 107, 128, 193, 225
Helms, Senator Jesse 29
Herald Sun 145, 146, 148, 151–2
heritage
   AIDS heritage 174–5, 195–200
   baroque 169–70, 179–82
   cinema 164, 166–7, 170–5, 195
   culture 170
   gaze 175–83, 188
   gothic 169, 179
   queer heritage 172, 186–7, 188

Index

Herkt, David 10
heteropolarity 92, 112–20
HEX (2014–15) 231–4
High Bid, The (1907) 187
Higson, Andrew 170–1
Hilderbrand, Lucas 167, 235
Hipsky, Martin 171
Hirsch, Marianne 234
HIV
    biopolitical management of 32, 132, 157–9
    chronic manageable illness 19
    disclosure of 102–3, 107–10, 154
    living with 19, 90, 109–10
    neoliberal management of 19, 23, 32, 102–3, 108, 120–1, 132–3, 157–9
    normalising of 10, 19–20
    temporal estrangement of 7, 223
    testing for 3–4, 47–8, 108
    treatment of 19
HIV Man 131, 147–51
HIV polarity 22, 92
HIV positive
    body 22, 101–11, 124
    character 44, 100–2, 223
Holding The Man (2015) 207
Hollinghurst, Alan 24, 25, 168–9, 196, 198
Hollywood 21, 24, 40, 51, 53, 55, 66, 72, 77, 83, 87, 209–13, 222
Holocaust 140, 228, 234
homographesis 35–6, 40
homonormativity 6, 7, 13, 33, 80, 85, 91, 99, 121, 228
homophobia 77, 79–80, 126, 139, 141–4, 184–6
homosexual panic 20

homosexuality
    inversion model of 35
    surveillance of 128, 153
horror genre 27, 45, 52, 125, 130, 245n.11
Hours, The (2002) 202
house, trope of 177, 189, 192, 199
How to Survive a Plague (2012) 24, 206–7, 226
Howard, John 158
Hubbard, Jim 208
Hudson, Rock 40–2, 72–3
Hunter, I. Q. 166–7, 195

identification 27–8
immunity 35, 62, 242.n96
immunology 16
Irreversible (2003) 153
Irvine, Janice 132, 153–4, 157

Jagose, Annemarie 32
James, Henry 163, 183, 184, 187–8, 195, 196, 198–9
Jameson, Frederic 172
Jarman, Derek 173
jouissance 44, 82
Junge, Benjamin 136

Kahan, Benjamin 59
Kaposi's Sarcoma (KS) 37, 40, 72
Kerr, Theodore 202, 208, 227
Kimmel, Michael 55, 64
kinship
    of choice 78
    queer 228–36
    representation of 87
kitsch 45, 49
Kohnen, Melanie 4, 6–7

Index

Kraft-Ebbing, Richard von 35
Kramer, Larry 207, 213–19
Kristeva, Julia 60, 61–3

Last of England, The (1987) 173
Laubenstein, Linda 218
leprosy 36–7
lesbian representation 95, 97
LGBTQI+ movement 5 22, 93, 121, 203, 205, 218–19
Liberace 40, 231
Line of Beauty, The (2004) 24, 25, 33, 163, 165–6, 168, 179, 185
Line of Beauty, The (BBC2, 2006), 2, 24–5, 164–200, 228
logic of epidemic 132, 157–9, 160, 192, 219
looking 175–82
Love, Heather 77, 85, 167, 174, 224, 234–5

Madonna 64–5, 66–72, 79
mainstream 11, 25
marriage 5, 92–3, 218
marriage plot 55
masculinity 38–9, 68, 143, 161
McGrath, Roberta 36
meaninglessness, 41, 43–4, 61–3, 68, 75
'Melancholia and Moralism' (2002) 203–5
melancholic disavowal 203–5, 208–9, 236
melodrama 22, 44–6, 49, 65–6, 67, 100, 120–4, 198
Melrose Place (1992–9) 47–9, 54
memory 196–7, 228–36
Mercury, Freddie 40, 231
metaphor 29–31

Meyer, Richard 40–2
migrants 26, 152, 158
Miller, James 43
Miller, Nancy K. 234
Miller, William 153
Monk, Claire 172
Morris, Paul 135
movie-of-the-week 91, 168, 211, 259n.11
Mowlabocus, Sharif 139
Mulvey, Laura 153
Muñoz, Jose 92, 235
Munt, Sally 94
Murphy, Ryan 207, 213, 218–19
muscular body 106, 110–14
My Best Friend's Wedding (1997) 53, 64

narcissism 41–2, 60, 81, 85, 128, 223
Neal, Michael John 131, 133, 145–63
Nelson, Robin 94
neoliberalism 22, 32
  experience of HIV/AIDS under 92–3, 185–6
  neoliberal sociality, 25, 32, 120–1
  social logics of 33, 123–4, 187–8, 193
  Thatcherite 33, 167, 171, 175, 185–6
New Gay Man 21, 46, 51, 55–60, 63, 94, 222–3
new relational modes 235
Next Best Thing, The 21–2, 52, 53, 60, 63–87, 187, 199, 201, 205, 222–3, 225
Noble, Bobby 97, 98
Normal Heart, The (2014) 25, 165, 207, 213–19, 228
nostalgia 25, 166, 171–3, 220–1, 227
  subcultural 167, 220–1, 227–36
Nureyev, Rudolf 40

Index

October 30–1
Odets, Walt 189
One Night Stand (1997) 45
Oprah Winfrey Show, The (1986–2011) 35
Orange, Donna M. 136
Orlando (1992) 173

paparazzi 181–2
party and play 125–30
passivity 38–9, 56, 72, 85, 98, 151, 188, 221
Patient Zero 42–3, 148, 150
Patton, Cindy 32, 36
Paulin, Scott 50, 53
Peeren, Esther 99
Person Living With HIV/AIDS (PLWHIV) 9, 45, 52, 80–3, 85, 109–11, 211–12
Persson, Asher 121
Philadelphia (1993) 44, 45–6, 52, 210, 214, 217
Picture of Dorian Gray, The 41–3, 149
Place for Annie, A (1994) 45
plague 29, 185, 211, 218
Plant, Aaron 141
pleasure 39, 59, 74, 81, 134–5, 216, 222, 223
Policing Desire (1987) 27
politics of representation 11–14, 21–2
popular culture 11
Potter, Sally 173
Portrait of a Lady, The (1881) 183
Portrait of a Lady, The (1996) 173
positive images 7, 11–14, 23, 44–6, 52–3, 55, 85, 202, 205
post-AIDS 9, 14–15

post-crisis
  conditions of 1, 7, 13–20, 9–10, 89
  dialectic of 19–20, 23, 28–29, 87, 93–100, 124, 132, 160–2, 236
post-feminism 52, 60
postmemory 228–36
poststructuralism 30–1
Powers of Horror (1982) 61
pre-exposure prophylaxis (PrEP) 16, 115, 130, 214
Pride (2014) 208
Pride and Prejudice 169, 179
Production (Hays) Code 67, 75
promiscuity 37–9, 49, 60, 65, 85, 94, 121, 126, 142–3, 214–18
Pronger, Brian 39
psychoanalysis 31, 60–3, 144, 224
punishment 40–1, 185, 218

quality TV 90, 91, 93–5, 121
Queer as Folk (2000–5), 2, 4, 22, 25, 33, 89–124, 205
queer as folk 99–100
Queer Eye for the Straight Guy 56–7, 74, 178
queer liberalism 12–13, 33
queer theory 13, 31–3
queerness
  as meaningless 43–4, 81–2, 87, 225

Race, Kane 15, 32, 103, 106, 108, 136–7
rapid testing 16
raw sex, 23
re-crisis 127, 131–3, 151–7
Reagan, Ronald 18, 202, 218
Reality Bites 47–51, 52
reckless infection 103, 130–1, 145–50, 154–5, 156, 158

Index

Rent (2005) 202
representation 14
reproduction 70, 81–2
resistance hypothesis 140–4
Retchy, John 216
retrovision 165–7, 195, 196–200, 205–19, 236
ribbon (AIDS) 44, 79, 154
Ridge, Damien 143
Riggs, Damien 92, 116–17
Riley, Benjamin 229–30
risk 102–3, 129
Rivkin, Julie 197
Rofes, Eric 139
romance narrative 55, 66, 71
Rubin, Gayle 137, 157
Russo, Vito 12, 206
Ryan, Benjamin 90
Ryan White Story, The 90

safe sex 15, 137–9, 217
sanitation 73–4
Savage, Dan, 82
Schatz, Thomas 169
Schulman, Sarah 206, 209
science, idealisation of 29–30
scopophilic gaze 68, 71, 175
Second Silence, the 18, 202–5, 223
secrets, 40, 178–9, 188, 190
Section 28 165, 186
Sedgwick, Eve 20, 59
semen 141
sentimentality 44–6, 49, 213
seroconversion 117, 119–20, 134, 145
serodiscord 22, 33, 92–3, 111–21
sero-melodrama 22, 92–3, 121–3
serosorting 136–7

sex panic 8, 23, 125–63, 131–3, 150–7, 192, 201
  emotions of 130, 153, 157
  language of 126, 155–6
sex work 26, 37–9
sexology 23, 27, 35, 148, 137–9, 153
Sexual Outlaw, The (1977) 216
Sheon, Nicolas 141
Shevory, Thomas 149
Shilts, Randy 42, 148
Shugart, Helene 51, 55–6, 67
Singer, Linda 132, 157–9
Single White Female (1992), 57
soap opera 44, 49, 54, 90–1, 93–5, 99, 120–2
Sontag, Susan 29, 34, 36, 40, 211–12
Sothern, Matthew 109–10
Spoils of Poynton (1896/7) 184, 261n.53
Spong, Rohan 230
Stacey, Jackie 33, 63
Stam, Robert 14
Stella Dallas 45
Stern-Wolfe, Mimi 230
stigma 101–2, 104–7
straight panic 21
Sullivan, Andrew 203–4
superspreader 42–3
Swaab, Peter 198–9
syphilis 37–9

TAG (Treatment Action Group) 206–7
Test (2014) 208
textual body discourse 34–6
Thatcher, Margaret
  government of 18, 24
  politics and culture under 165, 171, 174, 183–6, 199
tolerance 193–5, 213

Index

Tomso, Gregory 138, 294, 253n.12
Totem and Taboo (1913) 60
Tougaw, Jason, 234
transgender 210–11
traumatic memory 167, 204, 234
traumatic unremembering 18–19, 204–5
Treasure Island Media 135, 161
treatment as prevention (TasP) 16, 215
Treichler, Paula 8, 30, 31
Truvada 16, 134, 214
Turner, Victor 106

Ulrichs, Karl 35
UNAIDS 17
undetectable
   crisis 1, 10, 202
   representation of 108–11
United in Anger (2012) 24, 206
unspeakable 41, 50–2, 60, 61–3, 79, 134, 151–2, 191, 223

Vallée, Jean-Marc 212
vampires 149–50
Vice Media 125–30
viral load 16, 145, 150
viral sex 133
virology 16
Vito (2011) 24, 206–7
voyeurism 128, 153

Warner, Michael 157, 174, 250n.23
Watney, Simon 21, 28, 31
We Were Here (2011) 25, 206–7, 226, 228
Weeks, Jeffrey 9
Welsby, James 231–4
What Masie Knew (1897) 183
Whelahan, Imelda 166–7, 195
When We Rise (2017) 208, 227, 228
Wilde, Oscar 41–2, 149, 197, 199
Will and Grace (1998–2006) 54, 64
Williamson, Judith 43, 82
Wilton, Tamsin 92
Wood, Robin 52
Woodroof, Ron 210–13
work 67–72